MEMMLER'S

The Structure & Function of the Human Body

7th Edition

Barbara Janson Cohen

Dena Lin Wood

LIPPINCOTT WILLIAMS & WILKINS
A **Wolters Kluwer** Company
Philadelphia • Baltimore • New York • London
Buenos Aires • Hong Kong • Sydney • Tokyo

Acquisitions Editors: John P. Butler/Margaret Biblis
Editorial Assistant: Amy Amico
Managing Editor: Barbara Ryalls
Senior Production Manager: Helen Ewan
Production Coordinator: Mike Carcel
Art Director: Carolyn O'Brien
Indexer: Nancy Newman

7th Edition
Copyright © 2000 by Lippincott Williams & Wilkins

9 8 7 6 5 4 3 2 1

Library of Congress Cataloging-in-Publication Data

Cohen, Barbara J.
   Memmler's Structure & function of the human body / Barbara Janson Cohen,
Dena Lin Wood.—7th ed.
      p.   cm.
   Includes bibliographical references and index.
   ISBN 0–7817–2113–X (alk. paper) case bound ISBN 0–7817–2438–4 (softcover)
   1. Human physiology.   2. Human anatomy.   I. Wood, Dena Lin.
II. Memmler, Ruth Lundeen. Structure & funtion of the human body.
III. Title.   IV. Title: Structure and function of the human body.
   [DNLM: 1. Anatomy.   2. Physiology.   QS 4 C678s 2000]
   QP36.M54   2000
   612—dc21
   DNLM/DLC
   for Library of Congress   99–37062
                                                                    CIP

Care has been taken to confirm the accuracy of the information presented and to describe generally accepted practices. However, the authors, editors, and publisher are not responsible for errors or omissions or for any consequences from application of the information in this book and make no warranty, express or implied, with respect to the contents of the publication.

The authors, editors and publisher have exerted every effort to ensure that drug selection and dosage set forth in this text are in accordance with current recommendations and practice at the time of publication. However, in view of ongoing research, changes in government regulations, and the constant flow of information relating to drug therapy and drug reactions, the reader is urged to check the package insert for each drug for any change in indications and dosage and for added warnings and precautions. This is particularly important when the recommended agent is a new or infrequently employed drug.

Some drugs and medical devices presented in this publication have Food and Drug Administration (FDA) clearance for limited use in restricted research settings. It is the responsibility of the health care provider to ascertain the FDA status of each drug or device planned for use in their clinical practice.

In Memory of
Ruth L. Memmler

A mentor to ALL
She had confidence in each student's potential.

Preface

The seventh edition of *Memmler's Structure & Function of the Human Body* has built on the strong features of previous editions. It uses a systemic approach to study body.

1. Virtually all of the art has been redrawn to make the illustrations more appealing and modern. Figures have been revised for clarity and labeling has been enhanced. Some illustrations explaining physiologic concepts have been added.

2. The entire text has been updated and additional material on physiology has been added.

3. The text has been reorganized and information is presented in smaller segments.

4. Checkpoints have been inserted at intervals in the text. These short questions require the student to pause and think about the previous section of text and answer a question on some highlight of the section. The answers to the checkpoints are at the end of each chapter.

5. The Special Interest Boxes have been updated, and each chapter on the body systems now contains an additional box on a related health topic.

6. Summary charts have been added to aid in learning. Some of these incorporate figures to illustrate materials in the chart.

7. Information on aging and its effects on each body system has been added where appropriate.

AIDS TO LEARNING

Many valuable student aids have been retained from previous editions. These include:

1. Each chapter begins with Behavioral Objectives that state the learning goals for the chapter.

2. Selected Key Terms are listed at the start of each chapter.

3. New terms are emphasized when introduced with **boldface italic** type and a phonetic pronunciation is given.

4. Abundant illustrations are included.

5. Summary charts help to organize material and to aid in review.

6. Each chapter is followed by a Summary outline for review. These summaries now more closely parallel the headings in the text for easy reference.

7. Questions for Study and Review are included at the end of each chapter.

8. There is a complete Glossary with definitions and pronunciations of all key terms and other important words used in the text.

9. The chapters include Special Interest Boxes that expand on the text or add related information. One box in each chapter centers on normal structure and function. A second box in the systems chapters discusses a related health topic. Each type of the box is identified with a logo as follows:

    represents a box focusing on normal structure and function

    represents a health box

10. Appendices provide information on the metric system and temperature conversions.

11. A section on Biologic Terminology shows how scientific words are built from prefixes, roots, and suffixes. Learning these word parts will help the student remember terms and understand the meaning of new terms.

THE COMPLETE TEACHING–LEARNING PACKAGE INCLUDES

1. A Student Study Guide

   The Study Guide contains a variety of practice exercises that correlate directly with the text, including labeling exercises that correspond to illustrations.

2. The Instructor's Manual and Testbank includes:

   Chapter Overviews, Topics for Emphasis, Suggestions for Additional Studies, Supplementary Reading Assignments, a list of Web resources, and more than 1,000 multiple-choice-type Testbank questions. The printed version of Testbank questions is perforated and drilled for ease of use. Answers to the Study Guide and Testbank questions and answers to the chapter Questions for Study and Review are also provided in the Instructor's Manual.

3. Computerized Testbank

   Available upon adoption are the exact same questions mentioned above in an automatic, test-authoring, test-generating program that allows instructors to select questions electronically and prepare and print a test. The test is completely customized and includes test (or question) instructions and an answer key. This test-generator (ParTEST for Windows) provides the ability to add, change, or sort questions by chapter objective, subject area (structure or function), and question type. Additional features of the program include the ability to manipulate questions and produce different versions of the same test. It can also generate feedback reports.

4. Overhead Transparencies

   A set of color transparencies of key illustrations in the text is available for classroom instruction.

GUIDE TO PRONUNCIATION

The stressed syllable in each word is shown with capital letters. The vowel pronunciations are as follows:

Any vowel at the end of a syllable is given a long sound, as follows:

a as in say
e as in be
i as in nice
o as in go
u as in true

A vowel followed by a consonant and the letter e (as in rate) also is given a long pronunciation.

Any vowel followed by a consonant receives a short pronunciation, as follows:

a as in absent
e as in end
i as in bin
o as in not
u as in up

In some cases, the letter *h* is added to a syllable to make a short vowel sound.

FROM THE AUTHORS

A valuable text, like the body itself, requires feedback to remain healthy. Over many years of use, students, instructors, and reviewers have contributed to the development of *Structure & Function of the Human Body*. The authors appreciate all comments and weigh them carefully in the preparation of each edition. If you have any comments, questions, or criticism, please address them to the authors in care of the publisher, Lippincott Williams & Wilkins.

Acknowledgments

Above all, the authors wish to pay tribute to Dr. Ruth L. Memmler, the original author of *Structure and Function of the Human Body*. She first envisioned a book that would serve the needs of so many students preparing for Allied Health careers and over the years contributed to their training, not only with this book but in many personal and direct ways as well. This edition of *Structure and Function of the Human Body* is dedicated to Dr. Memmler.

We thank the Lippincott Williams & Wilkins staff members who have contributed their skills to this effort: the editors, Margaret Biblis and John P. Butler, Barbara Ryalls, Managing Editor, and for her extra contributions, editorial assistant Amy Amico. The art and design staff includes Brett Mac-Naughton, Carolyn O'Brien, and Kathy Luedtke. We appreciate the comments of reviewers and especially Jim Rosack, who reviewed sections of the text and contributed to the health boxes. Special thanks to Peg Waltner, Developmental Editor, who guided this book from start to finish, and to Darlene Pedersen, who consulted in the early stages of development.

Brief Contents

Contents

MEMMLER'S

The Structure &
Function of the
Human Body

Unit 1

THE BODY AS A WHOLE

This unit presents the basic levels of organization within the human body. Included is a description of the smallest units of life, called cells. Similar cells are grouped together as tissues, which are combined to form organs. Organs, in turn, work together in the various body systems, which together satisfy the needs of the entire organism. A short survey of chemistry, which deals with the composition of all matter and is important for the understanding of human physiology, is incorporated into this unit. These chapters should prepare the student for the more detailed study of individual body systems in the units that follow. The final chapter in the unit illustrates some of these basic principles, with a study of the skin and its associated structures that together make up the integumentary system.

Organization of the Human Body

SELECTED KEY TERMS

The following terms are defined in the Glossary:

anabolism

anatomy

ATP

catabolism

cell

gram

homeostasis

liter

metabolism

meter

negative feedback

organ

physiology

system

tissue

BEHAVIORAL OBJECTIVES

After careful study of this chapter, you should be able to:

1. Define the terms *anatomy* and *physiology*

2. Describe the organization of the body from chemicals to the whole organism

3. List 10 body systems and give the general function of each

4. Define *metabolism* and name the two phases of metabolism

5. Briefly explain the role of ATP in the body

6. Differentiate between extracellular and intracellular fluids

7. Define *homeostasis* and *negative feedback*

8. List and define the main directional terms for the body

9. List and define the three planes of division of the body

10. Name the subdivisions of the dorsal and ventral cavities

11. Name the basic metric units of length, weight, and volume

12. Name and locate the nine regions of the abdomen

13. Name the basic units of length, weight, and volume in the metric system

14. Define the metric prefixes *kilo-, centi-, milli-,* and *micro-*

STUDIES OF THE HUMAN BODY

Everyone is interested from the earliest age in the body and how it works. Picture an infant carefully examining his or her fingers and toes and exploring their uses. The scientific term for the study of body structure is *anatomy* (ah-NAT-o-me). Part of this word means "to cut," because a fundamental way to learn about the human body is to cut it apart, or *dissect* it. *Physiology* (fiz-e-OL-o-je) is the term for the study of how the body functions, and the two sciences are closely related. It is hoped that from these studies you will gain an appreciation for the design and balance of the human body and for living organisms in general.

Levels of Organization

All living things are organized from very simple levels to more complex levels (Fig. 1-1). Living matter begins with simple chemicals. These chemicals are formed into the complex substances that make living *cells*—the basic units of all life. Specialized groups of cells form *tissues,* and tissues may function together as *organs.* Organs functioning together for the same general purpose make up organ *systems*. The organ systems work together to maintain the body.

✔ CHECKPOINT **1**:

In studying the human body, one may concentrate on either its structure or its function. What are these two studies called?

BODY SYSTEMS

Most of the studies of the body as a whole are organized according to the individual systems, as follows:

- The *integumentary* (in-teg-u-MEN-tar-e) *system.* The word *integument* (in-TEG-u-ment) means skin. The skin with its associated structures is considered a separate body system. The structures associated with the skin include the hair, the nails, and the sweat and oil glands.
- The *skeletal system.* The basic framework of the body is a system of more than 200 bones and the joints between them, collectively known as the *skeleton.*
- The *muscular system.* Body movements result from the action of the skeletal muscles, which are attached to the bones. Other types of muscles are present in the walls of body organs, such as the intestine and the heart.
- The *nervous system.* The brain, the spinal cord, and the nerves make up this complex

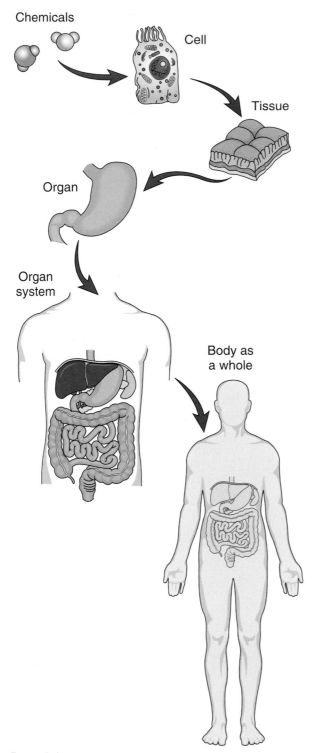

Chemicals

Cell

Tissue

Organ

Organ system

Body as a whole

FIGURE **1•1** Levels of organization.

system by which the body is controlled and coordinated. The organs of special sense (such as the eyes, ears, taste buds, and organs of smell), together with the receptors for touch and other senses, receive stimuli from the outside world. These stimuli are converted into impulses that are transmitted to the brain. The brain directs the body's responses to these outside messages and also to messages coming from within the body. Such higher functions as memory and reasoning also occur in the brain.

- The ***endocrine*** (EN-do-krin) ***system.*** The scattered organs known as ***endocrine glands*** are grouped together because they share a similar function. All produce special substances called ***hormones,*** which regulate such body activities as growth, food utilization within the cells, and reproduction. Examples of endocrine glands are the thyroid and the pituitary glands.

- The ***circulatory system.*** The heart and blood vessels make up the system that pumps blood to all the body tissues, bringing with it nutrients, oxygen, and other substances and carrying away waste materials. Lymphatic vessels play an important auxiliary role in circulation.

- The ***respiratory system.*** This system includes the lungs and the passages leading to the lungs. The purpose of this system is to take in air and conduct it to the areas designed for gas exchange. Oxygen passes from the air into the blood and is carried to all tissues by the circulatory system. In like manner, carbon dioxide, as a gaseous waste product, is taken by the circulation from the tissues back to the lungs to be expelled.

- The ***digestive system.*** This system comprises all the organs that are involved with taking in food and converting it into substances that body cells can use. Examples of these organs are the mouth, esophagus, stomach, intestine, liver, and pancreas.

- The ***urinary system.*** This system is also called the ***excretory system.*** Its main components are the kidneys, the ureters, the bladder, and the urethra. Its chief purpose is to rid the body of waste products and excess water. (Note that other waste products are removed by the digestive and respiratory systems and by the skin.)

- The ***reproductive system.*** This system includes the external sex organs and all related internal structures that are concerned with the production of offspring.

The number of systems may vary in different lists. Some, for example, show the sensory and lymphatic systems as separate entries. Others include the immune system, which protects the body from foreign matter. The immune system is identified by its function rather than its structure and includes elements of both the circulatory and lymphatic systems.

BODY PROCESSES

Metabolism

All the life-sustaining reactions that go on within the body systems together make up ***metabolism*** (meh-TAB-o-lizm). Metabolism can be divided into two types of activities:

- In ***catabolism*** (kah-TAB-o-lizm), complex substances are broken down into simpler compounds. The breakdown of the nutrients in food yields simple chemical building blocks and energy to power cell activities.
- In ***anabolism*** (ah-NAB-o-lizm), simple compounds are used to manufacture materials needed for growth, function, and repair of tissues. Anabolism is the building phase of metabolism.

The energy obtained from the breakdown of nutrients is used to form a compound often described as the "energy currency" of the cell. It has the long name of ***adenosine triphosphate*** (ah-DEN-o-sene tri-FOS-fate), but is commonly abbreviated ***ATP.*** Chapter 20 has more information on metabolism and ATP.

Fluid Balance

It is important to recognize that our bodies are composed of large amounts of fluids. The amount and composition of these fluids must be regulated at all times. Certain fluids bathe the cells, carry nutrient substances to and from the cells, and transport the nutrients into and out of the cells. This group of fluids is called ***extracellular fluid*** because it includes all body fluids outside the cells. A second type of fluid, ***intracellular fluid***, is contained within the cells. Extracellular and intracellular fluids account for about 60% of an adult's weight.

Homeostasis

The purpose of metabolism is to maintain a state of balance within the organism, an important characteristic of all living things. Such conditions as body temperature, the composition of body fluids, heart rate, respiration rate, and blood pressure must be kept within set limits to maintain health. This steady state within the organism is called ***homeostasis*** (ho-me-o-STA-sis), which literally means "staying (stasis) the same (homeo)."

Feedback

Homeostasis is maintained by the feedback of information. Sensors throughout the body monitor internal conditions and bring them back to normal when they shift, much as a thermostat regulates the temperature of a house to a set level. Because each change, up or down, must be reversed to restore the norm, this mechanism is described as ***negative feedback.*** The main controllers in this self-regulation are the nervous and endocrine systems. You will find many examples of negative feedback throughout this book.

✔ CHECKPOINT **2**:

Metabolism is divided into a breakdown phase and a building phase. What are these two phases called?

DIRECTIONS IN THE BODY

Because it would be awkward and inaccurate to speak of bandaging the "southwest part" of the chest, a number of terms are used to designate position and directions in the body. They refer to the body in the *anatomic position*—upright with face front, arms at the sides with palms forward, and feet parallel.

Directional Terms

The main terms for describing directions in the body are as follows (Fig. 1-2):

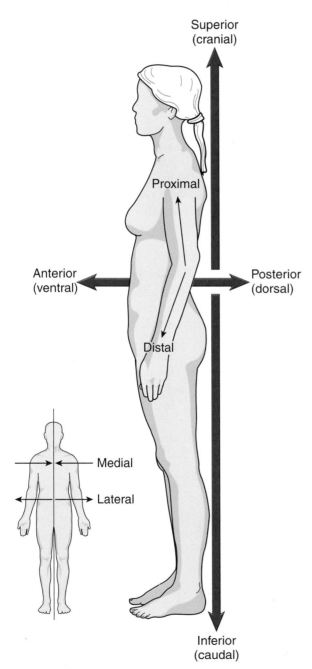

FIGURE **1•2** Directional terms.

- *Superior* is a term meaning above, or in a higher position. Its opposite, *inferior,* means below, or lower. The heart, for example, is superior to the intestine.
- *Ventral* and *anterior* mean the same thing in humans: located toward the belly surface or front of the body. Their corresponding opposites, *dorsal* and *posterior,* refer to locations nearer the back.
- *Cranial* means nearer to the head. *Caudal* means nearer to the sacral region of the spinal column (*i.e.,* where the tail is located in lower animals).
- *Medial* means nearer to an imaginary plane that passes through the midline of

A Map of the Body

The body's surface landmarks provide a good introduction to body structure. These landmarks are useful for orientation in surgery and other clinical procedures. For example, the lower tip of the sternum, the xiphoid process, is used as a reference point in the administration of CPR (cardiopulmonary resuscitation).

Feel for some of the other superficial markings to learn how your body is organized. The joint between the mandible and the temporal bone of the skull (the temporomandibular or TM, joint) can be felt in front of the ear canal as you move your lower jaw up and down. The pulse of the facial artery can be felt in a small depression about 1 inch in front of the angle of the lower jaw. The pulse of the carotid artery can be felt at the side of the neck.

Touch behind your neck for the spine of the 7th cervical vertebra, the prominent vertebra at the base of the neck. At the distal end of the forearm, you can feel the pulse of the radial artery at the lateral surface of the anterior wrist.

In the torso, you can feel the ribs and the lower margin of the rib cage. By placing your hands on your hips, you can feel the crest of the hip bone. When it hurts to sit on a hard chair, you become aware of the lower bone of the pelvic girdle on each side.

Many other features can be seen and felt at the surface to tell us about the structure and the condition of the body.

the body, dividing it into left and right portions. *Lateral,* its opposite, means farther away from the midline, toward the side.

- *Proximal* means nearer the origin of a structure; *distal,* farther from that point. For example, the part of your thumb where it joins your hand is its proximal region; the tip of the thumb is its distal region.

For additional information, see A Map of the Body.

Planes of Division

For convenience in visualizing the spatial relations of various body structures to each other, anatomists have divided the body into three imaginary planes, each of which is a cut through the body in a different direction (Fig. 1-3).

- The *sagittal* (SAJ-ih-tal) *plane.* If you were to cut the body in two from front to back, separating it into right and left portions, the sections you would see would be sagittal sections. A cut exactly down the midline of the body, separating it into equal right and left halves, is a *midsagittal* section.
- The *frontal plane.* If the cut were made in line with the ears and then down the middle of the body, creating a front and a rear portion, you would see a front (anterior or ventral) section and a rear (posterior or dorsal) section. Another name for this plane is *coronal plane.*
- The *transverse plane.* If the cut were made horizontally, across the other two planes, it would divide the body into an upper (superior) part and a lower (inferior) part. There could be many such cross-sections, each of which would be on a transverse plane, also called a *horizontal plane.*

✔ CHECKPOINT **3**:

What are the three planes in which the body can be cut? What kind of a plane divides the body into two equal halves?

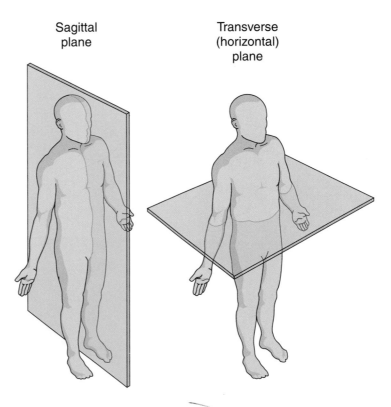

Frontal
(coronal)
plane

Sagittal
plane

Transverse
(horizontal)
plane

FIGURE **1•3** Planes of division.

1

BODY CAVITIES

The body contains a few large internal spaces, or **cavities,** within which various organs are located. There are two main cavities: **dorsal** and **ventral** (Fig. 1-4).

Dorsal Cavity

The dorsal body cavity has two regions: the **cranial cavity,** containing the brain, and the **spinal canal,** enclosing the spinal cord. These two areas form one continuous space.

Ventral Cavity

The ventral cavity is much larger than the dorsal cavity. It has two main regions, which are separated by the **diaphragm** (DI-ah-fram), a muscle used in breathing. The **thoracic** (tho-RAS-ik) **cavity** is located above the diaphragm. Its contents include the heart, the lungs, and the large blood vessels that join the heart. The

heart is contained in the pericardial sac; the lungs are in the pleural sacs (Fig. 1-5). The **abdominopelvic** (ab-dom-ih-no-PEL-vik) **cavity** is located below the diaphragm. This space is further subdivided into two regions. The uppermost **abdominal cavity** contains the stomach, most of the intestine, the kidneys, the liver, the gallbladder, the pancreas, and the spleen. The lower portion, set off by an imaginary line across the top of the hip bones, is the **pelvic cavity.** This cavity contains the urinary bladder, the rectum, and the internal parts of the reproductive system.

✔ CHECKPOINT **4**:

There are two main body cavities, one posterior and one anterior. Name these two cavities.

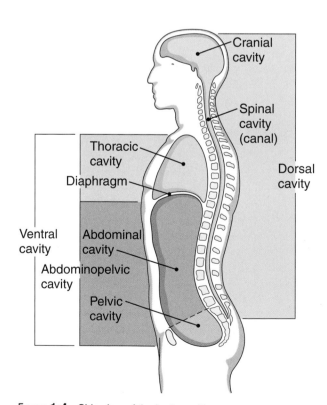

FIGURE **1•4** Side view of the body cavities.

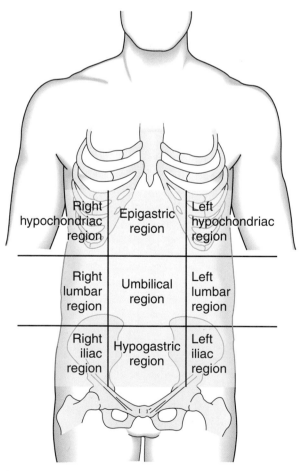

FIGURE **1•5** The nine regions of the abdomen.

Regions of the Abdomen

Because the abdomen is so large, it is helpful to divide it for examination and reference into nine regions (see Fig. 1-5). The three central regions are the **epigastric** (ep-ih-GAS-trik) **region,** located just below the breastbone; the **umbilical** (um-BIL-ih-kal) **region** around the umbilicus (um-BIL-ih-kus), commonly called the *navel;* and the **hypogastric** (hi-po-GAS-trik) **region,** the lowest of all the midline regions.

At each side are the right and left **hypochondriac** (hi-po-KON-dre-ak) **regions,** just below the ribs; then the right and left **lumbar regions;** and finally the right and left **iliac,** or **inguinal** (IN-gwih-nal), **regions.**

A simpler but less precise division into four quadrants is sometimes used. These are the right upper quadrant (RUQ), left upper quadrant (LUQ), right lower quadrant (RLQ), and left lower quadrant (LLQ) (Fig. 1-6).

 CHECKPOINT **5**:

Name the three central regions and the three lateral regions of the abdomen.

THE METRIC SYSTEM

Now that we have set the stage for further study of the body and its structure and processes, a look at the metric system is in order because this is the system used for all scientific measurements. The drug industry and the health care industry already have converted to the metric system, so anyone who plans a career in health care should be acquainted with metrics.

The metric system is like the monetary system in the United States. Both are decimal systems based on multiples of the number 10. One hundred cents equal one dollar; one hundred centimeters equal one meter. Each multiple in the decimal system is indicated by a prefix:

kilo = 1000
centi = 1/100
milli = 1/1000
micro = 1/1,000,000

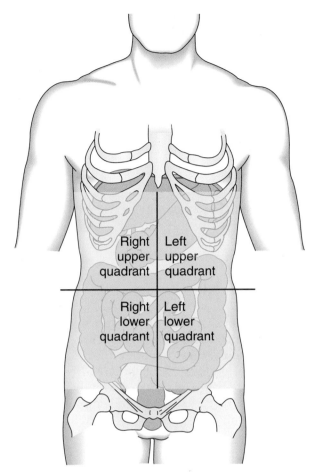

FIGURE 1•6 Quadrants of the abdomen showing the organs within each quadrant.

Units of Length

The basic unit of length in the metric system is the **meter.** Thus, 1 kilometer is equal to 1000 meters. A centimeter is 1/100 of a meter; stated another way, there are 100 centimeters in 1 meter. A changeover to the metric system has been slow in coming to the United States. Often, measurements on packages, bottles, and yard goods are now given according to both scales. In this text, equivalents in the more familiar units of inches, feet, and so forth are included along with the metric units for comparison. There are 2.5 centimeters (cm) or 25 millimeters (mm) in 1 inch, as shown in Figure 1-7. Some equivalents that may help you to appreciate the size of various body parts are as follows:

FIGURE **1•7**   Comparison of centimeters and inches.

1 mm = 0.04 inch, or 1 inch = 25 mm
1 cm = 0.4 inch, or 1 inch = 2.5 cm
1 m = 3.3 feet, or 1 foot = 30 cm

Units of Weight

The same prefixes used for linear measurements are used for weights and volumes. The *gram* is the basic unit of weight. Thirty grams are about equal to 1 ounce, and 1 kilogram to 2.2 pounds. Drug dosages are usually stated in grams or milligrams. One thousand milligrams equal 1 gram; a 500-milligram (mg) dose would be the equivalent of 0.5 gram (g), and 250 mg is equal to 0.25 g.

Units of Volume

The dosages of liquid medications are given in units of volume. The basic metric measurement for volume is the *liter* (LE-ter). There are 1000 milliliters (ml) in a liter. A liter is slightly greater than a quart, a liter being equal to 1.06 quarts. For smaller quantities, the milliliter is used most of the time. There are 5 ml in a teaspoon and 15 ml in a tablespoon. A fluid ounce contains 30 ml.

Temperature

The Celsius (centigrade) temperature scale, now in use by most countries and by scientists in this country, is discussed in Chapter 18.

A chart of all the common metric measurements and their equivalents is shown in Appendix 1. A Celsius-Fahrenheit temperature conversion scale appears in Appendix 2.

✔ CHECKPOINT **6**:

Name the basic units of length, weight, and volume in the metric system.

Summary

I. Studies of the human body
  1. Anatomy—study of structure
  2. Physiology—study of function
  A. Levels of organization—chemicals, cell, tissue, organ, organ system, whole organism

II. Body systems
  1. Integumentary system—skin and associated structures
  2. Skeletal system—support
  3. Muscular system—movement
  4. Nervous system—reception of stimuli and control of responses
  5. Endocrine system—production of hormones for regulation of growth, metabolism, reproduction
  6. Circulatory system (includes lymphatic system)—transport
  7. Respiratory system—intake of oxygen and release of carbon dioxide
  8. Digestive system—intake and breakdown of food
  9. Urinary system—elimination of waste and water
  10. Reproductive system—production of offspring

III. Body processes
  A. Metabolism—all the chemical reactions needed to sustain life
    1. Catabolism—breakdown of complex

substances into simpler substances; release of energy from nutrients
   a. ATP (adenosine triphosphate)—energy compound of cells
  2. Anabolism—building of body materials
B. Fluid balance
  1. Extracellular fluid—outside the cells
  2. Intracellular fluid—inside the cells
C. Homeostasis
  1. Steady state of body conditions
  2. Maintained by negative feedback

IV. Directions in the body
  1. Anatomic position—upright, palms forward, face front, feet parallel
A. Directional terms
  1. Superior—above or higher; inferior—below or lower
  2. Ventral (anterior)—toward belly or front surface; dorsal (posterior)—nearer to back surface
  3. Cranial—nearer to head; caudal—nearer to sacrum
  4. Medial—toward midline; lateral—toward side
  5. Proximal—nearer to point of origin; distal—farther from point of origin
B. Planes of division
  1. Sagittal—from front to back, dividing the body into left and right parts
    a. Midsagittal—exactly down the midline
  2. Frontal (coronal)—from left to right, dividing the body into anterior and posterior parts
  3. Transverse—horizontally, dividing the body into superior and inferior parts

V. Body cavities
A. Dorsal cavity—contains cranial and spinal cavities for brain and spinal cord
B. Ventral cavity
  1. Thoracic—chest cavity
    a. contains heart and lungs
    b. divided from abdominal cavity by diaphragm
  2. Abdominopelvic
    a. Abdominal—upper region containing stomach, most of intestine, kidneys, liver, spleen, and others
    b. Pelvic—lower region containing reproductive organs, urinary bladder, rectum
    c. Nine regions of the abdomen: epigastric, umbilical, hypogastric, right and left hypochondriac, right and left lumbar, right and left iliac (inguinal)
    d. Quadrants—abdomen divided into four regions

VI. The metric system—based on multiples of 10
  1. Basic units
    a. Meter—length
    b. Gram—weight
    c. Liter—volume
  2. Prefixes—indicate multiples of 10
    a. Kilo—1000 times
    b. Centi—1/100th (0.01)
    c. Milli—1/1000th (0.001)
    d. Micro—1/1,000,000 (0.000001)
A. Units of length
B. Units of weight
C. Units of volume
D. Temperature—measured in Celsius (centigrade) scale

Questions for Study and Review

1. List two types of study of the human body and define each.
2. List levels of organization in the body from the simplest to the most complex.
3. Define *cell, tissue, organ,* and *system.*
4. List 10 body systems and briefly describe the function of each.
5. Name and define the two phases of *metabolism.*
6. What is ATP?
7. Define the term *homeostasis* and give two examples. How is homeostasis maintained?
8. Stand in the anatomic position.
9. List the opposite term for each of the following body directions: *superior, ventral, anterior, cranial, medial,* and *proximal.* Define each term and its opposite.
10. Describe the location of the knee in relation to the ankle; in relation to the hip.
11. Describe the location of the stomach in relation to the heart; in relation to the urinary bladder.
12. Describe the location of the ears in relation to the nose.
13. What are the three main body planes? Explain the division each makes.
14. Name the cavities within the dorsal and ventral cavities. Name one organ found in each.
15. Make a rough sketch of the abdomen and label the nine divisions.
16. Name and locate the four quadrants of the abdomen.
17. Why should you learn the metric system? What are its advantages?

✔ ANSWERS TO CHECKPOINTS

1. Study of body structure is anatomy; study of body function is physiology.
2. The breakdown phase of metabolism is catabolism; the building phase of metabolism is anabolism.
3. The three planes in which the body can be cut are sagittal, frontal (coronal), and transverse (horizontal). The midsagittal plane divides the body into two equal halves.
4. The posterior cavity is the dorsal cavity; the anterior cavity is the ventral cavity.
5. The three central regions of the abdomen are the epigastric, umbilical, and hypogastric regions; the three lateral regions of the abdomen are the hypochondriac, lumbar, and iliac (inguinal) regions.
6. The basic unit of length in the metric system is the meter; of weight, the gram; of volume, the liter.

Chemistry, Matter, and Life

BEHAVIORAL OBJECTIVES

After careful study of this chapter, you should be able to:

1. Define an element
2. Describe the structure of an atom
3. Differentiate between molecules and compounds
4. Explain why water is so important to the body
5. Define *mixture*; list the three types of mixtures and give two examples of each
6. Differentiate between ionic and covalent bonds
7. Define the terms *acid, base,* and *salt*
8. Explain how the numbers on the pH scale relate to acidity and alkalinity
9. Define *buffer* and explain why buffers are important in the body
10. List three characteristics of organic compounds
11. Name the three main types of organic compounds and the building blocks of each
12. Define *enzyme*; describe how enzymes work

WHAT IS CHEMISTRY?

Great strides toward an understanding of living organisms, including humans, have come to us through *chemistry,* the science that deals with the composition of matter. Knowledge of chemistry and chemical changes helps us understand the normal and abnormal functioning of the body. The digestion of food in the intestinal tract, the production of urine by the kidneys, the regulation of breathing—all body processes—are based on chemical principles. Foods, vitamins, and minerals are chemicals, as are the various components of our bodies and the environment.

To provide some understanding of the importance of chemistry in the life sciences, this chapter briefly describes *elements, atoms* and *molecules, compounds,* and *mixtures,* which are fundamental forms of matter.

✔ CHECKPOINT **1**:

What is studied in the science of chemistry?

ELEMENTS

Elements are the substances from which all matter is made. Everything around us, everything we can see and touch, is made of ele-

ments—the food we eat, the atmosphere, all the water in the environment, the smoke coming out of a chimney. There are 92 naturally occurring elements. (Twenty additional elements have been created in the laboratory.) Examples of elements include various gases, such as hydrogen, oxygen, and nitrogen; liquids, such as the mercury used in thermometers and blood pressure instruments; and many solids, such as iron, aluminum, gold, silver, and carbon. Graphite (the so-called "lead" in a pencil), coal, charcoal, and diamonds are examples of the element carbon.

Elements can be identified by their names or their chemical symbols, which are abbreviations of the modern or Latin names of the element. Each element is also identified by its own number, which is based on the structure of the atoms that compose it. Table 2-1 lists some elements found in the human body along with their functions.

ATOMS

The subunits of elements are *atoms.* These are the smallest complete units of matter. They cannot be broken down or changed into another form by ordinary chemical and physical means. These subunits are so small that millions of them could fit on the sharpened end of a pencil.

Table 2•1	Some Common Chemical Elements*	

NAME	SYMBOL	FUNCTION
Oxygen	O	Part of water; needed to metabolize nutrients for energy
Carbon	C	Basis of all organic compounds; in carbon dioxide, the waste gas of metabolism
Hydrogen	H	Part of water; participates in energy metabolism, acid–base balance
Nitrogen	N	Present in all proteins, ATP (the energy compound), and nucleic acids (DNA and RNA)
Calcium	Ca	Builds bones and teeth; needed for muscle contraction, nerve impulse conduction, and blood clotting
Phosphorus	P	Active ingredient in the energy-storing compound ATP; builds bones and teeth; in cell membrane and nucleic acids
Potassium	K	Nerve impulse conduction; muscle contraction; water balance and acid–base balance
Sulfur	S	Part of many proteins
Sodium	Na	Active in water balance, nerve impulse conduction, and muscle contraction
Chlorine	Cl	Active in water balance and acid–base balance; found in stomach acid
Iron	Fe	Part of hemoglobin, the compound that carries oxygen in red blood cells

*The elements are listed in decreasing order by weight in the body.

Atomic Structure

Despite the fact that the atom is such a tiny particle, it has been carefully studied and has been found to have a definite structure. At the center of the atom is a nucleus, which contains positively charged electrical particles called **protons** and noncharged particles called **neutrons.** Together, the protons and neutrons contribute nearly all of the atom's weight.

Outside the nucleus, in regions called orbitals, are **electrons** (Fig. 2-1). These nearly weightless particles are negatively charged. The protons and electrons always are equal in number, so that the atom as a whole is electrically neutral. The atomic number of an element is equal to the number of protons that are present in the nucleus of each of its atoms. Because the number of protons is equal to the number of electrons, the atomic number also represents the number of electrons whirling around the nucleus.

The positively charged protons keep the negatively charged electrons in the orbital area around the nucleus by means of the opposite charges on the particles. Positively (+) charged protons attract negatively (–) charged electrons. It is the electrons that determine how the atom will react chemically.

Electron ———

Central nucleus
8 protons
8 neutrons

FIGURE **2•1**   Representation of the oxygen atom. Eight protons and eight neutrons are tightly bound in the central nucleus, around which the eight electrons revolve.

Energy Levels

Most atoms have several orbitals of electrons. Each orbital, however, can hold only two electrons. The orbitals are arranged into energy levels. Their distance from the nucleus of the atom identifies energy levels. The first energy level, the one closest to the nucleus, is composed of one orbital. The second energy level, the next in distance away from the nucleus, can have four orbitals. Because each orbital contains two electrons, the second energy level has the capacity to hold eight electrons.

The electrons farthest away from the nucleus are the particles that give the atom its chemical characteristics. If the outermost energy level has more than four electrons but less than its capacity of eight, the atom normally completes this level by gaining electrons. In the process, it becomes negatively charged because it has more electrons than protons. Such an atom is called a **nonmetal.** The oxygen atom illustrated in Figure 2-1 has six electrons in its second, or outermost, level. When oxygen enters into chemical reactions, it gains two electrons. The oxygen atom then has two more electrons than protons.

If the outermost shell has fewer than four electrons, the atom normally loses those electrons to attain a complete outer energy level. In so doing, it becomes positively charged. Such an atom is called a **metal**.

MOLECULES AND COMPOUNDS

When, on the basis of electron structure, two or more atoms unite, a **molecule** is formed. A molecule can be made of like atoms—the oxygen molecule is made of two identical atoms—but more often it is made of two or more different atoms. For example, a molecule of water (H_2O) contains 1 atom of oxygen (O) and 2 atoms of hydrogen (H) (Fig. 2-2).

Substances that contain molecules formed by the union of two or more different atoms are called **compounds.** Some compounds are made of a few elements in a simple combination. For example, the gas carbon monoxide (CO) contains 1 atom of carbon (C) and 1 atom of oxygen (O). Other compounds are very large and complex. Such complexity characterizes many of the compounds found in living organisms. Some proteins, for example, have thousands of atoms.

It is interesting to observe how different a compound is from any of its constituents. For example, a molecule of liquid water is formed from oxygen and hydrogen, both of which are gases. Another example is a crystal sugar, glucose ($C_6H_{12}O_6$). Its constituents include 12 atoms of the gas hydrogen, 6 atoms of the gas oxygen, and 6 atoms of the solid element carbon. In this case, the component gases and the solid carbon do not in any way resemble the glucose.

✔ CHECKPOINT **2**:

What is the difference between atoms and molecules?

More About Water

Water is the most abundant compound in the body. No plant or animal, including the human, can live very long without it. Water is of critical importance in all physiologic processes in body tissues. Water carries substances to and from the cells and makes possible the essential processes of absorption, exchange, secretion, and excretion. What are some of the properties of water that make it such an ideal medium for living cells?

- Water can dissolve many different substances in large amounts. For this reason, it is called the **universal solvent.** All the materials needed by the body, such as gases, minerals, and nutrients, dissolve in water to be carried from place to place.
- Water is stable as a liquid at ordinary temperatures. Water does not freeze until the temperature drops to 0°C (32°F) and does not boil until the temperature reaches 100°C (212°F). This stability provides a constant environment for body cells. Water can also be used to distribute heat through-

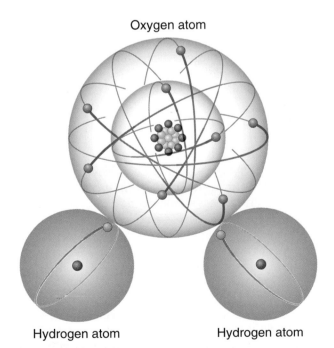

Oxygen atom

Hydrogen atom   Hydrogen atom

FIGURE **2•2**   Molecule of water.

out the body and to cool the body by evaporation of sweat from the body surface.

- Water participates in chemical reactions in the body. It is needed directly in the process of digestion and in many of the metabolic reactions that occur in the cells.

 CHECKPOINT **3**:

What is the most abundant compound in the body?

Mixtures: Solutions and Suspensions

Not all elements or compounds combine chemically when brought together. The air we breathe every day is a mixture of gases, largely nitrogen, oxygen, and carbon dioxide, along with smaller percentages of other substances. The constituents in the air maintain their identity, although the proportions of each may vary. Blood plasma is also a mixture in which the various components maintain their identity. The many valuable compounds in the plasma remain separate entities with their own properties. Such combinations are called *mixtures*—blends of two or more substances.

A mixture, such as salt water, in which the component substances remain evenly distributed, is called a *solution.* The dissolving substance, in this case water, is the *solvent;* the substance dissolved, in this case salt, is the *solute.* Solutions of glucose, salts, or both in water are used for intravenous fluid treatments.

In some mixtures, the material distributed in the solvent settles out unless the mixture is constantly shaken; this type of mixture is called a *suspension.* Settling occurs in a suspension because the particles in the mixture are large and heavy. Examples of suspensions are milk of magnesia, finger paints, and, in the body, red blood cells suspended in blood plasma.

One other type of mixture is of importance in the body. Some organic compounds form *colloidal suspensions,* in which the molecules do not dissolve yet remain distributed in the solvent. The particles have electrical charges that repel each other, and the molecules are small

enough to stay in suspension. The fluid that fills the cells (cytoplasm) is a colloidal suspension, as is blood plasma.

Many mixtures are complex, with properties of solutions, suspensions, and colloidal suspensions. Blood plasma has dissolved compounds, making it a solution. The red blood cells and other formed elements give blood the property of a suspension. The proteins in the plasma give it the property of a colloidal suspension. Chocolate milk also has all three properties.

 CHECKPOINT **4**:

Both solutions and suspensions are types of mixtures. What is the difference between them?

CHEMICAL BONDS

Ionic Bonds

When discussing the structure of the atom, we mentioned the positively charged (+) protons that are located in the nucleus, with the corresponding number of negatively charged (−) electrons found in the surrounding space that neutralize the protons. This neutrality is altered in chemical reactions. Atoms interact to reach a stable number of electrons in the outermost energy level. The sodium atom, for example, tends to lose the single electron in its outermost shell (Fig. 2-3A). Removal of a single electron from the sodium atom leaves one more proton than electrons, and the atom then has a single net positive charge. The sodium atom in this form is symbolized as Na^+.

Similarly, atoms can gain electrons so that there are more electrons than protons. Chlorine, which has seven electrons in its outermost energy level, tends to gain one electron to fill the level to its capacity. Such an atom of chlorine is negatively charged (Cl^-) (see Fig. 2-3A).

An atom or group of atoms with a positive or negative charge is called an *ion* (I-on). An ion that is positively charged is a *cation* (CAT-i-on), whereas a negatively charged ion is an *anion* (AN-i-on).

Let us imagine a sodium atom coming in contact with a chlorine atom. The chlorine atom

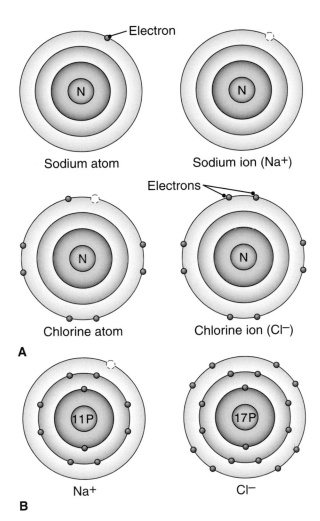

Figure **2•3** **(A)** Formation of sodium cation (Na⁺) and chlorine anion (Cl⁻). Only the electrons in the outermost energy level are shown. **(B)** A sodium ion with 11 protons in the nucleus and 10 electrons in orbitals is attracted to a chlorine ion with 17 protons in the nucleus and 18 electrons in oribitals to form the compound sodium chloride.

gains an electron from the sodium atom, and the two newly formed ions (Na⁺ and Cl⁻), because of their opposite charges, which attract each other, cling together and produce the compound sodium chloride, ordinary table salt. A bond formed by this method of electron transfer is called an ***ionic bond*** (see Fig. 2-3*B*).

Electrolytes

Ionically bonded molecules, when they go into solution, separate into charged particles. Compounds formed by ionic bonds that release ions when they are in solution are called ***electrolytes*** (e-LEK-tro-lites). (In practice, the term *electrolytes* is also used to refer to the ions themselves in body fluids.) Electrolytes are responsible for the acidity and the alkalinity of solutions. They also include a variety of salts, such as sodium chloride and potassium chloride. Electrolytes must be present in exactly the right quantities in the fluid within the cell (intracellular fluid) and the fluid outside the cell (extracellular fluid), or very damaging effects will result, preventing the cells in the body from functioning properly.

Ions in the Body

Many different ions are found in body fluids. Calcium ions (Ca⁺⁺) are necessary for the clotting of blood, the contraction of muscle, and the health of bone tissue. Bicarbonate ions (HCO_3^-) are required for the regulation of acidity and alkalinity of body fluids. The stable condition of the normal organism, homeostasis, is influenced by ions.

Because ions are charged particles, electrolyte solutions can conduct an electric current. Records of electric currents in tissues are valuable indications of the functioning or malfunctioning of tissues and organs. The ***electrocardiogram*** (e-lek-tro-KAR-de-o-gram) and the ***electroencephalogram*** (e-lek-tro-en-SEF-ah-lo-gram) are graphic tracings of the electric currents generated by the heart muscle and the brain, respectively (see Chaps. 9 and 13).

✔ CHECKPOINT **5**:

Ionically bonded substances are called electrolytes. What happens when an electrolyte goes into solution?

Covalent Bonds

Although ionic bonds form many chemical compounds, a much larger number of compounds are formed by another type of chemical bond. This bond involves not the exchange of electrons but a sharing of electrons between the atoms in the molecule and is called a ***covalent***

2

bond. The electrons orbit around both of the atoms, making both of them stable. Sometimes, the electrons are equally shared, as in the case of a hydrogen molecule (H_2), as well as other molecules composed of atoms of the same element. More commonly, the electrons are held closer to one atom than the other, as in the case of water (H_2O), shown in Figure 2-2. These bonds are called **covalent bonds.** Covalently bonded compounds do not conduct an electric current in solution. Carbon, the element that is the basis of organic chemistry, forms covalent bonds. Thus, the compounds that are characteristic of living things are covalently bonded compounds. These bonds may involve the sharing of one, two, or three pairs of electrons between atoms.

✔ CHECKPOINT **6**:

What type of chemical bond is formed by the sharing of electrons?

TYPES OF COMPOUNDS

Acids

An **acid** is a chemical substance capable of donating a hydrogen ion (H^+) to another substance. A common example is hydrochloric acid, the acid found in stomach juices:

HCl   → H$^+$ + Cl$^-$
(hydrochloric   (hydrogen ion)   (chlorine ion)
acid)

Bases

A **base** is a chemical substance, usually containing a hydroxide ion (OH^-), that can accept a hydrogen ion. Sodium hydroxide, which releases hydroxide ion in solution, is an example of a base:

NaOH   → Na$^+$ + OH$^-$
(sodium   (sodium ion)   (hydroxide
hydroxide)   ion)

Salts

A reaction between an acid and a base produces a **salt,** such as sodium chloride:

$$HCl \ + \ NaOH \ \rightarrow \ NaCl \ + \ H_2O$$

THE pH SCALE

The greater the concentration of hydrogen ions in a solution, the greater is the acidity of that solution. As the concentration of hydrogen ions becomes less than it is in pure water, the more alkaline (basic) the solution becomes. Acidity is indicated by **pH** units, which represent the concentration of hydrogen ions in a solution. These units are listed on a scale from 0 to 14, with 0 being the most acidic and 14 being the most basic (Fig. 2-4).

A pH of 7.0 is neutral, having an equal number of hydrogen and hydroxide ions. Solutions that measure less than 7.0 are acidic; those that measure above 7.0 are alkaline (basic).

Each pH unit on the scale represents a 10-fold change in the number of hydrogen and hydroxide ions present. A solution registering 5.0 on the scale has 10 times the number of hydrogen ions as a solution that registers 6.0. A solution registering 9.0 has one tenth the number of hydrogen ions and 10 times the number of hydroxide ions as one registering 8.0. Thus, the lower the pH rating, the greater is the acidity, and the higher the pH, the greater is the alkalinity. Blood and other body fluids are close to neutral but are slightly on the alkaline side,

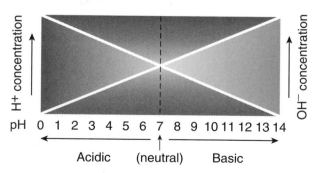

FIGURE **2•4**   The pH scale measures degree of acidity or alkalinity.

with a pH range of 7.35 to 7.45, or nearly neutral. Figure 2-5 shows the pH of some other common substances.

Buffers

A delicate balance exists in the acidity or alkalinity of body fluids. If a person is to remain healthy, these chemical characteristics must remain within narrow limits. This balanced chemical state is maintained in large part by *buffers.* Chemicals that serve as buffers form a system that prevents sharp changes in hydrogen ion concentration and thus maintains a relatively constant pH. Buffers are important in maintaining the stability of body fluids.

FIGURE **2•5**   The pH of some common substances.

✔ CHECKPOINT **7**:

The pH scale is used to measure acidity of fluids. What number is neutral on the pH scale? What kind of compound measures lower than this number? Higher?

CHEMISTRY OF LIVING MATTER

Of the 92 elements that exist in nature, only 26 have been found in living organisms. Most of these are the elements that are light in weight. Not all are present in large quantity. Hydrogen, oxygen, carbon, and nitrogen are the elements that make up about 96% of the cells. Calcium, sodium, potassium, phosphorus, sulfur, chlorine, and magnesium are the seven elements that make up most of the remaining 4% of the elements in living cells. A number of others are present in trace amounts, such as iron, copper, iodine, and fluorine (see Trace Elements).

Trace Elements

Trace elements are required in very small amounts by the body but are absolutely essential for health. Many are used in enzymes and vitamins.

Iodine is needed for the manufacture of thyroid hormones. Selenium is an antioxidant; that is, it helps to prevent damage to cells caused by the chemical process of oxidation. A deficiency of selenium leads to muscular disorders. Growth is impaired if the body lacks chromium. This element works with insulin, the hormone that helps the cells to take up glucose from the blood. Copper is needed for the proper use of iron, and cobalt is a part of vitamin B$_{12}$ needed for blood cell formation. Zinc is used in energy metabolism, protein manufacture, immunity, and wound healing.

Other elements that are needed in trace amounts include silicon, nickel, fluorine, tin, and manganese. The diet must contain adequate sources of trace elements, which may be missing in refined and processed foods. More information on trace elements may be discovered as nutrition studies continue.

2

Organic Compounds

The chemical compounds that characterize living things are called *organic compounds.* All of these contain the element *carbon.* Because carbon can combine with a variety of different elements and can even bond to other carbon atoms to form long chains, most organic compounds consist of large, complex molecules. The starch found in potatoes, the fat in the tissue under the skin, and many drugs are examples of organic compounds. These large molecules are often formed from simpler molecules called *building blocks,* which bond together in long chains. The main types of organic compounds are carbohydrates, lipids, and proteins. All three contain carbon, hydrogen, and oxygen as their main ingredients.

✔ CHECKPOINT **8**:

Where are organic compounds found?

Carbohydrates

Carbohydrates are the simple sugars, called *monosaccharides* (mon-o-SAK-ah-rides), or are molecules made from simple sugars linked together. Carbohydrates in the form of sugars and starches are important sources of energy in the diet. Examples of carbohydrates in the body are the glucose that circulates in the blood as a nutrient for the cells and a storage form of glucose called *glycogen* (GLI-ko-jen).

Lipids

Lipids are a class of organic compounds mainly found in the body as *fat.* Fats are made from a substance called *glycerol* (glycerin) in combination with fatty acids. Fats provide insulation for the body and protection for organs. In addition, they are the main form in which energy is stored.

A group of complex lipids, called *phospholipids* (fos-fo-LIP-ids) because they contain the element phosphorus, is of importance. Among other functions, phospholipids make up a major part of the membrane around living cells. *Cholesterol*, found in cell membranes and also needed for the metabolism of fats, is derived from lipid, as are certain hormones.

Proteins

All *proteins* contain, in addition to carbon, hydrogen, and oxygen, the element *nitrogen.* They may also contain sulfur or phosphorus. Proteins are composed of building blocks called *amino* (ah-ME-no) *acids.* Although there are only about 20 different amino acids found in the body, a vast number of proteins can be made by linking them together in different combinations.

Proteins are the structural materials of the body, found in muscle, bone, and connective tissue. They also make up the pigments that give hair, eyes, and skin their color. It is protein that makes each individual physically distinct from others. All three categories of organic compounds, in addition to minerals and vitamins, must be taken in as part of a normal diet. These compounds are discussed further in Chapters 17 and 18.

✔ CHECKPOINT **9**:

What are the three main categories of organic compounds?

Enzymes

Enzymes are proteins that are essential for metabolism. They serve as catalysts in the hundreds of reactions that take place within cells. Without these catalysts, which speed the rate of chemical reactions, metabolism would not occur at a fast enough rate to sustain life. Because each enzyme works only on a specific substance and does only one specific chemical job, many different enzymes are needed. Their production is determined by genes.

Like all catalysts, enzymes take part in reactions only temporarily; they are not used up or changed by the reaction. Therefore, they are needed in very small amounts. Many of the vitamins and minerals required in the diet are parts of enzymes.

The shape of the enzyme is important in its action. The form of the enzyme must match the shape of the substance or substances the enzyme combines with in much the same way as a key fits a lock. This so-called "lock-and-key"

FIGURE **2•6**   Diagram of enzyme action. The enzyme combines with substance 1 (S_1) and substance 2 (S_2). When a new product is formed, the enzyme is released unchanged.

mechanism is illustrated in Figure 2-6. Harsh conditions, such as extremes of temperature or pH, can alter the shape of an enzyme and stop its action. Such an event is always harmful to the cells.

You can usually recognize the names of enzymes because, with few exceptions, they end with the suffix *-ase*. Examples are amylase, lipase, and oxidase. The first part of the name usually refers to the substance acted on or the type of reaction in which the enzyme is involved.

✔ CHECKPOINT **10**:

Enzymes are proteins that act as catalysts. What is a catalyst?

Summary

I. What is chemistry?
  1. Science that deals with composition of matter
  2. Important in study of life sciences

II. Elements—substances from which all matter is made

III. Atoms—subunits of elements
  A. Atomic structure
   1. Protons—positively charged particles in the nucleus
   2. Neutrons—neutral particles in the nucleus
   3. Electrons—negatively charged particles in energy levels around the nucleus

IV. Molecules and compounds
  1. Molecules—combinations of two or more atoms
  2. Compounds—combinations of different atoms
  A. More about water—solvent; essential for metabolism
  B. Mixtures: solutions and suspensions
   1. Mixture: blend of two or more substances
   2. Solution—substance (solute) remains evenly distributed in solvent (*e.g.*, salt in water)
   3. Suspension—material settles out of mixture on standing (*e.g.*, red cells in blood plasma)
   4. Colloidal suspension—particles do not dissolve but remain suspended (*e.g.*, cytoplasm)

V. Chemical bonds
  A. Ionic bonds—formed by transfer of electrons from one atom to another
   1. Electrolytes
    a. Ionically bonded substances
    b. Separate in solution into charged particles (ions)
    c. Conduct electric current

B. Covalent bonds—formed by sharing of electrons between atoms

VI. Types of compounds
   A. Acids—donate hydrogen ions
   B. Bases—accept hydrogen ions
   C. Salts—formed by reaction between acid and base

VII. The pH scale
   1. Measure of acidity or alkalinity of a solution
   2. Scale goes from 0 to 14
      a. 7 is neutral; below 7 is acidic; above 7 is alkaline (basic)

A. Buffer—maintains constant pH of a solution

VIII. Chemistry of living matter
   A. Organic compounds—all contain carbon
      1. Carbohydrates (*e.g.,* sugars, starches)
      2. Lipids (*e.g.,* fats)
      3. Proteins (*e.g.,* structural materials, enzymes)
   B. Enzymes—organic catalysts

Questions for Study and Review

1. Define *chemistry* and tell something about what is included in this study.
2. Define an atom and describe the basic structure of an atom.
3. Define *molecule, element, compound,* and *mixture.*
4. What is an element and what are some examples of elements?
5. Why is water so important to life?
6. How does a mixture differ from a compound? Give two examples of each.
7. Dissolve a teaspoon of sugar in a cup of tea. Which is the solute? The solvent?
8. What are ions and how are they related to electrolytes? What are some examples of ions and of what importance are they in the body?
9. Explain how covalent bonds are formed. Give two examples of covalently bonded compounds.
10. What would a pH reading of 6.5 indicate about a solution? 8.5? 7.0?
11. What are organic compounds and what element is found in all of them?
12. What elements are found in the largest amounts in living cells?
13. What are the building blocks of carbohydrates? fats? proteins?
14. What are enzymes? What type of organic compound are they?
15. Why is the shape of an enzyme important to its action?

✔ ANSWERS TO CHECKPOINTS

1. The composition of matter is studied in the science of chemistry.
2. Atoms are the building blocks of elements; molecules are formed by the union of two or more atoms.
3. Water is the most abundant compound in the body.
4. In a solution, the components remain evenly distributed; in a suspension, the particles settle out unless the mixture is shaken.
5. When an electrolyte goes into solution, it separates into charged particles called ions.
6. A covalent bond is formed by the sharing of electrons.
7. A value of 7.0 is neutral on the pH scale. An acid measures lower than 7.0; a base measures higher than 7.0.
8. Organic compounds are found in living things.
9. The three main categories of organic compounds are carbohydrates, lipids, and proteins.
10. A catalyst is a compound that speeds up the rate of a chemical reaction.

3

Cells and Their Functions

SELECTED KEY TERMS

The following terms are defined in the Glossary:

active transport

cell membrane

centriole

chromosome

cytoplasm

diffusion

DNA

interphase

isotonic

micrometer

mitochondria

mitosis

nucleotide

nucleus

organelle

osmosis

phagocytosis

ribosome

RNA

BEHAVIORAL OBJECTIVES

After careful study of this chapter, you should be able to:

1. List three types of microscopes used to study cells

2. Describe the function and composition of the plasma membrane and the cytoplasm

3. Name and describe the main organelles in the cell

4. Give the composition, location, and function of DNA in the cell

5. Give the composition, location, and function of RNA in the cell

6. Explain briefly how cells make proteins

7. Name and briefly describe the stages in cell division

8. Define six methods by which substances enter and leave cells

9. Explain what will happen if cells are placed in solutions with the same or different concentrations than the cell fluids

STUDIES OF CELLS

The cell is the basic unit of all life. It is the simplest structure that shows all the characteristics of life, including organization, metabolism, responsiveness, homeostasis, growth, and reproduction. In fact, it is possible for a single cell to live independently of other cells. Examples of some free-living cells are microscopic organisms such as protozoa and bacteria, some of which produce disease. All the activities of the human body, which is composed of millions of cells, result from the activities of individual cells. Cells produce all the materials manufactured within the body.

Microscopes

The scientific study of cells began more than 300 years ago with the invention of the microscope by Anton van Leeuwenhoek. In time, his single-lens microscope was replaced by the modern compound light microscope, which has two sets of lenses. This is the type of microscope most commonly used in laboratories. A great boon to cell biologists has been the development of the *transmission electron microscope,* which uses an electron beam instead of visible light to magnify an image up to 1 million times (Fig. 3-1). Another type, the *scanning electron microscope,* does not magnify as much (×100,000) but gives a three-dimensional view of an object.

The metric unit used for microscopic measurements is the *micrometer* (MI-kro-me-ter). This unit is 1/1000 of a millimeter and is symbolized with the Greek letter for m, as μm.

Before they are examined under the microscope, cells and tissues usually are colored with special dyes called *stains* to aid in viewing. These stains produce the variety of colors you see when looking at pictures of cells and tissues taken under a microscope.

✔ CHECKPOINT **1**:

The cell is the basic unit of life. What characteristics of life does it show?

STRUCTURE OF THE CELL

Just as people may look different but still have certain features in common—two eyes, a nose, and a mouth, for example—all cells share certain characteristics. A typical animal cell is shown in Figure 3-2.

Plasma Membrane

The outer limit of the cell is the *plasma membrane,* also called the *cell membrane* (Fig. 3-3). A double layer of lipid molecules makes up the main substance of this membrane. Because

Liver

FIGURE **3•1** Liver tissue shown at three different magnifications. **(A)** Low power of the compound light microscope—100X. **(B)** Highest power of the compound light microscope—1000X. **(C)** Portion of a cell seen with a transmission electron microscope—48,000X.

these lipids contain the element phosphorus, they are called ***phospholipids.*** Some molecules of cholesterol, another type of lipid, are located between the phospholipids. Cholesterol strengthens the membrane.

A variety of different proteins float within the phospholipids. Some proteins act as receptors, that is, as points of attachment for materials coming to the cell in the blood or tissue fluid. Others are enzymes, participating in reactions occurring at the plasma membrane. Some are transporters, shuttling materials into or out of the cell, and some form channels through which selected substances can pass. The plasma membrane is important in regulating what can enter and leave the cell.

Carbohydrates are present in small amounts, combined either with proteins or with lipids. These carbohydrates help cells to recognize each other and to stick together (see Cell Junctions).

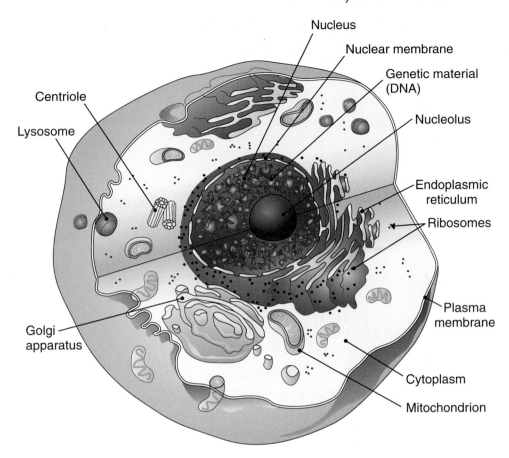

FIGURE **3•2** Diagram of a typical animal cell showing the main organelles.

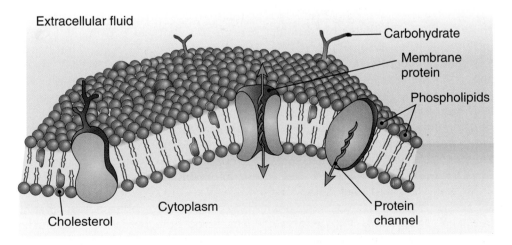

FIGURE **3•3** Current concept of the structure of the plasma membrane.

Cell Junctions

Some cells, for example, blood cells floating in plasma, are not in fixed contact with other cells. Most cells, however, are held in position with surrounding cells. What keeps cells together? First, the cell membranes contain complex substances that are sticky and tend to bind cells to each other. Second, there are special intercellular junctions, which vary according to the functions of the cells.

A *tight junction* is formed when the membranes of adjacent cells actually become fused. This type of junction is found in the lining of the digestive tract and acts to keep digestive juices and other harmful substances from damaging the organs. One substance that can seep through the tight junctions of the stomach and damage the deeper tissues is alcohol.

Connections can form between adjacent cells where tissues are under great stress, for example, in the skin. Protein filaments extend from the cells; bridging the space between the membranes and anchoring cells to each other. These junctions are called *desmosomes* (DES-mo-somz).

Gap junctions allow materials to pass between cells. Small tubes made of protein connect the cells and act as channels for exchange of chemicals. These are found where cells need to communicate easily, as in the nervous system.

Cytoplasm

The main substance that fills the cell and holds the cell contents is the *cytoplasm* (SI-to-plazm). This is a suspension of nutrients, minerals, enzymes, and other specialized materials in water. Although the composition of the cytoplasm has been analyzed, no one has been able to produce it in a laboratory; there must be something about the organization of these substances that has not yet been discovered.

✔ CHECKPOINT **2**:

The outer limit of the cell is a complex membrane. What are the three main ingredients in this plasma membrane?

Organelles

Just as the body has different organs to carry out special functions, the cell contains specialized subdivisions that perform different tasks. These structures are called *organelles,* which means "little organs." Each of these is examined next (see Fig. 3-2).

Nucleus

The largest organelle is the *nucleus* (NU-kle-us). This is often called the *control center* of the cell because it contains the genetic material, which governs all the activities of the cell, including protein manufacture and cell reproduction. Within the nucleus is a smaller globule called the *nucleolus* (nu-KLE-o-lus), which means "little nucleus." Its functions are not entirely understood, but it is believed to act in the manufacture of proteins within the cell.

Organelles in the Cytoplasm

The actual formation of proteins occurs on small bodies called *ribosomes* (RI-bo-somz). These are attached to a network of membranes throughout the cell called the *endoplasmic reticulum* (en-do-PLAS-mik re-TIK-u-lum). The name literally means "network" (reticulum) "within the cytoplasm" (endoplasmic), but for ease, it is almost always called simply the *ER*.

The *mitochondria* (mi-to-KON-dre-ah) are large organelles. They are round or bean-shaped structures with folded membranes on the inside. Within the mitochondria, the energy from nutrients is converted to energy for the cell in the form of ATP. These are the "power plants" of the cell. Active cells need lots of energy and thus have large numbers of mitochondria.

Other organelles in a typical cell include the *Golgi* (GOL-je) *apparatus,* which formulates special substances, such as mucus, released from cells; *lysosomes* (LI-so-somes), which contain digestive enzymes (see Lysosomes); and the *centrioles,* rod-shaped bodies near the nucleus that function in cell division. The features of all these cell structures are summarized in Table 3-1 for easy study.

Although the basic structure of all body cells is the same, individual cells may vary widely in

Table 3·1   Cell Structures

NAME	DESCRIPTION	FUNCTION
Cell membrane	Outer layer of the cell; composed mainly of lipids and proteins	Limits the cell; regulates what enters and leaves the cell
Cytoplasm	Colloidal suspension that fills cell	Holds cell contents
Nucleus	Large, dark-staining body near the center of the cell, composed of DNA and proteins	Contains the chromosomes with the genes (the hereditary material that directs all cell activities)
Nucleolus	Small body in the nucleus; composed of RNA, DNA, and protein	Needed for protein manufacture
Endoplasmic reticulum (ER)	Network of membranes in the cytoplasm	Used for storage and transport; holds ribosomes
Ribosomes	Small bodies attached to the ER; composed of RNA and protein	Manufacture proteins
Mitochondria	Large organelles with folded membranes inside	Convert energy from nutrients into ATP
Golgi apparatus	Layers of membranes	Put together special substances such as mucus
Lysosomes	Small sacs of digestive enzymes	Digest substances within the cell
Centrioles	Rod-shaped bodies (usually two) near the nucleus	Help separate the chromosomes in cell division
Cilia	Short, hairlike projections from the cell	Create movement around the cell
Flagellum	Long, whiplike extension from the cell	Moves the cell

size, shape, and composition according to the function of each. In size, they may range from the 7 µm of a red blood cell to the 200 µm or more of a muscle cell. A neuron with its long fibers is different in appearance from a muscle cell or from a transparent cell in the clear lens of the eye. Most human cells have all the organelles described, but these may vary in number.

Cilia and Flagellum

Some cells have small, hairlike projections from the surface called *cilia* (SIL-e-ah), which wave to create movement around the cell. Examples are the cells that line the passageways of the respiratory and reproductive tracts. A long, whiplike extension from the cell is a *flagellum* (flah-JEL-lum). Each human sperm cell has a flagellum that is used for locomotion. Thus, each cell is specialized for its particular function.

✔ CHECKPOINT **3**:

What are cell organelles?

✔ CHECKPOINT **4**:

What are the two types of organelles used for movement, and what do they look like?

CELL FUNCTIONS

Protein Synthesis

Because protein molecules play an indispensable part in the body's activities, we need to identify the cellular substances that direct the production of protein. In the cytoplasm and in the nucleus are chemicals called **nucleic** (nu-KLE-ik) **acids.** The two nucleic acids important in protein production are **deoxyribonucleic** (de-ok-se-RI-bo-nu-kle-ik) **acid,** or **DNA,** and **ribonucleic** (RI-bo-nu-kle-ik) **acid,** abbreviated **RNA.** Both of these are large, complex molecules composed of subunits called **nucleotides** (NU-kle-o-tides) (Fig. 3-4). There are four nucleotides in DNA and four in RNA, but only three of these are common to both.

DNA

DNA molecules are found mostly in the nucleus of the cell, where they make up the **chromosomes** (KRO-mo-somes), which are dark-staining, threadlike bodies. Looking at Figure 3-4, you can see that DNA exists as a double strand. The two strands are matched according to the pattern of the nucleotides. The adenine (A) nucleotide always pairs with the thymine (T) nucleotide; the guanine (G) nucleotide always

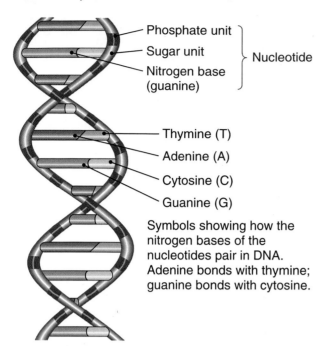

Phosphate unit
Sugar unit
Nitrogen base
(guanine)
⎫ Nucleotide

Thymine (T)
Adenine (A)
Cytosine (C)
Guanine (G)

Symbols showing how the nitrogen bases of the nucleotides pair in DNA. Adenine bonds with thymine; guanine bonds with cytosine.

FIGURE **3•4**   Schematic representation of the basic structure of a DNA molecule. Each structural unit, or nucleotide, consists of a phosphorus-containing unit and a sugar unit to which is attached a nitrogen base. There are four different nucleotides. Their arrangement "spells out" the genetic instructions that control all activities of the cell. The symbols in the upper right show how the nucleotides pair in DNA.

✔ CHECKPOINT **5**:

What category of compounds does DNA code for in the cell?

pairs with the cytosine (C) nucleotide. The two strands of DNA are held together by weak bonds. The doubled strands then coil into a spiral, giving DNA the descriptive name of the *double helix.*

Specific regions of the DNA in the chromosomes make up the **genes,** the hereditary factors of each cell. It is the genes that carry the messages for the development of particular inherited characteristics, such as brown eyes, curly hair, or blood type. Their message is actually contained in the pattern of the four nucleotides in the DNA (see DNA Fingerprinting in Chapter 5, page 57). These subunits code for the building of amino acids into the various cellular proteins. Remember that all enzymes are proteins, and enzymes are essential for cellular reactions. DNA is thus considered the master blueprint for the cell.

The Role of RNA

A blueprint is only a map. The information it illustrates must be translated by appropriate actions. RNA is the substance needed for this step. RNA is much like DNA except that it is a single strand and has a nucleotide called *thymine* (T) instead of cytosine (C). By pairing of nucleotides, RNA picks up the message of the DNA, which has by now broken its weak bonds and uncoiled into single strands. This *messenger RNA* travels into the cytoplasm to the ribosomes attached to the ER. Ribosomes are the organelles responsible for protein manufacture. They are so named because they are composed mainly of RNA. At the ribosomes, the genetic message is decoded to build amino acids into the long chains that form proteins.

Cell Division

For growth, repair, and reproduction, cells must multiply to increase their numbers. To ensure that every cell in the body has the same genetic information, cell division must be precise. In this process of cell division, or mitosis (mi-TO-sis), each original parent cell divides to form two identical daughter cells. Before mitosis can occur, however, the genetic information (DNA) in the parent cell must be doubled. DNA duplicates during interphase, the period between one mitosis and the next. While DNA is uncoiled from its double-stranded form, each strand duplicates itself according to the pattern of the nucleotides.

Stages of Mitosis

Mitosis itself is described as occurring in four stages, during which distinct changes can be seen in the dividing cell (Fig. 3-5).

* In **prophase** (PRO-faze), the doubled strands return to their spiral organization

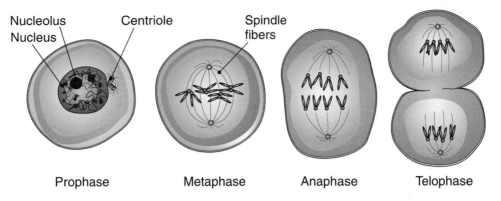

FIGURE **3•5**   The stages of mitosis. The cell shown is for illustration only. It is not a human cell, which has 46 chromosomes.

and become visible under the microscope as dark, threadlike chromosomes. Meanwhile, in the cytoplasm, the two centrioles move to opposite ends of the cell, trailing thin, threadlike substances that form a structure resembling a spindle stretched across the cell.

- In *metaphase* (MET-ah-faze), the chromosomes line up across the threadlike spindle.
- Then, in *anaphase* (AN-ah-faze), the duplicated chromosomes separate and begin to move toward opposite ends of the cell.
- As mitosis continues into *telophase* (TEL-o-faze), the nuclear area becomes pinched in the middle until two new nuclei have formed.

A similar pinching off occurs in the plasma membrane during telophase, making the cell resemble a dumbbell. The midsection between the two halves of the dumbbell becomes progressively smaller until, finally, the cell splits in two. There are now two identical daughter cells, which are themselves identical to, but smaller than, the parent cell. The two new cells grow and mature and continue to carry out life functions.

During mitosis, all the organelles, except those needed for the division process, temporarily disappear. After the cell splits, these organelles reappear in each daughter cell. Also at this time, the centrioles usually duplicate in preparation for the next cell division.

Body cells differ in the rate at which they reproduce. Some, such as nerve cells and muscle cells, stop dividing at some point in development and are not replaced if they die. They remain in interphase. Others, such as skin cells, multiply rapidly to replace cells destroyed by injury, disease, or natural wear-and-tear. As a person ages, characteristic changes in the overall activity of his or her body cells take place. One example of these changes is the slowing down of repair processes. A bone fracture, for example, takes considerably longer to heal in an aged person than in a young person.

✔ CHECKPOINT **6**:

Cells must divide to allow for growth, repair, and reproduction. What is the scientific name for cell division?

Movement of Substances Across the Plasma Membrane

Cells constantly need nutrients and other materials from their environment to function. How to receive these nutrients would seem to be a problem because a protective membrane surrounds cells. However, if a cell is bathed in water containing dissolved nutrients, an interesting thing happens: the water with the dissolved nutrient particles passes through the plasma membrane. Not only do these molecules pass in, but also waste products pass out of the cell in the opposite direction, enabling the cell

3

to perform the function of elimination. Thus, exchanges of some substances can occur between the cell and its environment through the plasma membrane. For this reason, the plasma membrane is described as ***semipermeable*** (sem-e-PER-me-ah-bl). It is permeable or passable to some molecules but impassable to others. Some particles, for example, proteins, are simply too large to travel through the membrane unaided.

Water, a tiny molecule, is always able to penetrate the membrane with ease. Foods, however, must be split into small molecules by the process of digestion so that they can travel through the plasma membrane. For example, sucrose (table sugar) is converted to glucose, a smaller molecule that enters the cell to serve as a major source of energy.

Various physical processes are responsible for exchanges through plasma membranes. These are grouped according to whether they require cellular energy.

Movement That Does Not Require Cellular Energy

- ***Diffusion*** is the constant movement of molecules from a region of relatively higher concentration to one of lower concentration. Molecules, especially those in solution, tend to spread throughout an area until

FIGURE **3•7** Diffusion of a solid in a liquid. Here, a solid diffuses into water. The molecules of the solid tend to spread evenly throughout the water.

they are equally concentrated in all parts of a container (Figs. 3-6 and 3-7). When substances diffuse through a membrane, such as the intact plasma membrane, passage is limited to those particles small enough to pass through spaces in the membrane. A large-scale example is shown in Figure 3-8.

- ***Osmosis.*** Of all substances, water moves most rapidly through the cell membrane. The term *osmosis* means specifically the diffusion of water through a semipermeable membrane. The water molecules move, as expected, from an area where they are in higher number to an area where they are in lower number. That is, they move from a more dilute solution into a more concentrated solution. The tendency of a solution to draw water into it is called the ***osmotic pressure*** of the solution. This force is directly related to concentration: the higher the concentration of a solution, the greater is its tendency to draw water in.
- ***Filtration*** is the passage of water containing dissolved materials through a membrane as a result of a mechanical ("pushing") force on one side (Fig. 3-9). One example of filtration in the body is the formation of urine in the kidney (see Chap. 19). Another is the movement of materials out of the capillaries under the force of blood pressure (see Chap. 14).

These three processes are described as *passive* because they do not require cellular energy. They depend on the natural energy of the molecules for movement.

FIGURE **3•6** Diffusion of gaseous molecules throughout a given space. When a solution vaporizes, the molecules tend to spread throughout the area. Common examples are the diffusion of perfumes, oils, and cleaning solutions.

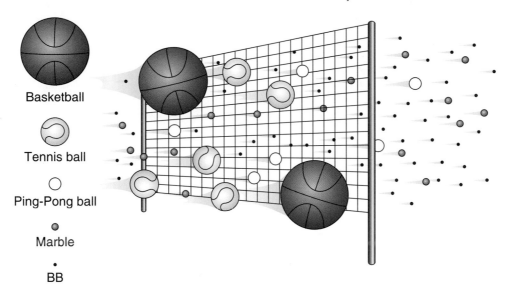

FIGURE **3•8** Diffusion through a semipermeable membrane. In this example, large objects (basketballs and tennis balls) cannot pass through the net. In the human body, large particles (proteins and blood cells) do not pass through intact membranes, such as the walls of the blood capillaries.

Movement That Requires Cellular Energy

- *Active transport.* Molecules often move into or out of a living cell in a direction opposite to the way they would normally flow by diffusion. That is, they move from an area where they are in relatively lower concentration to an area where they are in higher concentration. This movement, because it is against the natural flow, requires energy in the form of ATP. It also requires proteins in the cell membrane that act as *transporters* for the molecules. This process, called *active transport,* is a function of the living cell membrane. It allows the cell to take in what it needs from the surrounding fluids and to release materials from the cell. Because the cell membrane can carry on active transport, it is most accurately described as *selectively permeable.* It regulates what can enter and leave the cell based on its needs.

- *Phagocytosis* (fag-o-si-TO-sis) is the engulfing of relatively large particles by the cell membrane and the movement of these particles into the cell. Certain white blood cells carry out phagocytosis to rid the body of foreign material and dead cells.

- In *pinocytosis* (pi-no-si-TO-sis), droplets of fluid are engulfed by the cell membrane. This is a way for large protein molecules in suspension to travel into the cell. The word *pinocytosis* means "cell drinking."

✔ CHECKPOINT **7**:

Substances are constantly moving into and out of cells through the plasma membrane. What types of movement do not require cellular energy and what types of movement do require cellular energy?

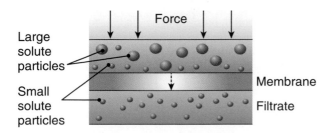

FIGURE **3•9** Filtration. A mechanical force pushes a substance through a membrane.

Large solute particles

Small solute particles

Force

Membrane

Filtrate

How Osmosis Affects Cells

As stated earlier, water moves easily through the cell membrane. Therefore, for a normal fluid balance to be maintained, all cells must be

Isotonic solution
(normal)

Hypotonic solution
(dilute)

Hypertonic solution
(concentrated)

Water —

Solute —

Normal red
blood cell

Swollen/ruptured
red blood cell

Shrunken red
blood cell

<small>FIGURE **3•10**   Osmosis. Water moving through a red blood cell membrane in solutions with three different concentrations of solute. *(Left)* The isotonic (normal) solution has the same concentration as the cell, and the water moves into and out of the cell at the same rate. *(Center)* The hypotonic (dilute) solution causes the cell to swell and eventually hemolyze (burst) because of the large amount of water moving into the cell. *(Right)* The hypertonic (concentrated) solution draws water out of the cell, causing it to shrink.</small>

kept in solutions that have the same concentration of dissolved substances (solutes) as the fluids within the cell (Fig. 3-10). If not, water will move rapidly into or out of the cell by osmotic pressure. Solutions with concentrations equal to the concentration of the cytoplasm are described as ***isotonic.***

Tissue fluids and blood plasma are isotonic for body cells. Manufactured solutions that are isotonic for the cells and can thus be used to replace body fluids include 0.9% salt or ***normal saline*** and 5% dextrose (glucose).

A solution that is less concentrated than the intracellular fluid is described as ***hypotonic.*** A cell placed in a hypotonic solution draws water in, swells, and may burst. When a red blood cell draws in water and bursts in this way, the cell is said to ***hemolyze*** (HE-mo-lize). If a cell is placed in a ***hypertonic*** solution, which is more concen-

trated than the cell fluid, it loses water to the surrounding fluids and shrinks (see Fig. 3-10).

Fluid balance is an important facet of homeostasis and must be properly regulated for health. You can figure out in which direction water will move through the plasma membrane if you remember the saying "water follows salt," salt meaning any dissolved material (solute). The total amount and distribution of body fluids is discussed in Chapter 19.

 CHECKPOINT **8**:

The concentration of fluids in and around the cell is important in homeostasis. What term describes a fluid that is the same concentration as the fluid within the cell (intracellular fluid)? What type of fluid is less concentrated? More concentrated?

Summary

I. Studies of cells
1. Cell is basic unit of life
   a. Has all characteristics of life
   b. Is responsible for all body activities
   A. Microscopes
   1. Types
      a. Compound light microscope
      b. Transmission electron microscope—magnifies up to 1 million times
      c. Scanning electron microscope—gives three-dimensional image
   2. Micrometer—metric unit commonly used for microscopic measurements
   3. Stains—dyes used to aid in viewing cells under the microscope

II. Structure of the cell
A. Plasma membrane—regulates what enters and leaves cell
B. Cytoplasm—colloidal suspension that holds organelles
C. Organelles—subdivisions that carry out special functions
   1. Nucleus
      a. Controls cell activities
      b. Contains nucleolus
   2. Ribosomes, ER, mitochondria, Golgi apparatus, lysosomes, centrioles
   3. Cilia, flagellum—used for movement

III. Cell functions
A. Protein synthesis—carried out by nucleic acids
   1. DNA
      a. Double strand of nucleotides
      b. Located in the nucleus
      c. Carries the genetic message
   2. RNA
      a. Single strand of nucleotides
      b. Located in the cytoplasm
      c. Translates DNA message into proteins
      d. Ribosomes—site of protein synthesis
B. Cell division
   1. Duplication of chromosomes during interphase
   2. Mitosis
      a. Separation of chromosomes
      b. Division of cell into two identical daughter cells
      c. Four stages—prophase, metaphase, anaphase, telophase
C. Movement of substances across plasma membrane
   1. Movement that does not require cellular energy
      a. Diffusion—molecules move from area of higher concentration to area of lower concentration
      b. Osmosis—diffusion of water through semipermeable membrane
      c. Filtration—movement of materials through cell membrane under mechanical force
   2. Movement that requires cellular energy
      a. Active transport—movement of molecules from area of lower concentration to area of higher concentration
      b. Phagocytosis—engulfing of large particles by plasma membrane
      c. Pinocytosis—intake of droplets of fluid
   3. How osmosis affects cells
      a. Isotonic solution—same concentration as cell fluids; cell remains the same
      b. Hypotonic solution—lower concentration than cell fluids; cell swells and may hemolyze (burst)
      c. Hypertonic solution—higher concentration than cell fluids; cell shrinks

Questions for Study and Review

1. Why is the study of cells so important in the study of the body?
2. Why is the plasma membrane so important to the cell?
3. Define the term *organelle.* List 10 organelles found in cells and give the function of each.
4. Compare DNA and RNA with respect to location in the cell and composition.
5. What are chromosomes? Where are they located in the cell and what is their function?
6. Explain the role of each of the following in protein synthesis: DNA, nucleotide, RNA, ribosomes.
7. Name the stage between one mitosis and the next.
8. Name the process of cell division. Name the stages of cell division and describe what happens during each.
9. Explain why it is necessary to reduce large molecules to smaller molecules by the process of digestion.
10. List and define six methods by which materials cross the cell membrane. Which of these requires cellular energy?
11. What substance moves most rapidly through the cell membrane?
12. Why is the cell membrane described as selectively permeable?
13. What is meant by the term *isotonic*? Name four isotonic solutions.
14. What will happen to a red blood cell placed in a 5.0% salt solution? in distilled water?

✔ ANSWERS TO CHECKPOINTS

1. The cell shows organization, metabolism, responsiveness, homeostasis, growth, and reproduction.
2. The three main ingredients in the plasma membrane are phospholipids (lipids), proteins, and carbohydrates.
3. The cell organelles are specialized subdivisions that perform different tasks.
4. The two types of organelles used for movement are the cilia, which are small and hairlike, and the flagellum, which is long and whiplike.
5. DNA codes for proteins in the cell.
6. Mitosis is the scientific name for cell division.
7. Diffusion, osmosis, and filtration do not require cellular energy; active transport, phagocytosis, and pinocytosis require cellular energy.
8. An isotonic solution is the same concentration as the fluid within the cell; a hypotonic solution is less concentrated; a hypertonic solution is more concentrated.

4

Tissues, Glands, and Membranes

SELECTED KEY TERMS

The following terms are defined in the Glossary:

adipose

areolar

cartilage

collagen

endocrine

epithelium

exocrine

fascia

histology

matrix

membrane

mucosa

myelin

neuroglia

neuron

serosa

BEHAVIORAL OBJECTIVES

After careful study of this chapter, you should be able to:

1. Name the four main groups of tissues and give the location and general characteristics of each

2. Describe the difference between exocrine and endocrine glands and give examples of each

3. Give examples of soft, fibrous, hard, and liquid connective tissues

4. Describe three types of epithelial membranes

5. List several types of connective tissue membranes

Tissues are groups of cells similar in structure, arranged in a characteristic pattern, and specialized for the performance of specific tasks. The study of tissues is known as **histology** (his-TOL-o-je). The tissues in our bodies might be compared with the different materials used to construct a building. Think for a moment of the great variety of building materials used according to need—wood, stone, steel, plaster, insulation, and so forth. Each of these has different properties, but together they contribute to the building as a whole. The same may be said of tissues in the body.

TISSUE CLASSIFICATION

The four main groups of tissue are the following:

- **Epithelial** (ep-ih-THE-le-al) **tissue** covers surfaces, lines cavities, and forms glands.
- **Connective tissue** supports and forms the framework of all parts of the body.
- **Muscle tissue** contracts and produces movement.
- **Nervous tissue** conducts nerve impulses.

This chapter concentrates mainly on epithelial and connective tissues; muscle and nervous tissues receive more attention in later chapters.

Epithelial Tissue

Epithelial tissue, or **epithelium** (ep-ih-THE-le-um), forms a protective covering for the body and all the organs. It is the main tissue of the outer layer of the skin. It forms the lining of the intestinal tract, the respiratory and urinary passages, the blood vessels, the uterus, and other body cavities.

Structure of Epithelial Tissue

Epithelium has many forms and many purposes, and the cells of which it is composed vary accordingly. Epithelial tissue is classified according to the shape and the arrangement of its cells (Fig. 4-1). In shape, the cells may be referred to as follows:

- **Squamous** (SKWA-mus)—flat and irregular
- **Cuboidal**—square
- **Columnar**—long and narrow.

The cells may be arranged in a single layer, described as **simple,** or in many layers, termed **stratified.** Thus, a single layer of flat, irregular cells would be described as *simple squamous epithelium,* whereas tissue with many layers of these same cells would be described as *stratified squamous epithelium.*

Some organs, such as the urinary bladder, must vary a great deal in size during the course

4

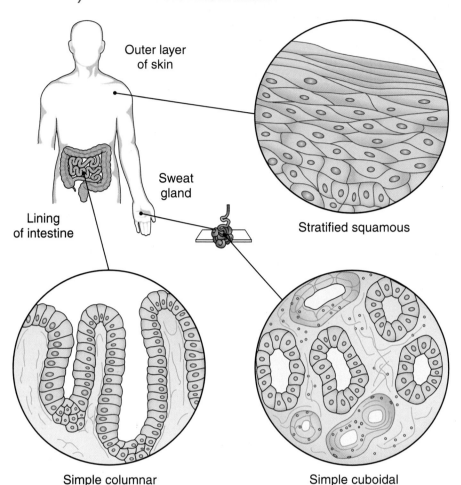

Outer layer
of skin

Sweat
gland

Lining
of intestine

Stratified squamous

Simple columnar

Simple cuboidal

Figure **4•1** Three types of epithelium.

of their work. For this purpose, there is a special wrinkled, crepe-like tissue, called ***transitional epithelium,*** which is capable of great expansion yet returns to its original form once tension is relaxed—as when, in this case, the bladder is emptied.

Functions of Epithelial Tissue

The cells of some kinds of epithelium produce secretions, such as ***mucus*** (MU-kus) (a clear, sticky fluid), digestive juices, sweat, and other substances. The digestive tract is lined with a special kind of epithelium, the cells of which not only produce secretions but also are designed to absorb digested foods. The air that we breathe passes over yet another form of epithelium that lines the passageways of the respiratory (breathing) system. This lining secretes mucus and is provided with tiny hairlike projections

called ***cilia.*** Together, the mucus and the cilia help trap bits of dust and other foreign particles that could otherwise reach the lungs and damage them.

Certain areas of the epithelium that form the outer layer of the skin are capable of modifying themselves for greater strength whenever they are subjected to unusual wear and tear; the growth of calluses is a good example of this response.

Epithelium repairs itself quickly after it is injured. If, for example, there is a cut, the cells near and around the wound immediately form daughter cells, which grow until the cut is closed. Epithelial tissue reproduces frequently in areas of the body subject to normal wear and tear, such as the skin, the inside of the mouth, and the lining of the intestinal tract.

> ✔ CHECKPOINT **1**:
>
> Epithelium is classified according to cell shape. What are the three basic shapes?

Glands

The active cells of many glands are epithelial cells. A gland is an organ specialized to produce a substance that is sent out to other parts of the body. These secretions are manufactured from blood constituents.

Glands are divided into two categories:

- *Exocrine* (EK-so-krin) *glands* have ducts or tubes to carry secretions away from the gland. The secretions may be carried to another organ, to a body cavity, or to the body surface. They are effective in a limited area near their source. Examples include the digestive juices, the secretions from the sebaceous (oil) glands of the skin, and tears from the lacrimal glands. These glands are discussed in the chapters on specific systems.
- *Endocrine* (EN-do-krin) *glands* depend on blood flowing through the gland to carry the secretion to another organ. These substances, called **hormones,** have specific effects on other tissues. Endocrine glands are the so-called ductless glands.

Exocrine glands vary in design from simple depressions resembling tiny dimples to more complex structures. Simple, tubelike glands are found in the stomach wall and in the intestinal lining. Complex glands composed of treelike groups of ducts are found in the liver, the pancreas, and the salivary glands. Most glands are made largely of epithelial tissue with a framework of connective tissue. There may be a tough connective tissue capsule (a fibrous envelope) enclosing the gland, with extensions into the organ that form partitions. Between the partitions are groups of cells that unite to form lobes.

Endocrine glands produce secretions that are carried to all parts of the body by the blood. These substances often affect tissues at a considerable distance from the point of origin. En-

docrine glands, because they secrete directly into the blood stream, have an extensive blood vessel network. The organs believed to have the richest blood supply in the body are the tiny adrenal glands located near the upper part of the kidneys. Some glands, such as the pancreas, have both endocrine and exocrine functions and therefore have both ducts and a rich blood supply. Hormones and the glands that produce them are discussed in Chapter 11.

> ✔ CHECKPOINT **2**:
>
> Glands are classified according to whether or not they secrete through ducts. What are the two types of glands called?

CONNECTIVE TISSUE

The supporting fabric of all parts of the body is connective tissue (Fig. 4-2). This is so extensive and widely distributed that if we were able to dissolve all the tissues except connective tissue, we would still be able to recognize the contours of the entire body.

Connective tissue has large amounts of non-living material between the cells. This intercellular background material or **matrix** (MA-trix) contains varying amounts of water, fibers, and hard minerals. Connective tissue may be classified simply according to its degree of hardness:

- Soft connective tissue—loosely held together with semi-liquid material between the cells; includes adipose (fat) tissue and areolar (loose) connective tissue
- Fibrous connective tissue—most connective tissue contains some fibers, but this type is densely packed with them. Cells called fibroblasts produce the fibers in connective tissue. (The word ending *-blast* refers to a young and active cell). Examples of structures composed of fibrous connective tissue are ligaments, tendons, and the capsules (coverings) around certain organs.
- Hard connective tissue—has a very firm consistency, as in cartilage, or is hardened by minerals in the matrix, as in bone.

4

SOFT AND LIQUID CONNECTIVE TISSUE

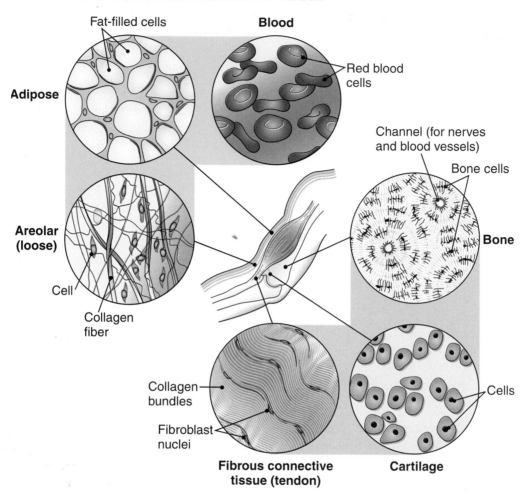

FIGURE **4•2** Connective tissue.

- Liquid connective tissue—Blood and lymph (the fluid that circulates in the lymphatic system) are examples of liquid connective tissues. The cells in liquid connective tissue are suspended in a fluid environment.

> ✔ CHECKPOINT **3**:
>
> Connective tissue varies according to the composition of the material that is between the cells. What is the general name for this intercellular material?

Soft Connective Tissue

The ***areolar*** (ah-RE-o-lar) or loose form of connective tissue (see Fig. 4-2) is found in membranes around vessels and organs, between muscles, and under the skin. It is the most common type of connective tissue in the body. It contains cells and fibers in a very loose, jellylike background material.

Adipose (AD-ih-pose) ***tissue*** (see Fig. 4-2) contains cells that are able to store large amounts of fat. The fat in this tissue is used as a reserve energy supply for the body. Adipose tissue also serves as a heat insulator and as protective padding for organs and joints.

Fibrous Connective Tissue

Fibrous connective tissue (see Fig. 4-2) is very dense and has large numbers of fibers that give it strength and flexibility. The main type of fiber in this and other connective tissues is *collagen* (KOL-ah-jen), a flexible white protein (see Collagen: The Body's Scaffolding).

Some fibrous connective tissue contains large amounts of elastic fibers that allow the tissue to stretch and then return to its original length. This type of elastic connective tissue appears in the vocal cords, the passageways of the respiratory tract, and the walls of the large arteries (blood vessels).

This tissue makes up the fibrous membranes that cover various organs, as described later in this chapter. Particularly strong forms make up the tough *capsules* around certain organs, such as the kidneys, liver, and glands. If the fibers in the connective tissue are all arranged in the same direction, like the strands of a cable, the tissue can pull in one direction. Examples are the cordlike *tendons,* which connect muscles to bones, and the *ligaments,* which connect bones to other bones.

Tissue Repair

Like epithelial tissue, fibrous connective tissue can repair itself easily. Repair begins after blood has clotted and a scab has formed at the surface to protect underlying tissue. From damaged capillaries, new vessels branch and grow into the injured tissue. Fibroblasts (cells that produce fibers) manufacture collagen to close the gap made by the wound. A large wound requires extensive growth of new connective tissue, which forms a *scar*. After the upper layer of epithelium has regenerated, the scab is released. The underlying scar tissue may then continue to show at the surface as a white line.

Suturing (sewing) the edges of a clean wound together, as is done in the case of operative wounds, decreases the amount of connective tissue needed for repair and thus reduces the size of the resulting scar. Scar tissue is strong but is not as flexible as normal tissue and does not function like the tissue it replaces.

Excess production of collagen in the formation of a scar may result in the development of *keloids* (KE-loyds), sharply raised areas on the surface of the skin. These are not dangerous but may be removed for the sake of appearance.

Hard Connective Tissue

The hard connective tissues, which as the name suggests are more solid than the other groups, include cartilage and bone (see Fig. 4-2).

Cartilage

Because of its strength and flexibility, cartilage is used as a shock absorber and as a bearing surface that reduces friction between moving parts. A common form of cartilage is the tough, elastic, translucent material, popularly called *gristle*, that covers the ends of the long bones. Another form of cartilage is found between segments of the spine. Cartilage is also used as structural material and reinforcement, such as at the tip of

Collagen: The Body's Scaffolding

The most abundant protein in the body, making up about 25% of total protein, is the tough, flexible, white material known as *collagen*. Its name comes from a Greek word meaning "glue," indicating that it is the main structural substance in the body. Collagen is the major ingredient in all connective tissue.

The arrangement of the fibers in collagen gives this substance its different properties. It may form a fibrous connective tissue, as in the heart valves; a cord of great strength, as in tendons and ligaments; or a tough, transparent tissue, as in the cornea of the eye. It is collagen that gives strength and resilience to the skin.

The varied properties of collagen are evident in the preparation of a gelatin dessert. Gelatin is a collagen extract made by boiling animal bones and other connective tissue. It is a viscous (thick) liquid in hot water but forms a semisolid gel on cooling.

the nose, the outer ear, and parts of the larynx ("voicebox") and trachea ("windpipe").

Bone

The tissue of which bones are made, called **osseous** (OS-e-us) **tissue,** is much like cartilage in its cellular structure (see Fig. 4-2). In fact, the skeleton of the fetus in the early stages of development is made almost entirely of cartilage. This tissue gradually becomes impregnated with salts of calcium and phosphorus that make bone characteristically solid and hard. Within the bones are nerves, blood vessels, bone-forming cells, and a special form of tissue, bone marrow, in which blood cells are manufactured.

The liquid connective tissues, blood and lymph, are discussed in Chapters 12 and 15, respectively.

 CHECKPOINT **4**:

Connective tissue is the supportive and protective material found throughout the body. What are some examples of soft, fibrous, hard, and liquid connective tissue?

MUSCLE TISSUE

Muscle tissue is designed to produce movement by contraction of its cells, which are called **muscle fibers** because most of them are long and threadlike. If a piece of well-cooked meat is pulled apart, small groups of these muscle fibers may be seen. Muscle tissue is usually classified as follows (Fig. 4-3):

- **Skeletal muscle,** which works with tendons and bones to move the body. This type of tissue is also known as **voluntary muscle** because it can be made to contract by conscious thought.

The next two types of muscle tissue are described as **involuntary muscle** because they typically contract independently of thought. Most of the time we are not aware of their actions at all.

- **Cardiac muscle,** which forms the bulk of the heart wall and is known also as **myocardium** (mi-o-KAR-de-um). This is the muscle that produces the regular contractions known as *heartbeats.*
- **Smooth muscle,** known also as **visceral muscle,** which forms the walls of the **viscera** (VIS-er-ah), or organs of the ventral body cavities (with the exception of the heart). Some examples of visceral muscles are those that move food and waste materials along the digestive tract. Visceral muscle is also found in the walls of many tubular structures, such as the blood vessels and the tubes that carry urine from the kidneys. A smooth muscle is attached to the base of each body hair. Contraction of these muscles causes the skin condition we call *gooseflesh.* Other structures containing visceral muscle are discussed under the various body systems.

Muscle tissue, like nervous tissue, repairs itself only with difficulty or not at all once an injury has been sustained. When injured, muscle tissue is frequently replaced with connective tissue.

Chapter 7 has more detail on muscles.

 CHECKPOINT **5**:

What are the three types of muscle tissue?

NERVOUS TISSUE

The human body is made up of countless structures, both large and small, each of which contributes something to the action of the whole organism. This aggregation of structures might be compared to an army. For all the members of the army to work together, there must be a central coordinating and order-giving agency somewhere; otherwise, chaos would ensue. In the body, this central agency is the **brain.** Each structure of the body is in direct communication with the brain by means of its own set of "wires," called **nerves.** The nerves from even the most remote parts of the body all come together and form a great trunk cable called the

4

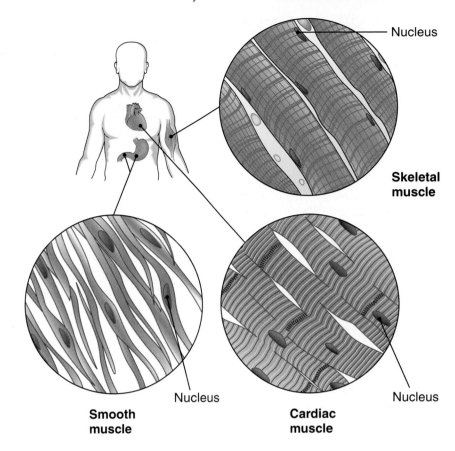

Skeletal muscle

Nucleus

Nucleus

Smooth muscle

Cardiac muscle

Nucleus

FIGURE **4•3**   Muscle tissue.

spinal cord, which in turn leads directly into the central switchboard of the brain. Here, messages come in and orders go out 24 hours a day. This entire communication system, brain and all, is made of nervous tissue.

The Neuron

The basic unit of nervous tissue is the ***neuron*** (NU-ron), or nerve cell (Fig. 4-4). A neuron consists of a nerve cell body plus small branches, like those of a tree, called *fibers.* One type of fiber, the ***dendrite*** (DEN-drite), carries nerve impulses, or messages, to the nerve cell body. A single fiber, the ***axon*** (AK-son), carries impulses away from the nerve cell body. Neurons may be quite long; their fibers can extend for several feet. A nerve is a bundle of nerve cell fibers held together with connective tissue.

Just as wires are insulated to keep them from being short-circuited, some axons are insulated

and protected by a coating of material called ***myelin*** (MI-eh-lin). Groups of myelinated fibers form "white matter," so called because of the color of the myelin, which is much like fat in appearance and consistency. Not all neurons have myelin, however; some axons are unmyelinated, as are all dendrites and all cell bodies. These areas appear gray in color. Because the outer layer of the brain has large collections of cell bodies and unmyelinated fibers, the brain is popularly termed *gray matter.*

Neuroglia

Nervous tissue is supported by special connective tissue cells known as ***neuroglia*** (nu-ROG-le-ah) or *glial* (GLI-al) *cells,* which are named from the Greek word *glia* meaning "glue." Some of these cells protect the brain from harmful substances; others get rid of foreign organisms and cellular debris; still others form the myelin

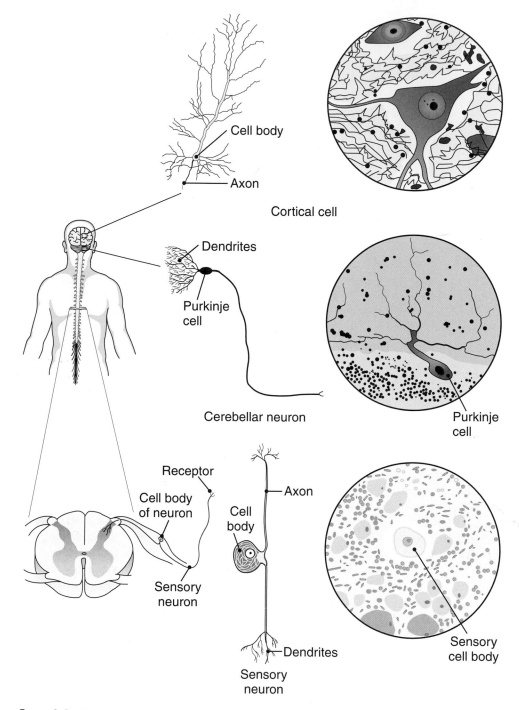

FIGURE **4•4** Nervous tissue.

sheath around axons. They do not, however, transmit nerve impulses.

A more detailed discussion of nervous tissue and the nervous system can be found in Chapters 8 and 9.

✔ CHECKPOINT **6**:

What is the basic cellular unit of the nervous system and what is its function?

✔ CHECKPOINT **7**:

What are the nonconducting support cells of the nervous system called?

MEMBRANES

Membranes are thin sheets of tissue. Their properties vary: some are fragile, others tough; some are transparent, others opaque (*i.e.,* they cannot be seen through). Membranes may cover a surface, may serve as a dividing partition, may line a hollow organ or body cavity, or may anchor an organ. They may contain cells that secrete lubricants to ease the movement of organs, such as the heart and lung, and the movement of joints.

Epithelial Membranes

An *epithelial membrane* is so named because its outer surface is made of epithelium. Underneath, however, there is a layer of connective tissue that strengthens the membrane, and in some cases, there is a thin layer of smooth muscle under that. Epithelial membranes are made of closely packed active cells that manufacture lubricants and protect the deeper tissues from invasion by microorganisms. Epithelial membranes are of several types:

- *Serous* (SE-rus) *membranes* line the walls of body cavities and are folded back onto the surface of internal organs, forming their outermost layer.
- *Mucous* (MU-kus) *membranes* line tubes and other spaces that open to the outside of the body.
- The *cutaneous* (ku-TA-ne-us) *membrane,* commonly known as the *skin*, has an outer layer of epithelium. This membrane is complex and is discussed in detail in Chapter 6 on the integumentary system.

Because they consist mainly of epithelial and connective tissue, serous and mucous membranes are described here.

Serous Membranes

Serous membranes line the closed ventral body cavities and do not communicate with the outside of the body. They secrete a thin, watery lubricant that allows organs to move with a minimum of friction. The thin epithelium of serous membranes is a smooth, glistening kind of tissue called *mesothelium* (mes-o-THE-le-um). The membrane itself may be referred to as the *serosa* (se-RO-sah).

There are three serous membranes:

- The *pleurae* (PLU-re) or *pleuras* (PLU-rahs) line the thoracic cavity and cover each lung.
- The *pericardium* (per-ih-KAR-de-um) is a sac that encloses the heart, which is located in the chest between the lungs.
- The *peritoneum* (per-ih-to-NE-um) is the largest serous membrane. It lines the walls of the abdominal cavity, covers the organs of the abdomen, and forms supporting and protective structures within the abdomen (see Fig. 17-3 in Chap. 17).

Serous membranes are so arranged that one portion forms the lining of the closed cavity while another part folds back to cover the surface of an organ. The serous membrane attached to the wall of a cavity or sac is known as the *parietal* (pah-RI-eh-tal) *layer;* the word *parietal* refers to a wall. Parietal pleura lines the chest wall, and parietal pericardium lines the sac that encloses the heart. Because internal organs are called *viscera,* the membrane attached to the organs is the *visceral layer.* On the surface of the heart is visceral pericardium, and each lung surface is covered by visceral pleura. To visualize this, think of pushing your hand into a soft balloon. The balloon is continuous, but has been folded into two layers. The outer layer is the parietal layer; the inner layer, against your hand, is the visceral layer.

The area between the layers of a serous membrane is a *potential space.* It is *possible* for a space to exist there, but normally the membrane surfaces are in direct contact, with a minimal amount of lubricant between them. Only if substances accumulate between the layers, as when inflammation causes the production of excessive amounts of fluid, is there an actual space.

Mucous Membranes

Mucous membranes are so named because they produce a thick and sticky substance called **mucus** (MU-kus). (Note that the adjective *mucous* contains an "o," whereas the noun *mucus* does not). These membranes form extensive continuous linings in the digestive, respiratory, urinary, and reproductive systems, all of which are connected with the outside of the body. They vary somewhat in both structure and function. The cells that line the nasal cavities and the passageways of the respiratory tract are supplied with tiny, hairlike extensions called *cilia,* as described in Chapter 3. The microscopic cilia move in waves that force secretions outward. In this way, foreign particles, such as bacteria, dust, and other impurities trapped in the sticky mucus, are prevented from entering the lungs and causing harm. Ciliated epithelium is also found in certain tubes of both the male and the female reproductive systems.

The mucous membranes that line the digestive tract have special functions. For example, the mucous membrane of the stomach serves to protect the deeper tissues from the action of powerful digestive juices. If for some reason a portion of this membrane is injured, these juices begin to digest a part of the stomach itself—as in the case of peptic ulcers. Mucous membranes located farther along in the digestive system are designed to absorb food materials, which are then transported to all the cells of the body.

The noun **mucosa** (mu-KO-sah) is used in referring to the mucous membrane of an organ.

> ✔ CHECKPOINT **8**:
>
> Epithelial membranes have an outer layer of epithelium. Which are the three type of epithelial membranes?

Connective Tissue Membranes

The following list is an overview of membranes that consist of connective tissue with no epithelium. These membranes are described in greater detail in later chapters.

- **Synovial** (sin-O-ve-al) **membranes** are thin connective tissue membranes that line the joint cavities. They secrete a lubricating fluid that reduces friction between the ends of bones, thus permitting free movement of the joints. Synovial membranes also line small cushioning sacs near the joints called **bursae** (BUR-se).
- The **meninges** (men-IN-jeze) are several layers of membranes covering the brain and the spinal cord.

Fascia (FASH-e-ah) refers to fibrous bands or sheets that support organs and hold them in place. Fascia is found in two regions:

- **Superficial fascia** is the continuous sheet of tissue that underlies the skin and contains adipose (fat) tissue to insulate and protect the skin.
- **Deep fascia** covers, separates, and protects skeletal muscles.

Finally, there are membranes whose names all start with the prefix *peri-* because they are around organs:

- The **pericardium** (per-e-KAR-de-um) is the fibrous sac that encloses the heart.
- **Periosteum** (per-e-OS-te-um) is around bones.
- **Perichondrium** (per-e-KON-dre-um) is around cartilage (*chondro* is the word root for cartilage).

Summary

I. **Tissue classification**—epithelial tissue, connective tissue, muscle tissue, nervous tissue
   A. Epithelial tissue—covers surfaces, lines cavities
      1. Cells—squamous, cuboidal, columnar
      2. Arrangement—simple or stratified
   B. Glands—active cells are epithelial cells
      1. Exocrine
         a. Secrete through ducts
         b. Produce external secretions
      2. Endocrine
         a. Secrete into bloodstream
         b. Produce hormones

II. **Connective tissue**—supports, binds, forms framework of body
   A. Soft—jellylike intercellular material
      1. Areolar (loose)
      2. Adipose—stores fat
   B. Fibrous—dense tissue with collagenous or elastic fibers between cells
      1. Examples
         a. Tendons—attach muscle to bone
         b. Ligaments—connect bones
         c. Capsules—around organs
         d. Fascia—bands or sheets that support organs
      2. Tissue repair—epithelium and fibrous connective tissue repair easily
   C. Hard—firm and solid
      1. Cartilage—found at ends of bones, nose, outer ear, trachea, etc.
      2. Bone—contains mineral salts
   D. Liquid
      1. Blood
      2. Lymph

III. **Muscle tissue**—contracts to produce movement
      1. Skeletal muscle—voluntary; moves skeleton

2. Cardiac muscle—forms the heart
3. Smooth muscle—involuntary; forms visceral organs

IV. **Nervous tissue**
   A. Neuron—nerve cell
      1. Cell body—contains nucleus
      2. Dendrite—fiber carrying impulses toward cell body
      3. Axon—fiber carrying impulses away from cell body
         a. Myelin—fatty material that insulates some axons
            (1) Myelinated fibers—make up white matter
            (2) Unmyelinated cells and fibers—make up gray matter
   B. Neuroglia—support and protect nervous tissue

V. **Membranes**—thin sheets of tissue
   A. Epithelial membranes—outer layer epithelium
      1. Serous membrane—secretes watery fluid
         a. Parietal layer—lines body cavity
         b. Visceral layer—covers internal organs
         c. Examples—pleurae, pericardium, peritoneum
      2. Mucous membrane
         a. Secretes mucus
         b Lines tube or space that opens to the outside (*e.g.,* respiratory, digestive, reproductive tracts)
      3. Cutaneous membrane—skin
   B. Connective tissue membranes
      1. Synovial membrane—lines joint cavity
      2. Meninges—around brain and spinal cord
      3. Fascia—under skin and around muscles
      4. Pericardium—around heart
      5. Periosteum—around bone
      6. Perichondrium—around cartilage

Questions for Study and Review

1. Define *tissue.* Give a few general characteristics of tissues.
2. Define *epithelium* and give three examples of epithelium.
3. Describe the difference between endocrine and exocrine glands and give examples of each.
4. Define *connective tissue.* Name the main kinds of connective tissue and give an example of each.
5. What kinds of fibers are found in connective tissue?
6. Name three kinds of muscle tissue and give an example of each.
7. What is the difference between voluntary and involuntary muscle?
8. What is the main purpose of nervous tissue? What is its basic structural unit called?
9. Define *myelin.* Where is it found?
10. What are some general characteristics of epithelial membranes?
11. Compare serous and mucous membranes.
12. Name and describe the two layers of serous membranes.
13. List five examples of connective tissue membranes.

✔ ANSWERS TO CHECKPOINTS

1. The three basic shapes of epithelium are squamous (flat and irregular), cuboidal (square), and columnar (long and narrow).
2. Exocrine glands secrete through ducts; endocrine glands do not have ducts and secrete directly into the bloodstream.
3. The intercellular material in connective tissue is the matrix.
4. Examples of soft connective tissue are areolar (loose) and adipose tissue; fibrous connective tissue makes up capsules, tendons, and ligaments; hard connective tissue is cartilage and bone; liquid connective tissue is blood and lymph.
5. The three types of muscle tissue are skeletal (voluntary), cardiac, and smooth (visceral) muscle.
6. The basic cellular unit of the nervous system is the neuron and it carries nerve impulses.
7. The nonconducting support cells of the nervous system are neuroglia (glial cells).
8. The three types of epithelial membranes are the cutaneous membrane (skin), serous membranes, and mucous membranes.

5

The Skin

SELECTED KEY TERMS

The following terms are defined in the Glossary:

dermis

epidermis

integument

keratin

melanin

sebaceous

sebum

subcutaneous

sudoriferous

BEHAVIORAL OBJECTIVES

After careful study of this chapter, you should be able to:

1. Name and describe the layers of the skin

2. Describe the subcutaneous tissue

3. Give the location and function of the appendages of the skin

4. List the main functions of the skin

5. Summarize the information to be gained by observation of the skin

The skin is easily observed. It gives clues to its own health and reflects the health of other body systems. Although the skin may be viewed simply as a membrane enveloping the body, it is far more complex than the other epithelial membranes described in Chapter 4.

The skin is associated with structures known as *appendages*, which include glands, hair, and nails. Together with blood vessels, nerves, and sensory organs, the skin and its appendages form the **integumentary** (in-teg-u-MEN-tar-e) **system.** This name is from the word *integument* (in-TEG-u-ment), which means "covering." The term *cutaneous* (ku-TA-ne-us) also refers to the skin. The functions of this system are discussed later in the chapter after a description of its structure.

STRUCTURE OF THE SKIN

The skin consists of two layers (Fig. 5-1):

- The **epidermis** (ep-ih-DER-mis), the outermost portion, which itself is subdivided into thin layers called **strata** (STRA-tah). The epidermis is composed entirely of epithelial cells and contains no blood vessels.
- The **dermis,** or "true skin," which has a framework of connective tissue and con-

tains many blood vessels, nerve endings, and glands.

Epidermis

The epidermis is the surface layer of the skin, the outermost cells of which are constantly lost through wear and tear. Because there are no blood vessels in the epidermis, the only living cells are in its deepest layer, the **stratum germinativum** (jer-min-a-TI-vum), where nourishment is provided by capillaries in the underlying dermis. The cells in this layer are constantly dividing and producing daughter cells, which are pushed upward toward the surface. As the surface cells die from the gradual loss of nourishment, they undergo changes. Mainly, they develop large amounts of a protein called **keratin** (KER-ah-tin), which serves to thicken and protect the skin.

By the time epidermal cells reach the surface, they have become flat and horny, forming the uppermost layer of the epidermis, the **stratum corneum** (KOR-ne-um). Between the stratum germinativum and the stratum corneum there are additional layers that vary in number and quantity depending on the thickness of the skin. Cells in the deepest layer of the epidermis produce **melanin** (MEL-ah-nin), a dark pigment that colors the skin; irregular patches of melanin are called *freckles*.

5

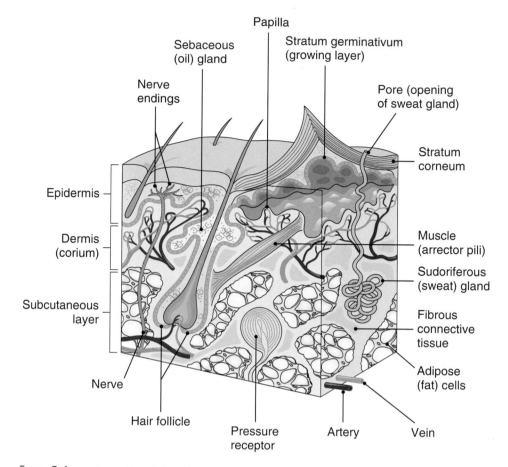

Papilla
Sebaceous (oil) gland
Stratum germinativum (growing layer)
Nerve endings
Pore (opening of sweat gland)
Stratum corneum
Epidermis
Dermis (corium)
Muscle (arrector pili)
Sudoriferous (sweat) gland
Subcutaneous layer
Fibrous connective tissue
Adipose (fat) cells
Nerve
Hair follicle
Pressure receptor
Artery
Vein

FIGURE 5•1   Cross section of the skin.

Dermis

The ***dermis,*** or ***corium*** (KO-re-um), the so-called true skin, has a framework of elastic connective tissue and is well supplied with blood vessels and nerves. Because of its elasticity, the skin can stretch, even dramatically as in pregnancy, with little damage. Most of the appendages of the skin, including the sweat glands, the oil glands, and the hair, are located in the dermis and may extend into the subcutaneous layer under the skin.

The thickness of the dermis also varies in different areas. Some places, such as the soles of the feet and the palms of the hands, are covered with very thick layers of skin, whereas others, such as the eyelids, are covered with very thin and delicate layers.

Portions of the dermis extend upward into the epidermis, allowing blood vessels to get closer to the surface cells (see Fig. 5-1). These extensions, or ***papillae,*** form a distinct pattern of ridges on the surface of thick skin, which help to prevent slipping, such as when grasping an object. The unchanging patterns of the ridges are determined by heredity. Because they are unique to each person, fingerprints and footprints can be used for identification (see DNA Fingerprinting).

Subcutaneous Layer

The dermis rests on the subcutaneous (sub-ku-TA-ne-us) layer, sometimes referred to as the *hypodermis* or the *superficial fascia* (see Fig. 5-1). This layer connects the skin to the surface muscles. It consists of loose connective tissue and large amounts of adipose (fat) tissue. The fat serves as insulation and as a reserve supply for energy. Continuous bundles of elastic fibers connect the subcutaneous tissue with the der-

DNA Fingerprinting

Alike only in name, DNA fingerprinting is totally different from the traditional method of identification using raised patterns of the skin on the fingertips. This newer method starts with any tissue specimen, such as a sample of skin, hair, blood, or semen, and analyzes the pattern of the DNA (the genetic material) in the cells. Even very small quantities suffice because the DNA can be multiplied in the laboratory for the test. The DNA is first extracted from the cells. Enzymes are then used to cut the DNA into fragments based on specific patterns of bases (subunits) of the molecules. After the fragments are marked with radioactive labels, their picture can be taken with x-ray film. When these fragments are sorted and organized by length, they give a unique pattern that looks much like a labeling bar code.

DNA fingerprinting has been used to link suspects to the scene of a crime. When the DNA pattern of an unknown sample matches that of the suspect, the chances are extremely low that they came from different individuals. The method can also be used to identify missing persons or to analyze the closeness of relationship, as in establishing paternity of a child. The DNA patterns of related individuals show many matching bars.

mis, so there is no clear boundary between the two.

The blood vessels that supply the skin and help to regulate body temperature run through the subcutaneous layer. This tissue is also rich in nerves and nerve endings, including those that supply the dermis and epidermis. The thickness of the subcutaneous layer varies in different parts of the body; it is thinnest on the eyelids and thickest on the abdomen.

Figure 5-2 is a photograph of the skin and its appendages as seen through a microscope.

✔ CHECKPOINT **1**:

The skin and all its associated structures comprise a body system. What is the name of this system?

✔ CHECKPOINT **2**:

The skin itself is composed of two layers. Moving from the superficial to the deeper layer, what are the names of these layers?

APPENDAGES OF THE SKIN

Sweat Glands

The **sudoriferous** (su-do-RIF-er-us) **glands,** or sweat glands, are coiled, tubelike structures located in the dermis and the subcutaneous tissue (see Fig. 5-1). Each gland has an excretory tube that extends to the surface and opens at a pore. The slant at which the excretory tube joins the skin serves as a valve. Sudoriferous glands function to regulate body temperature through the evaporation of sweat from the body surface. Sweat consists of water with small amounts of mineral salts and other wastes.

Another type of sweat gland is located mainly in the armpits and the groin area. These glands release their secretions through the hair follicles in response to emotional stress and sexual stimulation. The secretions contain cellular material that is broken down by bacteria, producing body odor.

Several types of glands associated with the skin are modified sweat glands. These are the **ceruminous** (seh-RU-min-us) **glands** in the ear canal that produce ear wax, or **cerumen;** the **ciliary** (SIL-e-er-e) **glands** at the edges of the eyelids; and the **mammary glands.**

Sebaceous Glands

The **sebaceous** (se-BA-shus) **glands** are sac-like in structure, and their oily secretion, **sebum** (SE-bum), lubricates the skin and hair and prevents drying. The ducts of the sebaceous glands open into the hair follicles.

Babies are born with a covering produced by these glands that resembles cream cheese; this secretion is called the **vernix caseosa** (VER-niks ka-se-O-sah).

Blackheads consist of a mixture of dried

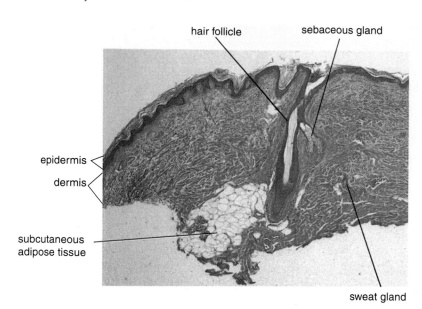

hair follicle   sebaceous gland

epidermis

dermis

subcutaneous
adipose tissue

sweat gland

FIGURE **5•2** Microscopic view of thin skin showing tissue layers and some appendages. (Adapted from Cormack DH: Essential Histology, Plate 12-1B. Philadelphia, JB Lippincott, 1993)

sebum and keratin that may collect at the openings of the sebaceous glands. If these glands become infected, pimples result. If sebaceous glands become blocked by accumulated sebum, a sac of this secretion may form and gradually increase in size. These sacs are referred to as ***sebaceous cysts.*** Usually, it is not difficult to remove such tumorlike cysts by surgery.

✔ CHECKPOINT **3**:

What is the scientific name for the sweat glands?

✔ CHECKPOINT **4**:

Some skin glands produce an oily secretion called sebum. What is the name of these glands?

Hair

Almost all of the body is covered with hair, which in most areas is soft and fine. Hair is composed mainly of keratin and is not living. Each hair develops within a sheath called a ***follicle,*** and new hair is formed from cells at the bottom of the follicles (see Fig. 5-1). Attached to most hair follicles is a thin band of involuntary muscle. When this muscle contracts, the hair is

raised, forming "goose bumps" on the skin. (The name of this muscle is *arrector pili*, which literally means "hair raiser.") This response is of no importance to humans but helps animals with furry coats to conserve heat. As this muscle contracts, it presses on the sebaceous gland associated with the hair follicle, causing the release of sebum to lubricate the skin.

Nails

Nails are protective structures made of hard keratin produced by cells that originate in the outer layer of the epidermis (stratum corneum). New cells form continuously at the proximal end of the nail in an area called the ***nail root.***

Nails of both the toes and the fingers are affected by general health. Changes in nails, including abnormal color, thickness, shape, or texture (*e.g.,* grooves or splitting), occur in chronic diseases such as heart disease, peripheral vascular disease, malnutrition, and anemia.

✔ CHECKPOINT **5**:

Each hair develops within a sheath. What is this sheath called?

FUNCTIONS OF THE SKIN

Although the skin has many functions, the following are its four major functions:

- Protection against infection
- Protection against dehydration (drying)
- Regulation of body temperature
- Collection of sensory information

Protection Against Infection

Intact skin forms a primary barrier against invasion of pathogens. The cells of the stratum corneum, the outermost layer of the epidermis, form a tight interlocking pattern that is resistant to penetration. The surface cells are constantly being shed, causing the mechanical removal of pathogens. Rupture of this barrier, as in cases of wounds or burns, invites infection of deep tissues. The skin also protects against bacterial toxins (poisons) and other harmful chemicals in the environment.

Protection Against Dehydration

The function of the epidermis in preventing water loss is vital to maintenance of the wet environment required by all cells. In addition to keratin, the sebum that serves as a lubricant for the skin is also waterproof and helps to prevent loss by evaporation.

Regulation of Body Temperature

Both the loss of excess heat and protection from cold are important functions of the skin. Indeed, most of the blood supply to the skin is concerned with temperature regulation. The skin forms a large surface for radiating body heat to the surrounding air. When the blood vessels dilate (widen), more blood is brought to the surface so that heat can be dissipated.

The other mechanism for cooling the body involves the sweat glands. The evaporation of perspiration from the surface of the skin draws heat from the body. A person feels uncomfortable on a hot and humid day because water does not evaporate as readily from the skin into the surrounding air. A dehumidifier makes one more comfortable even though the temperature remains high.

In cold conditions, vessels in the skin become narrower (constrict) to reduce the flow of blood to the surface and diminish heat loss. The skin may become visibly pale under these conditions. Special vessels that directly connect arteries and veins in the skin of the ears, nose, and other exposed locations provide the volume of blood flow needed to prevent freezing. As is the case with so many body functions, temperature regulation is complex and involves several parts of the body, including certain centers in the brain.

Collection of Sensory Information

Because of the many nerve endings and other special receptors for pain, touch, pressure, and temperature, which are located mostly in the dermis, the skin may be regarded as one of the chief sensory organs of the body. Many of the reflexes that make it possible for humans to adjust themselves to the environment begin as sensory impulses from the skin. Here, too, the skin works with the brain and the spinal cord to make these important functions possible.

Other Activities of the Skin

Substances can be absorbed through the skin in limited amounts. Some drugs, for example, estrogens and medications to control motion sickness, can be absorbed from patches placed on the skin (see Using Medication Patches). Most medicated ointments used on the skin, however, are for the treatment of local conditions only. Injection of medication into the subcutaneous tissues is limited by the slow absorption that occurs here.

There is also a minimal amount of excretion through the skin. A mixture of water and electrolytes (salts) is excreted in perspiration. Some nitrogen-containing wastes are also eliminated through the skin, but even in disease, the amount of waste products excreted by the skin is small.

Vitamin D needed for the development and maintenance of bone tissue is manufactured in the skin under the effects of ultraviolet radiation in sunlight (see Vitamin D in Chap. 6).

Note that the human skin does not "breathe." The pores of the epidermis serve only as outlets for perspiration from the sweat glands and sebum (oil) from the sebaceous glands. They are not used for exchange of gases.

✔ CHECKPOINT **6**:

What two mechanisms are used to regulate temperature through the skin?

OBSERVATION OF THE SKIN

What can the skin tell you? What do its color, texture, and other attributes indicate? Is there any damage? Much can be learned by an astute observer. In fact, the first indication of a serious systemic disease (such as syphilis) may be a skin disorder.

Color

The color of the skin depends on a number of factors, including the following:

- Amount of pigment in the epidermis
- Quantity of blood circulating in the surface blood vessels
- Composition of the circulating blood
  ○ Quantity of oxygen
  ○ Concentration of hemoglobin
  ○ Presence of bile, silver compounds, or other chemicals

Pigment
The main pigment of the skin, as we have noted, is called ***melanin.*** This pigment is also found in the hair, the middle coat of the eyeball, the iris of the eye, and certain tumors. Melanin is common to all races, but darker people have a much larger quantity in their tissues. The melanin in the skin helps to protect against damaging ultraviolet radiation from the sun. Thus, skin that is exposed to the sun shows a normal increase in this pigment, a response we call *tanning.*

✔ CHECKPOINT **7**:

What is the name for any substance that gives color to the skin?

Effects of Aging on the Integumentary System

As people age, wrinkles, or crow's feet, develop around the eyes and mouth owing to the loss of fat and collagen in the underlying tissues. The dermis becomes thinner, and the skin may become transparent and lose its elasticity, the effect of which is sometimes called "parchment skin." The formation of pigment decreases with age. However, there may be localized areas of extra pigmentation in the skin with the formation of brown spots ("liver spots"), especially on areas exposed to the sun (*e.g.* the back of the hands).

The hair does not replace itself as rapidly as before and thus becomes thinner. Lack of pigment causes the hair to become gray or white. The sweat glands decrease in number, so there is less output of perspiration and lowered ability to withstand heat. The elderly are also more sensitive to cold because of less fat in the skin and poor circulation. Lack of sebum causes dryness of the hair and skin. The fingernails may flake, become brittle, or develop ridges, and toenails may become discolored or abnormally thickened.

CARE OF THE SKIN

The most important factors in caring for the skin are those that ensure good general health. Proper nutrition and adequate circulation are vital to the maintenance of the skin. Regular cleansing removes dirt and dead skin debris and sustains the slightly acid environment that inhibits bacterial growth on the skin. Careful handwashing with soap and water, with attention to the undernail areas, is a simple measure that reduces the spread of disease.

The skin needs protection from continued exposure to sunlight to prevent premature aging and cancerous changes. Appropriate applications of sunscreens before and during time spent in the sun can prevent skin damage (see Protection From the Sun).

Protection From the Sun

Each of the three most common forms of skin cancer, basal cell carcinoma, squamous cell carcinoma, and malignant melanoma, share a common risk factor—exposure to the ultraviolet radiation found in sunlight. Excessive exposure to the sun may not only cause cancer, it may also cause premature aging of the skin, including the production of wrinkles, discoloration, and changes in texture.

The damaging radiation found in sunlight occurs in two different forms, ultraviolet-A (UVA) and ultraviolet-B (UVB). UVA damages the deeper layers of the skin, resulting in a loss of elasticity and a general decrease in blood flow to the skin. UVA also causes damage to the skin cells' ability to repair themselves, thereby increasing the risk of the cells becoming cancerous. UVB damages the outermost layers of the skin. Exposure leads to the redness, swelling, and peeling common to the average "sunburn." Repeated, excessive exposure leads to changes in the texture of the skin such as wrinkling and thickening, as well as a change in texture most often referred to as "leathery skin."

The best way to reduce the risks of damage caused by UVA and UVB is to limit exposure to them. This is especially important between the hours of 10 AM and 4 PM when the level of radiation from the sun is at its highest. You can significantly reduce your exposure to UVA and UVB even during exposure to the midday sun, by doing the following:

- Always apply a sunscreen with an SPF (sun protection factor) of at least 15. The SPF generally indicates the amount of time you are protected relative to using no sunscreen at all (therefore, an SPF of 15 allows you to stay in the sun 15 times longer than without SPF-related protection.) Always follow the specific products' directions. However, generally, all sunscreens should be applied at least 15–20 minutes before exposure and should be reapplied periodically during continued exposure.
- Take advantage of the protection offered by clothing. Hats, long pants, and long-sleeve shirts can protect much of the skin. Special fabrics continue to be developed that effectively block both UVA and UVB.
- Take advantage of the shade. Although shaded areas are still exposed to both UVA and UVB, shade can significantly decrease overall exposure.
- Drink plenty of fluids during and after prolonged exposure to the sun. This can help keep the skin fully hydrated, which promotes the skin's own natural defenses.

Summary

I. Structure of the skin
  A. Epidermis—surface layer of the skin
  B. Dermis—deeper layer of the skin
    1. Subcutaneous layer—under the skin

II. Appendages of the skin
  A. Sweat glands—sudoriferous glands
  B. Sebaceous glands—oil glands
  C. Hair
  D. Nails

III. Functions of the skin
    1. Protection against infection
    2. Protection against dehydration
    3. Regulation of body temperature
    4. Collection of sensory information
    5. Other activities of the skin—absorption, excretion, manufacture of vitamin D

IV. Observation of the skin
  A. Color
    1. Pigment—main one is melanin

V. Effects of aging on the integumentary system

VI. Care of the skin

Questions for Study and Review

1. Of what type of cells is the epidermis composed? Name the deepest and the uppermost layers.
2. Explain how the outermost cells of the epidermis are replaced.
3. Describe the structure of the dermis.
4. Describe the contents and functions of the subcutaneous layer.
5. Describe the location and function of the two types of skin glands.
6. Explain the four most important functions of the skin.
7. What are the most important contributors to the color of the skin, normally?
8. Define melanin and explain its function.
9. What changes may occur in the skin with age?
10. List some factors involved in proper care of the skin.
11. What are the dangers of overexposure to the sun, and what precautions against it need to be considered?

✔ ANSWERS TO CHECKPOINTS

1. The skin and all its associated structures make up the integumentary system.
2. The superficial layer of the skin is the epidermis; the deeper layer is the dermis.
3. The sweat glands are the sudoriferous glands.
4. The sebaceous glands produce an oily secretion called sebum.
5. Each hair develops within a sheath called the follicle.
6. Temperature is regulated through the skin by changes in the size of blood vessels and by evaporation of perspiration from the surface of the body.
7. Any substance that gives color to the skin is a pigment.

This unit deals with the skeletal and muscular systems. It covers the functions of the skeletal system, going beyond support purposes and including those purposes related to blood formation and to the storage and metabolism of certain mineral salts. The important muscles and their functions in various movements, as well as their ability to produce heat and to aid in the circulation of body fluids, are noted in Chapter 7, The Muscular System.

Unit II

MOVEMENT AND SUPPORT

The Skeleton: Bones and Joints

Selected Key Terms

The following terms are defined in the Glossary:

amphiarthrosis

bursa

circumduction

diaphysis

diarthrosis

endosteum

epiphysis

fontanel

joint

osteoblast

osteoclast

osteocyte

periosteum

resorption

synarthrosis

synovial

Behavioral Objectives

After careful study of this chapter, you should be able to:

1. List the functions of bones
2. Describe the structure of a long bone
3. Differentiate between compact bone and spongy bone with respect to structure and location
4. Differentiate between red and yellow marrow with respect to function and location
5. Name the three different types of bone cells and describe the functions of each
6. Explain how a long bone grows
7. Name and describe various markings found on bones
8. List the bones in the axial skeleton
9. List the bones in the appendicular skeleton
10. Describe the normal curves of the spine
11. Describe how the skeleton changes with age
12. Describe the three types of joints
13. Describe the structure of a synovial joint and give six examples of synovial joints
14. Define six types of movement that occur at synovial joints

The skeleton is the framework on which the body is constructed. Much like the frame of a building, the skeleton must be strong enough to support and protect all the body structures. Bones work with muscles to produce movement at the joints. The bones and joints, together with supporting connective tissue, form the skeletal system.

BONES

Main Functions of Bones

Bones have a number of functions, several of which are not evident in looking at the skeleton. Some of these are listed below:

- To serve as a firm framework for the entire body
- To protect such delicate structures as the brain and the spinal cord
- To serve as levers, working with attached muscles to produce movement
- To serve as a storehouse for calcium salts, which may be resorbed into the blood if there is not enough calcium in the diet
- To produce blood cells (in the red marrow)

Bone Structure

The complete bony framework of the body, known as the **skeleton** (Fig. 6-1), consists of 206 bones. These bones have several different shapes. They may be flat (rib, skull), cube shaped (wrist, ankle), or irregular (vertebrae, face). The most familiar shape, however, is the **long bone,** the type of bone that makes up almost all of the arms and legs. This bone has a long narrow shaft, called the **diaphysis** (di-AF-ih-sis), which has a central marrow cavity, and two irregular ends, each called an **epiphysis** (eh-PIF-ih-sis) (Fig. 6-2).

Bone Tissue

Bones are not lifeless. Even though the spaces between the cells of bone tissue are permeated with stony deposits of calcium salts, the bone cells themselves are very much alive. Bones are organs, with their own system of blood vessels, lymphatic vessels, and nerves.

There are two types of bone tissue, known as **osseous** (OS-e-us) **tissue** (see Fig. 6-2).

One type is **compact bone,** which is hard and dense. This makes up the main shaft of a long bone and the outer layer of other bones. The cells (osteocytes) in this type of bone are located in rings of bone tissue around a central **haversian** (ha-VER-shan) **canal** containing nerves and blood vessels. The second type,

6

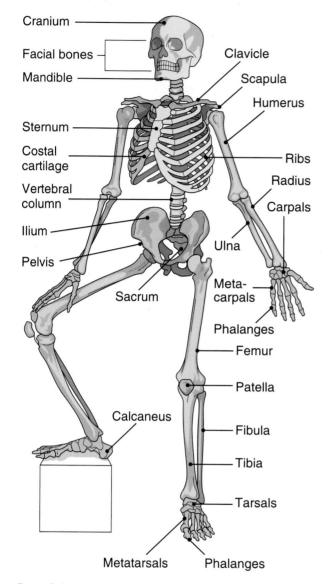

FIGURE **6•1** The skeleton.

bones. Yellow marrow is composed largely of fat.

Bone Membranes

Bones are covered on the outside (except at the joint region) by a membrane called the ***periosteum*** (per-e-OS-te-um). The inner layer of this membrane contains cells (osteoblasts), which are essential in bone formation, not only during growth but also in the repair of fractures. Blood vessels and lymphatic vessels in the periosteum play an important role in the nourishment of bone tissue. Nerve fibers in the periosteum make their presence known when one suffers a fracture, or when one receives a blow, such as on the shinbone. A thinner membrane, the ***endosteum*** (en-DOS-te-um), lines the marrow cavity of a bone; it too contains cells that aid in the growth and repair of bone tissue.

> ✔ CHECKPOINT **1**:
>
> A long bone has a long narrow shaft and two irregular ends. What are the scientific names for the shaft and the ends of a long bone?

> ✔ CHECKPOINT **2**:
>
> What are the two types of osseous (bone) tissue and where is each type found?

Bone Growth and Repair

Bone Cells and Their Actions

In the embryo (the early developmental stage of a baby), most of the "bones to be" are composed of cartilage. (Portions of the skull develop from fibrous connective tissue.) Bone formation, known as ***ossification,*** begins during the second and third months of embryonic life. At this time, bone-building cells, called ***osteoblasts*** (OS-te-o-blasts), become active. First, they begin to manufacture the ***matrix,*** which is the material located between the cells. This intercellular substance contains large quantities of ***collagen,*** a fibrous protein that gives strength and resilience to the tissue. Then, with the help of enzymes, calcium compounds are deposited

called ***spongy bone,*** has more spaces than compact bone. It is made of a meshwork of small, bony plates filled with red marrow and is found at the ends of the long bones and at the center of other bones.

Bone Marrow

Bones contain two kinds of marrow. ***Red marrow*** is found at the ends of the long bones and at the center of other bones. Red bone marrow manufactures blood cells. ***Yellow marrow*** is found chiefly in the central cavities of the long

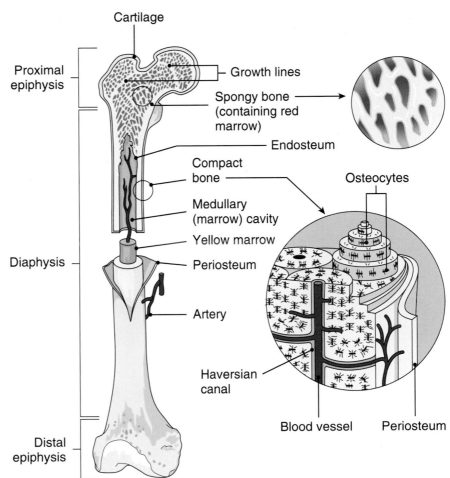

FIGURE **6•2** The structure of a long bone; the composition of compact bone.

within the matrix. Once this intercellular material has hardened around the cells, they are known as *osteocytes* (OS-te-o-sites). These cells are still living and continue to maintain the bone, but they do not produce new bone tissue. Other cells, called *osteoclasts* (OS-te-o-klasts), are responsible for the process of *resorption,* or the breakdown of bone, which is necessary for remodeling and repair. The formation and resorption of bone tissue are regulated by several hormones, including vitamin D (see Vitamin D).

Formation of a Long Bone

In a long bone, the transformation of cartilage into bone begins at the center of the shaft. Later, secondary bone-forming centers develop across the ends of the bones. The long bones continue to grow in length at these centers through childhood and into the late teens. Finally, by the late teens or early 20s, the bones

stop growing in length. Each bone-forming region hardens and can be seen in x-ray films as a thin line across the end of the bone. Physicians can judge the future growth of a bone by the appearance of these lines on x-ray films.

As a bone grows in length, the shaft is remodeled so that it grows wider as the central marrow cavity increases in size. Thus, alterations in the shape of the bone are a result of the addition of bone tissue to some surfaces and its resorption from others.

The processes of bone resorption and bone formation continue throughout life, more actively in some places than in others, as bones are subjected to "wear and tear" or injuries. The bones of small children are relatively pliable because they contain a larger proportion of cartilage and are undergoing active bone formation. In elderly people, there is a slowing of the processes that continually renew bone tissue.

6

Vitamin D

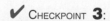

Vitamin D is necessary for the formation and maintenance of bone. This "vitamin" is actually a group of related fat-soluble compounds that aids in the intestinal absorption of calcium from foods. It is manufactured from a substance in the skin that is activated by the ultraviolet (UV) radiation in sunlight. Enzymes in the liver and kidneys then modify it into its most active form. Because it is manufactured in the body and carried in the blood to the tissues on which it acts, vitamin D is now considered to be a hormone.

A lack of vitamin D results in bone malformation. This condition is called rickets in children and osteomalacia (literally, "bone softening") in adults. The requirement for vitamin D is easily met by even moderate exposure to sunlight. Exposure of the arms and face fo only 1 hour per week is enough to avoid a deficiency. As a safeguard, all milk sold in the United States is fortified with vitamin D. Only people who stay mostly indoors and drink little or no milk are at risk for developing a deficiency in this vitamin.

As a result, the bones are weaker and more fragile. Elderly people also have a decreased ability to form the protein framework on which calcium salts are deposited. Fractures in elderly people heal more slowly because of these decreases in bone metabolism.

✔ CHECKPOINT **3**:

As the embryonic skeleton is converted from cartilage to bone, the intercellular matrix becomes hardened. What compounds are deposited in the matrix to harden it?

Bone Markings

In addition to their general shape, bones have other distinguishing features, or **bone markings.** These markings include raised areas and depressions that help to form joints or serve as points for muscle attachments and various holes that allow the passage of nerves and blood vessels. Some of these identifying features are described next.

Projections

- **Head**—a rounded, knoblike end separated from the rest of the bone by a slender region, the neck
- **Process**—a large projection of a bone, such as the upper part of the ulna in the forearm that creates the elbow
- **Crest**—a distinct border or ridge, often rough, such as over the top of the hip bone
- **Spine**—a sharp projection from the surface of a bone, such as the spine of the scapula (shoulder blade)

Depressions or Holes

- **Foramen** (fo-RA-men)—a hole that allows a vessel or a nerve to pass through or between bones. The plural is **foramina** (fo-RAM-ih-nah).
- **Sinus** (SI-nus)—an air space found in some skull bones
- **Fossa** (FOS-sah)—a depression on a bone surface. The plural is fossae (FOS-se).
- **Meatus** (me-A-tus)—a short channel or passageway, such as the channel in the temporal bone of the skull that leads to the inner ear

---

✔ CHECKPOINT **4**:

Bones have a number of projections, depressions, and holes. What are the purposes of these markings?

Examples of these and other markings can be seen on the bones illustrated in this chapter.

DIVISIONS OF THE SKELETON

The skeleton may be divided into two main groups of bones (see Fig. 6-1):

- The **axial** (AK-se-al) **skeleton** consists of 80 bones and includes the bony framework of the head and the trunk.

- The **appendicular** (ap-en-DIK-u-lar) **skeleton** consists of 126 bones and forms the framework for the **extremities** (limbs) and for the shoulders and hips.

We describe the axial skeleton first and then proceed to the appendicular skeleton. Table 6-1 provides an outline of all the bones included in this discussion.

Bones of the Axial Skeleton

Framework of the Skull

The bony framework of the head, called the **skull,** is subdivided into two parts: the cranium and the facial portion. Refer to Figures 6-3 through 6-6, which show different views of the skull, as you study the following descriptions.

Cranium

This rounded chamber that encloses the brain is composed of eight distinct cranial bones.

- The **frontal bone** forms the forehead, the front of the skull's roof, and the roof of the eye socket. The **frontal sinuses** (air spaces) communicate with the nasal cavities. These sinuses and others near the nose are described as **paranasal sinuses.**
- The two **parietal** (pah-RI-eh-tal) bones form most of the top and the side walls of the cranium.
- The two **temporal bones** form part of the sides and some of the base of the skull. Each one contains **mastoid sinuses** as well as the ear canal, the eardrum, and the entire middle and internal ears. The **mastoid process** of the temporal bone projects downward immediately behind the external part of the ear. It contains the mastoid

Table 6•1 Bones of the Skeleton

REGION	BONES	DESCRIPTION
Axial Skeleton		
Skull		
Cranium	Cranial bones	Chamber enclosing the brain; houses the ear and forms part of the eye socket
Facial portion	Facial bones	Form the face and chambers for sensory organs
Hyoid		U-shaped bone under lower jaw; used for muscle attachments
Ossicles	Ear bones	Transmit sound waves in inner ear
Trunk		
Vertebral column	Vertebrae	Encloses the spinal cord
Thorax	Sternum	Anterior bone of the thorax
	Ribs (12 pair)	Enclose the organs of the thorax
Appendicular Skeleton		
Upper Division		
Shoulder girdle	Clavicle	Anterior; between sternum and scapula
	Scapula	Posterior, anchors muscles that move arm
Upper extremity	Humerus	Proximal arm bone
	Ulna	Medial bone of forearm
	Radius	Lateral bone of forearm
	Carpals	Wrist bones
	Metacarpals	Bones of palm
	Phalanges	Bones of fingers
Lower Division		
Pelvis	Os coxae	Join sacrum and coccyx to form the bony pelvis
Lower extremity	Femur	Thigh bone
	Patella	Kneecap
	Tibia	Medial bone of leg
	Fibula	Lateral bone of leg
	Tarsal bones	Ankle bones
	Metatarsals	Bones of instep
	Phalanges	Bones of toes

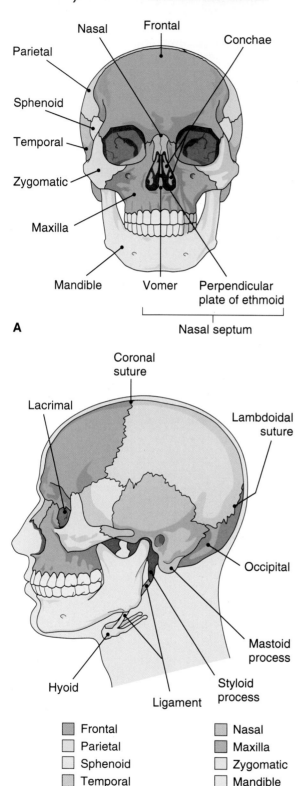

A

B

Legend	
Frontal	Nasal
Parietal	Maxilla
Sphenoid	Zygomatic
Temporal	Mandible

FIGURE **6•3** The skull **(A)** from the front and **(B)** from the left.

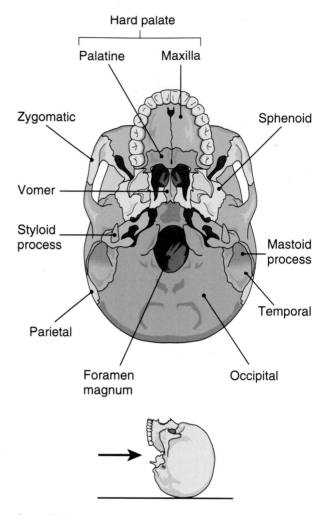

FIGURE **6•4** The skull from below, lower jaw removed.

air cells and serves as a place for muscle attachment.

- The ***ethmoid*** (ETH-moyd) ***bone*** is a light, fragile bone located between the eyes. It forms a part of the medial wall of the eye sockets, a small portion of the cranial floor, and most of the nasal cavity roof. It contains several air spaces, comprising some of the paranasal sinuses. A thin, platelike, downward extension of this bone (the perpendicular plate) forms much of the nasal septum, a midline partition in the nose.

- The ***sphenoid*** (SFE-noyd) ***bone,*** when seen from above, resembles a bat with its wings extended. It lies at the base of the skull in front of the temporal bones and forms part of the eye socket. The sphenoid

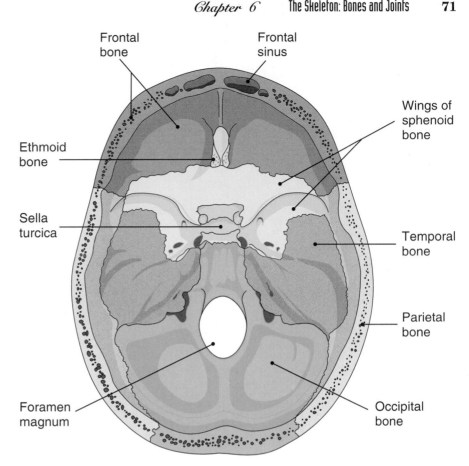

FIGURE **6•5** Floor of cranium showing the internal surfaces of some of the cranial bones.

contains a saddlelike depression, the ***sella turcica*** (SEL-a-TUR-sih-ka), that holds and protects the pituitary gland (see Fig. 6-5).

- The ***occipital*** (ok-SIP-ih-tal) ***bone*** forms the back and a part of the base of the skull. The ***foramen magnum,*** located at the base of the occipital bone, is a large opening through which the spinal cord communicates with the brain (see Figs. 6-4 and 6-5).

Facial Bones

The facial portion of the skull is composed of 14 bones (see Fig. 6-3).

- The ***mandible*** (MAN-dih-bl), or lower jaw bone, is the only movable bone of the skull.
- The two ***maxillae*** (mak-SIL-e) fuse in the midline to form the upper jaw bone, including the front part of the hard palate

(roof of the mouth). Each maxilla contains a large air space, called the ***maxillary sinus,*** that communicates with the nasal cavity.

- The two ***zygomatic*** (zi-go-MAT-ik) ***bones,*** one on each side, form the prominences of the cheeks.
- Two slender ***nasal bones*** lie side by side, forming the bridge of the nose.
- The two ***lacrimal*** (LAK-rih-mal) ***bones,*** each about the size of a fingernail, lie near the inside corner of the eye in the front part of the medial wall of the orbital cavity.
- The ***vomer*** (VO-mer), shaped like the blade of a plow, forms the lower part of the nasal septum (see Fig. 6-4).
- The paired ***palatine bones*** form the back part of the hard palate (see Figs. 6-4 and 6-6).
- The two ***inferior nasal conchae*** (KON-ke) extend horizontally along the lateral wall (sides) of the nasal cavities. The

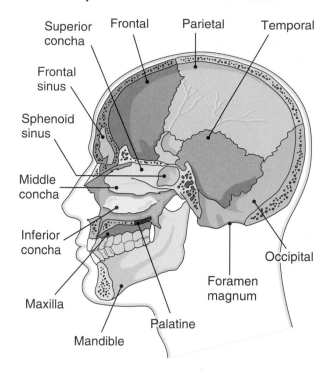

Superior concha · Frontal · Parietal · Temporal
Frontal sinus
Sphenoid sinus
Middle concha
Inferior concha
Maxilla
Mandible · Palatine · Foramen magnum · Occipital

FIGURE **6•6** The skull, internal view.

paired superior and middle conchae are part of the ethmoid bone (see Figs. 6-3*A* and 6-6).

In addition to the bones of the cranium and the facial bones, there are three tiny bones, or **ossicles** (OS-sik-ls), in each middle ear (see Chap. 10) and a single horseshoe, or U-shaped, bone just below the skull proper, called the **hyoid** (HI-oyd) **bone,** to which the tongue and other muscles are attached.

Openings in the base of the skull provide spaces for the entrance and exit of many blood vessels, nerves, and other structures. Projections and slightly elevated portions of the bones provide for the attachment of muscles. Some portions contain delicate structures, such as the part of the temporal bone that encloses the middle and internal sections of the ear. The sinuses

provide lightness and serve as resonating chambers for the voice (which is why your voice sounds better to you as you are speaking than it sounds when you hear it played back as a recording).

Infant Skull
The skull of the infant has areas in which the bone formation is incomplete, leaving so-called soft spots, properly called **fontanels** (fon-tah-NELS). Although there are a number of these, the largest and best known is near the front of the skull at the junction of the two parietal bones and the frontal bone. This **anterior fontanel** usually does not close until the child is about 18 months old (Fig. 6-7).

Framework of the Trunk
The bones of the trunk include the spine, or **vertebral** (VER-teh-bral) **column,** and the bones of the chest, or **thorax** (THO-raks).

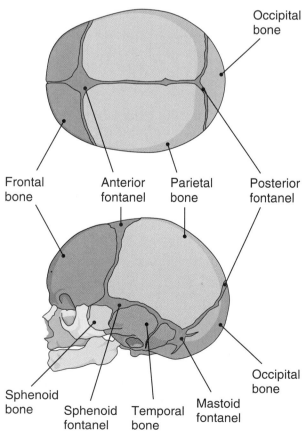

Occipital bone · Frontal bone · Anterior fontanel · Parietal bone · Posterior fontanel · Sphenoid bone · Sphenoid fontanel · Temporal bone · Mastoid fontanel · Occipital bone

FIGURE **6•7** Infant skull showing fontanels.

Vertebral Column

This bony sheath for the spinal cord is made of a series of irregularly shaped bones. These number 33 or 34 in the child, but because of fusions that occur later in the lower part of the spine, there usually are just 26 separate bones in the adult spinal column (Figs. 6-8 and 6-9).

The *vertebrae* (VER-teh-bre) have a drum-shaped body (centrum) located toward the front (anteriorly) that serves as the weight-bearing part; disks of cartilage between the vertebral bodies act as shock absorbers and provide flexibility.

In the center of each vertebra is a large hole, or foramen (see Fig. 6-9). When all the vertebrae are linked in series by strong connective tissue bands (ligaments), these spaces form the spinal canal, a bony cylinder that protects the spinal cord. Projecting backward from the bony arch that encircles the spinal cord is the *spinous process,* which usually can be felt just under the skin of the back. When viewed from the side, the vertebral column can be seen to have a series of *intervertebral foramina* through which spinal nerves emerge as they leave the spinal cord.

The bones of the vertebral column are named and numbered from above downward, on the basis of location:

- The *cervical* (SER-vih-kal) *vertebrae,* seven in number, are located in the neck. The first vertebra, called the *atlas,* supports the head; when one nods the head, the skull rocks on the atlas at the occipital bone. The second cervical vertebra, called the *axis,* serves as a pivot when the head is turned from side to side. The absence of a body in these vertebrae allows for the extra movement.
- The *thoracic vertebrae,* 12 in number, are located in the chest. The posterior ends of the 12 pairs of ribs are attached to these vertebrae.
- The *lumbar vertebrae,* five in number, are located in the small of the back. They are larger and heavier than the other vertebrae to support more weight.
- The *sacral* (SA-kral) *vertebrae* are five separate bones in the child. They eventually fuse to form a single bone, called the *sacrum* (SA-krum), in the adult. Wedged between the two hip bones, the sacrum completes the posterior part of the bony pelvis.
- The *coccyx* (KOK-siks), or tail bone, consists of four or five tiny bones in the child. These fuse to form a single bone in the adult.

Curves of the Spine

When viewed from the side, the vertebral column can be seen to have four curves, corresponding to the four groups of vertebrae (see Fig. 6-8). In the newborn infant, the entire column is concave forward (curves away from a

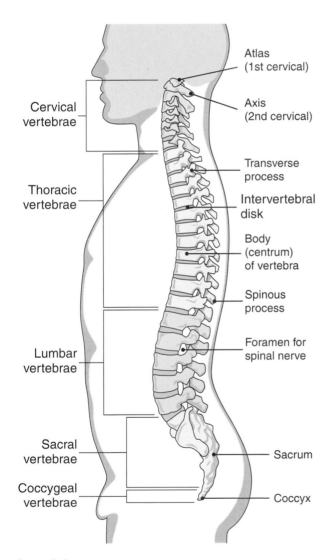

Cervical vertebrae

Thoracic vertebrae

Lumbar vertebrae

Sacral vertebrae

Coccygeal vertebrae

Atlas (1st cervical)

Axis (2nd cervical)

Transverse process

Intervertebral disk

Body (centrum) of vertebra

Spinous process

Foramen for spinal nerve

Sacrum

Coccyx

FIGURE **6•8**   Vertebral column from the side.

6

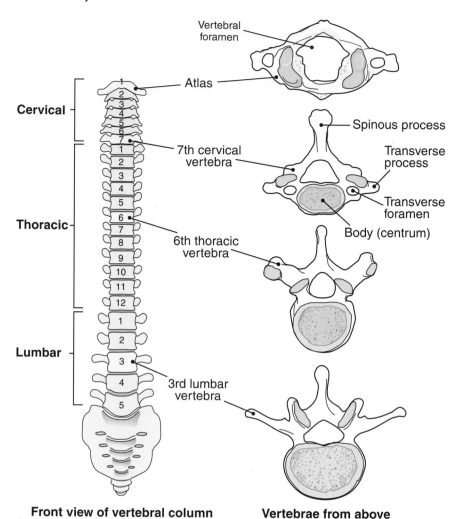

Vertebral foramen

Atlas

Cervical

7th cervical vertebra

Spinous process

Transverse process

Transverse foramen

Body (centrum)

Thoracic

6th thoracic vertebra

Lumbar

3rd lumbar vertebra

Front view of vertebral column

Vertebrae from above

FIGURE **6•9** Front view of the vertebral column; vertebrae from above.

viewer facing the infant), as seen in Figure 6-10. This is the primary curve.

When the infant begins to assume an erect posture, secondary curves develop. These curves are convex (curve toward the viewer). The cervical curve appears when the head is held up at about 3 months of age; the lumbar curve appears when the child begins to walk. The thoracic and sacral curves remain the two primary curves. These curves of the vertebral column provide some of the resilience and spring so essential in balance and movement.

Thorax

The bones of the **thorax** (Fig. 6-11) form a cone-shaped cage. Twelve pairs of **ribs** form the bars

of this cage, completed by the **sternum** (STER-num), or breastbone, anteriorly. These bones enclose and protect the heart and lungs and other organs of the thorax.

The top portion of the sternum is the broadly T-shaped **manubrium** (mah-NU-bre-um) that joins at the top on each side with the clavicle (collarbone) and joins laterally with the first pair of ribs. The **body** of the sternum is long and bladelike. It joins along each side with ribs two through seven. Where the manubrium joins the body of the sternum, there is a slight elevation, the **sternal angle,** which easily can be felt as a surface landmark.

The lower end of the sternum consists of a small tip that is made of cartilage in youth but

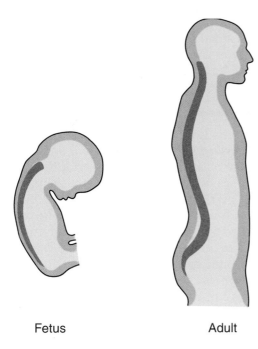

Fetus

Adult

FIGURE **6•10** Curves of the infant spine and adult spine.

becomes bone in the adult. This is the ***xiphoid*** (ZIF-oyd) ***process.*** It is used as a landmark for CPR (cardiopulmonary resuscitation) to locate the region for chest compression. The thorax protects the heart, lungs, and other organs.

All 12 of the ribs on each side are attached to the vertebral column posteriorly. However, variations in the *anterior* attachment of these slender, curved bones have led to the following classification:

- ***True ribs,*** the first seven pairs, are those that attach directly to the sternum by means of individual extensions called ***costal*** (KOS-tal) ***cartilages.***
- ***False ribs*** are the remaining five pairs. Of these, the 8th, 9th, and 10th pairs attach to the cartilage of the rib above. The last two pairs have no anterior attachment at all and are known as ***floating ribs.***

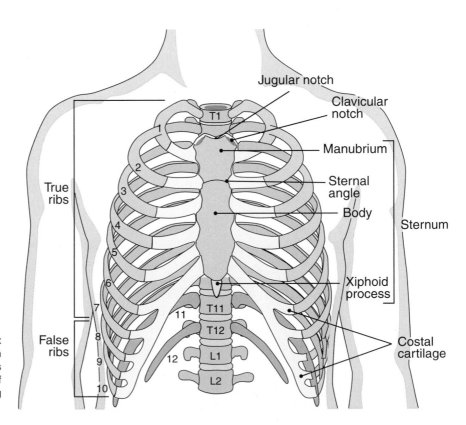

FIGURE **6•11** Bones of the thorax (anterior view). The first seven pairs of ribs are the true ribs; pairs 8 through 12 are the false ribs, of which the last two pairs are floating ribs.

6

The spaces between the ribs, called ***intercostal spaces,*** contain muscles, blood vessels, and nerves.

> ✔ CHECKPOINT **5**:
>
> What division of the skeleton consists of the bones of the skull and trunk?

Bones of the Appendicular Skeleton

The appendicular skeleton may be considered in two divisions: upper and lower. The upper division on each side includes the shoulder, the arm (between the shoulder and the elbow), the forearm (between the elbow and the wrist), the wrist, the hand, and the fingers. The lower division includes the hip (part of the pelvic girdle), the thigh (between the hip and the knee), the leg (between the knee and the ankle), the ankle, the foot, and the toes.

The Upper Division of the Appendicular Skeleton

The bones of the upper division may be divided into two groups:

The Shoulder Girdle
The shoulder girdle consists of two bones (Fig. 6-12):

- The ***clavicle*** (KLAV-ih-kl), or collarbone, is a slender bone with two shallow curves. It joins the sternum anteriorly and the scapula laterally and helps to support the shoulder. Because it often receives the full force of falls on outstretched arms or of blows to the shoulder, it is the most frequently broken bone.
- The ***scapula*** (SKAP-u-lah), or shoulder blade, is shown from a posterior view in Figure 6-12*B*. The ***spine*** of the scapula is the raised ridge that can be felt behind the shoulder in the upper portion of the back. Muscles that move the arm attach to the fossae (depressions) above and below the scapular spine. The ***acromion*** (ah-KRO-me-on) is the process that joins the clavicle. This can be felt as the highest point of the shoulder. Below the acromion there is a shallow socket, the ***glenoid cavity,*** that forms a ball-and-socket joint with the arm bone (humerus). Medial to the glenoid cavity is the ***coracoid process,*** to which muscles attach.

The Upper Extremity
Also referred to as the upper limb, or simply the arm, the upper extremity consists of the following bones:

- The proximal bone, the ***humerus*** (HU-mer-us), or arm bone, forms a joint with

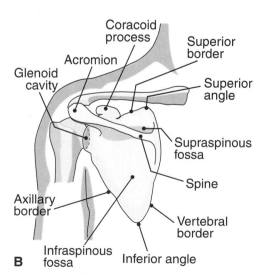

FIGURE **6•12**   **(A)** Bones of the shoulder girdle. **(B)** Left scapula (posterior view)

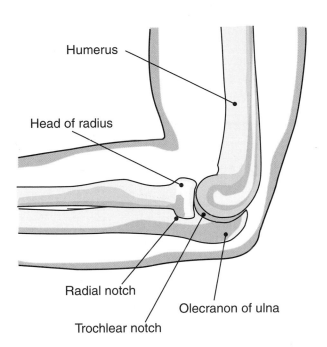

FIGURE **6•13** Lateral view of the right elbow.

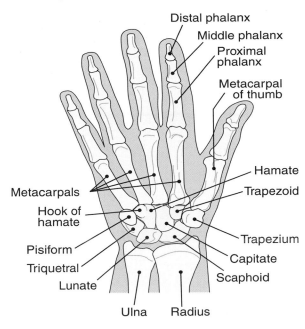

FIGURE **6•14** Bones of the right hand, anterior view.

the scapula above and with the two fore-arm bones at the elbow (Fig. 6-13).

- The forearm bones are the ***ulna*** (UL-nah), which lies on the medial side, in line with the little finger, and the ***radius*** (RA-de-us), on the lateral side, above the thumb. When the palm is up, or forward, the two bones are parallel; when the palm is turned down, or back, the lower end of the radius rotates around the ulna so that the shafts of the two bones are crossed. In this posi-tion, a distal projection of the ulna (the sty-loid process) pops up at the outside of the wrist.
- The top of the ulna has the large ***olecra-non*** (o-LEK-rah-non) that forms the point of the elbow (see Fig. 6-13). The pulley-shaped ***trochlea*** (TROK-le-ah) of the distal humerus fits into the deep ***trochlear notch*** of the ulna, allowing a hinge action at the elbow joint. This depression, because of its deep half-moon shape, is also known as the *semilunar notch*.
- The wrist contains eight small ***carpal*** (KAR-pal) ***bones*** arranged in two rows of four each. The names of these eight differ-ent bones are given in Figure 6-14.

- Five ***metacarpal bones*** are the frame-work for the palm of each hand. Their rounded distal ends form the knuckles.
- There are 14 ***phalanges*** (fah-LAN-jeze), or finger bones, in each hand, two for the thumb and three for each finger. Each of these bones is called a ***phalanx*** (FA-lanx). They are identified as the first, or proxi-mal, which is attached to a metacarpal; the second, or middle; and the third, or distal. Note that the thumb has only two pha-langes, a proximal and a distal (see Fig. 6-14).

The Lower Division of the Appendicular Skeleton

The bones of the lower division are grouped to-gether in a similar fashion.

The Pelvic Bones

The hip bone, or ***os coxae,*** begins its develop-ment as three separate bones that later fuse (Fig. 6-15):

- The ***ilium*** (IL-e-um), which forms the upper, flared portion. The ***iliac*** (IL-e-ak) ***crest*** is the curved rim along the upper

6

A Anterior view

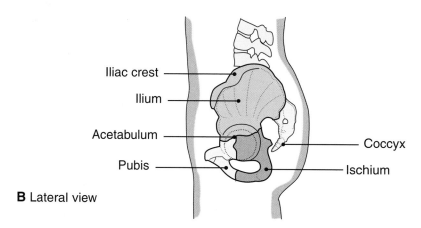

B Lateral view

FIGURE **6•15** The pelvic bones. **(A)** Anterior view. **(B)** Lateral view, shows joining of the three bones to form acetabulum.

border of the ilium. It can be felt just below the waist. At either end of the crest are two bony projections. The most prominent of these is the *anterior superior iliac spine,* which is often used as a surface landmark in diagnosis and treatment.

• The *ischium* (IS-ke-um), which is the lowest and strongest part. The *ischial* (IS-ke-al) *spine* at the back of the pelvic outlet is used as a point of reference during childbirth to indicate the progress of the presenting part (usually the baby's head) down the birth canal. Just below this spine is the large *ischial tuberosity,* which helps support the weight of the trunk when one sits down.

• The *pubis* (PU-bis), which forms the anterior part. The joint formed by the union of the two hip bones anteriorly is called the *pubic symphysis* (SIM-fih-sis).

Portions of all three bones contribute to the formation of the *acetabulum* (as-eh-TAB-u-lum), the deep socket that holds the head of the femur (thigh bone) to form the hip joint.

The largest foramina in the entire body are found near the front of each hip bone, one on each side of the pubic symphysis. These openings are partially covered by a membrane and are called the *obturator* (OB-tu-ra-tor) *foramina* (see Fig. 6-15B).

The two ossa coxae join in forming the pelvis,

a strong bony girdle completed by the sacrum and coccyx of the spine at the back (posteriorly). The pelvis supports the trunk and the organs in the lower abdomen, or pelvic cavity, including the urinary bladder, the internal reproductive organs, and parts of the intestine. The female pelvis is adapted for pregnancy and childbirth; it is broader and lighter than the male pelvis (Fig. 6-16).

The Lower Extremity

Also referred to as the lower limb, or simply the leg, the lower extremity consists of the following bones:

- The thigh bone, called the **femur** (FE-mer), is the longest and strongest bone in the body. Proximally, it has a large ball-shaped head that joins the os coxae (Fig. 6-17). The large lateral projection at the top of the femur is the **greater trochanter** (tro-KAN-ter), used as a surface landmark. The **lesser trochanter,** a smaller elevation, is located on the medial side.

- The **patella** (pah-TEL-lah), or kneecap, is embedded in the tendon of the large anterior thigh muscle, the quadriceps femoris, where it crosses the knee joint. It is an example of a **sesamoid** (SES-ah-moyd) **bone,** a type of bone that develops within a tendon or a joint capsule.

- There are two bones in the lower leg. Medially (on the great toe side), the **tibia,** or shin bone, is the longer, weight-bearing bone. It has a sharp anterior ridge that can be felt at the surface of the leg. Laterally, the slender **fibula** (FIB-u-lah) does not reach the knee joint; thus, it is not a weight-bearing bone. The **medial malleolus** (mal-LE-o-lus) is a downward projection at the lower end of the tibia; it forms the prominence on the inner aspect of the ankle (Fig. 6-18). The **lateral malleolus,** at the lower end of the fibula, forms the prominence on the outer aspect of the ankle.

- The structure of the foot is similar to that of the hand. However, the foot supports the weight of the body, so it is stronger and less mobile than the hand. There are seven **tarsal bones** associated with the ankle and foot. These are named and illustrated in Figure 18. The largest of these is the **calcaneus** (kal-KA-ne-us), or heel bone.

- Five **metatarsal bones** form the framework of the instep, and the heads of these bones form the ball of the foot.

- The **phalanges** of the toes are counterparts of those in the fingers. There are three of these in each toe except for the great toe, which has only two.

male pelvis

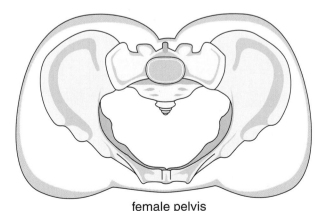

female pelvis

FIGURE **6•16** Comparison of the male pelvis and female pelvis seen from above.

✔ CHECKPOINT **6**:

What division of the skeleton consists of the bones of the shoulder girdle, hip, and extremities?

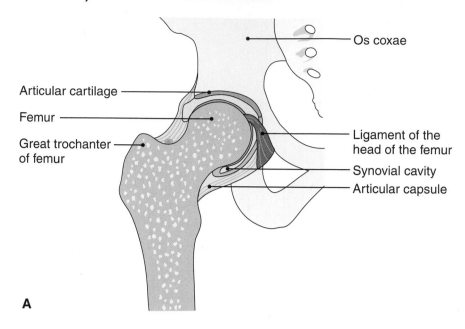

Os coxae

Articular cartilage

Femur

Great trochanter of femur

Ligament of the head of the femur

Synovial cavity

Articular capsule

A

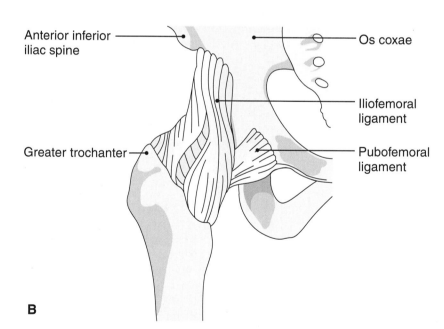

Anterior inferior iliac spine

Os coxae

Iliofemoral ligament

Greater trochanter

Pubofemoral ligament

B

FIGURE **6•17**   Hip joint. **(A)** Frontal section through right hip joint. **(B)** Anterior view showing ligaments.

Skeletal Changes in the Aging

The aging process includes significant changes in all connective tissues including bone. There is a loss of calcium salts and a decrease in the amount of protein formed in bone tissue. The reduction of collagen in bone and in tendons, ligaments, and skin contributes to the stiffness so often found in older people. Muscle tissue is also lost throughout adult life. Thus, there is a tendency to decrease the exercise that is so important to the maintenance of bone tissue.

Changes in the vertebral column with age lead to a loss in height. About 1.2 cm (about 0.5 inches) are lost each 20 years beginning at 40 years of age, owing primarily to a thinning of the intervertebral disks (between the bodies of the vertebrae). Even the vertebral bodies them-

Fibula

Lateral malleous

Cuboid

Cuneiforms

Tibia

Medial malleolus

Talus

Calcaneus

Navicular

Metatarsals

Phalanges

FIGURE **6•18**   Bones of the right foot.

6

A Strong and Healthy Skeleton

The development of strong, healthy bones throughout the skeleton must begin early in childhood. The maintenance of a healthy skeleton is a lifelong effort. The process of building sound bone tissue requires certain dietary components along with consistent, periodic exercise.

The physical strength of bone tissue is derived from the presence of calcium phosphate in the bone's matrix or anatomic scaffolding. The higher the calcium phosphate content, the stronger and healthier the bone is. For calcium phosphate to be deposited in the bones' matrix, it must first be absorbed into the bloodstream from the foods we eat. The presence of calcium in the blood stream is needed not only for bone growth and development but also for blood clotting, nerve and muscle signaling, and other processes. Typically, blood calcium is used for these processes before it is stored in the bones. Because many of us do not take in enough dietary calcium, the bones generally do not receive enough calcium for storage. In fact, if not enough dietary calcium is available, the body pulls stored calcium out of the bones to ensure muscle, nerve, and clotting function.

Overall, the amount of calcium in the bloodstream and the amount available to the bones for storage is dependent upon complex hormonal mechanisms, as well as the presence of adequate blood levels of vitamins A and D. However, the storage of calcium in bone tissue is also directly affected by exercise. Physical stress on the bones as occurs during strenuous exercise, especially during periods of growth, causes a direct increase in deposition of calcium at points where the bone is under stress. The long bones of the arms and legs build lines of strength along the direction force simply through everyday exercise. All bones respond to exercise by increasing in size and strength.

The health and strength of an individual's bones is dependent on both good nutrition and exercise, beginning in early childhood and continuing throughout life.

selves may lose height in later years. The costal (rib) cartilages become calcified and less flexible, and the chest may decrease in diameter by 2 to 3 cm (about 1 inch), mostly in the lower part. To learn about how to keep bones strong, see A Strong and Healthy Skeleton.

THE JOINTS

An *articulation*, or *joint*, is an area of junction or union between two or more bones.

Kinds of Joints

Joints are classified into three main types on the basis of the material between the bones. They may also be classified according to the degree of movement permitted (Table 6-2):

- *Fibrous joint.* The bones in this type of joint are held together by fibrous connective tissue. An example is a *suture* (SU-chur) between bones of the skull. This type of joint is immovable and is termed a *synarthrosis* (sin-ar-THRO-sis).
- *Cartilaginous joint.* The bones in this type of joint are connected by cartilage. Ex-

amples are the joint between the pubic bones of the pelvis—the pubic symphysis— and the joints between the bodies of the vertebrae. This type of joint is slightly movable and is termed an *amphiarthrosis* (am-fe-ar-THRO-sis).

6

Table 6•2 Types of Joints

Name	Movement	Material between the bones	Examples
Fibrous	Immovable (Synarthrosis)	No joint cavity; fibrous connective tissue between bones	Sutures between bones of skull
Cartilaginous	Slightly movable (Amphiarthrosis)	No joint cavity; cartilage between bones	Pubic symphysis; joints between bodies of vertebrae
Synovial	Freely movable (Diarthrosis)	Joint cavity containing synovial fluid	Gliding, hinge, pivot, condyloid, saddle, ball-and-socket joints

fibrous joint
(suture)

cartilaginous joint
(symphysis)

synovial joint

- **Synovial** (sin-O-ve-al) **joint.** The bones in this type of joint have a potential space between them called the **joint cavity,** which contains a small amount of thick, colorless fluid. This lubricant, **synovial fluid,** re-sembles uncooked egg white (*ov* is the root meaning "egg") and is secreted by the membrane that lines the joint cavity. The synovial joint is freely movable and is termed a **diarthrosis** (di-ar-THRO-sis). Most joints

Table 6•3 Synovial Joints

Type	Description	Examples	
Gliding joint	Bone surfaces slide over one another	Joints in the wrist and ankles. (See Figs. 6-14 and 6-18)	
Hinge joint	Allows movement in one direction, changing the angle of the bones at the joint.	Elbow joint, joints between phalanges of fingers and toes. (See Figs. 6-13, 6-14 and 6-18)	
Pivot joint	Allows rotation around the length of the bone.	Joint between first and second cervical vertebrae, joint at proximal ends of the radius and ulna. (See Figs. 6-8 and 6-13)	
Condyloid joint	Allows movement in two directions	Joint between the metacarpal and the first phalanx of the finger (knuckle) (See Fig. 6-14); joint between the occipital bone of the skull and the first cervical vertebra (Atlas) (See Fig. 6-8)	
Saddle joint	Like a condyloid joint, but with deeper articulating surfaces	Joint between the wrist and the metacarpal bone of the thumb. (See Fig. 6-14)	
Ball-and-socket joint	Allows movement in many directions around a central point. Gives the greatest freedom of movement	Shoulder joint and hip joint (See Figs. 6-12a and 6-17)	

are synovial joints; they are described in more detail next.

✔ CHECKPOINT **7**:

What are the three types of joints classified according to the type of material between the bones?

More About Synovial Joints

Structure of Synovial Joints

The bones in freely movable joints are held together by *ligaments,* bands of fibrous connective tissue. Additional ligaments reinforce and help stabilize the joints at various points (see Fig. 6-17). Also, for strength and protection, there is a *joint capsule* of connective tissue that encloses each joint and is continuous with the periosteum of the bones. The bone surfaces in freely movable joints are protected by a smooth layer of hyaline cartilage called the *articular* (ar-TIK-u-lar) *cartilage.*

FIGURE **6•19**   The knee joint (sagittal section).

Near some joints are small sacs called *bursae* (BER-se), which are filled with synovial fluid. These lie in areas subject to stress and help ease movement over and around the joints. Inflammation of a bursa, as a result of injury or irritation, is called *bursitis.*

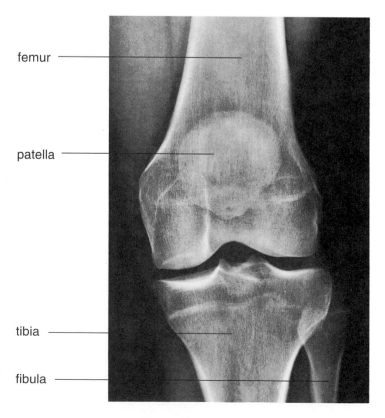

FIGURE **6•20**   X-ray (radiograph) of the knee joint showing the articulating bones. (Greenspan A: Orthopedic Radiology, p. 6.2. New York, Gower, 1988)

Types of Synovial Joints

Synovial joints may be classified according to the types of movement they allow (Table 6-3).

The knee is illustrated as an example of a synovial joint in Figure 6-19. Although basically a hinge joint, the knee is complex and has some of the properties of a gliding joint as well. An x-ray picture of the knee is shown in Figure 6-20.

Movement at Synovial Joints

The chief function of the freely movable joints is to allow for changes of position and so provide

for motion. These movements are named to describe changes in the positions of body parts (Fig. 6-21). For example, there are four kinds of angular movement, or movement that changes the angle between bones, as listed below:

- *Flexion* (FLEK-shun) is a bending motion that decreases the angle between bones, as in bending the fingers to close the hand.
- *Extension* is a straightening motion that increases the angle between bones, as in straightening the fingers to open the hand.

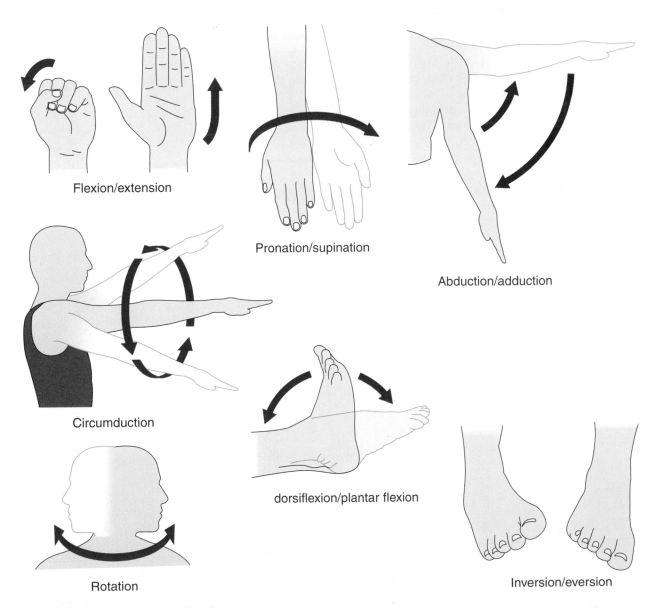

Flexion/extension

Pronation/supination

Abduction/adduction

Circumduction

dorsiflexion/plantar flexion

Rotation

Inversion/eversion

FIGURE **6•21** Movements at synovial joints.

- *Abduction* (ab-DUK-shun) is movement away from the midline of the body, as in moving the arms straight out to the sides.
- *Adduction* is movement toward the midline of the body, as in bringing the arms back to their original position beside the body.

A combination of these angular movements enables one to execute a movement referred to as *circumduction* (ser-kum-DUK-shun). To perform this movement, stand with your arm outstretched and draw a large imaginary circle in the air. Note the smooth combination of flexion, abduction, extension, and adduction that makes circumduction possible.

Rotation refers to a twisting or turning of a bone on its own axis, as in turning the head from side to side to say "no," or rotating the forearm to turn the palm up and down.

There are special movements that are characteristic of the forearm and the ankle:

- *Supination* (su-pin-A-shun) is the act of turning the palm up or forward; *pronation* (pro-NA-shun) turns the palm down or backward.
- *Inversion* (in-VER-zhun) is the act of turning the sole inward, so that it faces the opposite foot; *eversion* (e-VER-zhun) turns the sole outward, away from the body.
- In *dorsiflexion* (dor-sih-FLEK-shun), the foot is bent upward at the ankle, narrowing the angle between the leg and the top of the foot; in *plantar flexion*, the toes point downward, as in toe dancing, flexing the arch of the foot.

 CHECKPOINT **8**:

What is the most freely movable type of joint?

Summary

I. Bones

- **A. Main functions of bones**—serve as body framework; protect organs; serve as levers; store calcium salts; form blood cells
- **B. Bone structure**
  1. Long bone
     - a. Diaphysis—shaft
     - b. Epiphysis—end
  2. Bone tissue
     - a. Compact—shaft of long bones; outside of other bones
     - b. Spongy—end of long bones; center of other bones
  3. Bone marrow
     - a. Red—in spongy bone
     - b. Yellow—in central cavity of long bones
  4. Membranes—contain bone-forming cells
     - a. Periosteum—covers bone
     - b. Endosteum—lines marrow cavity
- **C. Bone growth and repair**
  1. Cells
     - a. Osteoblasts—bone-forming cells
     - b. Osteocytes—mature bone cells that maintain bone
     - c. Osteoclasts—bone cells that break down (resorb) bone
  2. Formation of a long bone—begins in center of shaft and continues at ends of bone; growing area forms line across epiphysis
- **D. Bone markings**
  1. Projections—head, process, crest, spine
  2. Depressions and holes—foramen, sinus, fossa, meatus

II. Divisions of the skeleton

- **A. Bones of the axial skeleton**
  1. Skull
     - a. Cranial—frontal, parietal, temporal, ethmoid, sphenoid, occipital

b. Facial—mandible, maxilla, zygomatic, nasal, lacrimal, vomer,
palatine, inferior nasal conchae
c. Other—ossicles (of ear), hyoid
d. Infant skull—fontanels (soft
spots)
2. Trunk
a. Vertebral column—divisions: cervical, thoracic, lumbar, sacral,
coccygeal
b. Thorax
(1) Sternum—manubrium, body,
xiphoid process
(2) Ribs
(a) True—first seven pairs
(b) False—remaining five
pairs, including two floating ribs
B. Bones of the appendicular skeleton
1. Shoulder girdle—clavicle, scapula
2. Upper extremity—humerus, ulna,
radius, carpals, metacarpals, phalanges
3. Pelvic bones—os coxae (hip bone):
ilium, ischium, pubis
4. Lower extremity—femur, patella,
tibia, fibula, tarsals, metatarsals,
phalanges

III. Skeletal changes in aging—loss of calcium salts, decreased production of collagen, thinning of intervertebral disks, loss
of flexibility

IV. Joints (articulations)
A. Kinds of joints
1. Fibrous—immovable (synarthrosis)
2. Cartilaginous—slightly movable
(amphiarthrosis)
3. Synovial—freely movable (diarthrosis)
B. More about synovial joints
1. Structure of synovial joints
a. Joint cavity—contains synovial
fluid
b. Ligaments—hold joint together
c. Joint capsule—strengthens and
protects joint
d. Articular cartilage—covers ends
of bones
e. Bursae—fluid-filled sacs near
joints; cushion and protect joints
and surrounding tissue
2. Types of synovial joints—gliding,
hinge, pivot, condyloid, saddle, ball-
and-socket
3. Movement at synovial joints—flexion, extension, abduction, adduction, circumduction, rotation,
supination, pronation, inversion,
eversion, dorsiflexion, plantar flexion

Questions for Study and Review

1. List five functions of bones.
2. Explain the difference between the terms in each of the following pairs:
   a. *osteoblast* and *osteoclast*
   b. *red marrow* and *yellow marrow*
   c. *periosteum* and *endosteum*
   d. *compact bone* and *spongy bone*
   e. *epiphysis* and *diaphysis*
3. What is an osteocyte and where are osteocytes located?
4. Define *resorption* as it applies to bone.
5. Name the two divisions of the skeleton. What parts of the skeleton are in each?
6. Name the main cranial and facial bones.

7. What is a sinus? Name several bones in which there are sinuses.
8. Define *fontanel* and name the largest fontanel.
9. What are the main divisions of the vertebral column? the ribs?
10. Name the bones of the upper and lower appendicular skeleton.
11. Name the bones on which you would find the following bone markings: mastoid process, acromion, olecranon, iliac crest, trochanter, medial malleolus, lateral malleolus, trochlea, ischial tuberosity, acetabulum, glenoid cavity, xiphoid process.
12. What is a foramen? Give at least two examples of foramina.
13. Name three effects of aging on the skeletal system.
14. List three types of joints. Describe the amount of movement that occurs at each type. Find an example of each type in the chapter illustrations.
15. Describe where each of the following is found in a synovial joint: joint capsule, articular cartilage, and synovial fluid.
16. Name six types of synovial joints and give one example of the location of each. Find one example of each in the chapter illustrations.
17. Differentiate between the terms in each of the following pairs:
    a. *flexion* and *extension*
    b. *abduction* and *adduction*
    c. *supination* and *pronation*
    d. *inversion* and *eversion*
    e. *circumduction* and *rotation*
    f. *dorsiflexion* and *plantar flexion*

✔ Answers to Checkpoints

1. Compact bone makes up the main shaft of long bones and the outer layer of other bones; spongy bone makes up the ends of the long bones and the center of other bones.
2. The shaft of the long bone is the diaphysis; the end of a long bone is the epiphysis.
3. Calcium compounds are deposited in the matrix of bone to harden it.
4. The markings on bones help to form joints, serve as points for muscle attachments, and allow passage of nerves and blood vessels.
5. The axial skeleton consists of bones of the skull and trunk.
6. The appendicular skeleton consists of bones of the shoulder girdle, hip, and extremities.
7. The three types of joints classified according to the material between the bones are fibrous, cartilaginous, and synovial.
8. The most freely movable type of joint is a synovial joint or diarthrosis.

The Muscular System

SELECTED KEY TERMS

The following terms are defined in the Glossary:

acetylcholine

actin

antagonist

aponeurosis

fascicle

glycogen

insertion

lactic acid

myoglobin

myosin

neuromuscular junction

neurotransmitter

origin

oxygen debt

prime mover

synapse

tendon

tonus

BEHAVIORAL OBJECTIVES

After careful study of this chapter, you should be able to:

1. Compare the three types of muscle tissue

2. Describe three functions of skeletal muscle

3. Briefly describe how skeletal muscles contract

4. List the substances needed in muscle contraction and describe the function of each

5. Define the term *oxygen debt*

6. List several compounds that delay the onset of oxygen debt

7. Cite the effects of exercise on muscles

8. Compare isotonic and isometric contractions

9. Explain how muscles work in pairs to produce movement

10. Compare the workings of muscles and bones to lever systems

11. Explain how muscles are named

12. Name some of the major muscles in each muscle group and describe the main function of each

13. Describe how muscles change with age

TYPES OF MUSCLE

There are three kinds of muscle tissue: smooth, cardiac, and skeletal muscle, as introduced in Chapter 4. After a brief description of all three types (Table 7-1), this chapter concentrates on skeletal muscle, which has been studied the most.

Smooth Muscle

Smooth muscle makes up the walls of the hollow body organs as well as those of the blood vessels and respiratory passageways. It moves involuntarily, producing the wavelike motions of peristalsis that move substances through a system. Smooth muscle fibers (cells) are tapered at each end and have a single, central nucleus. The cells appear smooth under the microscope because they do not contain the visible bands, or *striations*, that are seen in the other types of muscle cells. Smooth muscle may contract in response to a nerve impulse, hormonal stimulation, stretching, and other stimuli. The muscle contracts and relaxes slowly and can remain contracted for a long time.

Cardiac Muscle

Cardiac muscle, also involuntary, makes up the wall of the heart and creates the pulsing action of that organ. The cells of cardiac muscle are striated, like those of skeletal muscle. They differ in having one nucleus per cell and branching interconnections. The electrical impulse that produces contraction of cardiac muscle is generated within the muscle but can be modified by nervous stimuli and hormones.

When viewed under the microscope, skeletal muscle cells appear heavily striated (Fig. 7-1). The arrangement of protein threads within the cell that produces these striations is described later. The cells are very long and cylindrical and have multiple nuclei per cell. Skeletal muscle is stimulated to contract by the nervous system, and it usually contracts and relaxes rapidly. Because it is under conscious control, skeletal muscle is described as voluntary.

Skeletal Muscle

Skeletal muscle is attached to bones and produces movement at the joints. These muscles constitute the largest amount of muscle tissue of the body, making up about 40% of the total body weight. This muscular system is composed of almost 700 individual skeletal muscles. Although each one is a distinct structure, muscles usually act in groups to execute body movements.

✔ CHECKPOINT **1**:

What are the three types of muscle?

Table 7•1 **Comparison of the Different Types of Muscle**

	SMOOTH	CARDIAC	SKELETAL
Location	Wall of hollow organs, vessels, respiratory passageways	Wall of heart	Attached to bones
Cell characteristics	Tapered at each end, single nucleus, nonstriated	Branching networks, single nucleus, lightly striated	Long and cylindrical; multinucleated; heavily striated
Control	Involuntary	Involuntary	Voluntary
Action	Produces peristalsis; contracts and relaxes slowly; may sustain contraction	Pumps blood out of heart; self-excitatory but influenced by nervous system and hormones	Produces movement at joints; stimulated by nervous system; contracts and relaxes rapidly

muscle fiber nuclei (peripheral)   striations

FIGURE **7•1** Microscopic view of skeletal muscle fibers (cells) showing multiple nuclei and striations. (Cormack DH: Essential Histology. Philadelphia, JB Lippincott, 1993)

MUSCULAR SYSTEM

Functions

The three primary functions of skeletal muscles are:

- Movement of the skeleton. Muscles are attached to bones and contract to change the position of the bones at a joint.
- Maintenance of posture. A steady partial contraction of muscle, known as **muscle tone,** keeps the body in position. Some of the muscles involved in maintaining posture are the large muscles of the thighs, back, neck, and shoulders as well as the abdominal muscles.
- Generation of heat. Most of the heat needed to keep the body at 37°C (98.6°F) is generated by muscles. Heat is a natural byproduct of muscle cell metabolism. When we are cold, muscles can boost their heat output by the rapid small contractions we know of as *shivering*.

✔ CHECKPOINT **2**:

What are the three main functions of skeletal muscle?

Structure of a Muscle

In forming whole muscles, individual muscle fibers are arranged in bundles, or *fascicles* (FAS-ih-kls), held together by connective tissue (Fig. 7-2). Deeper layers of connective tissue surround each individual fiber in the bundle. The entire muscle is then encased in a tough connective tissue sheath that is part of the *deep fascia.* All these supporting tissues merge to form the tendon that attaches the muscle to a bone. Each muscle also has a rich supply of blood vessels and nerves.

Muscle Cells in Action

Skeletal muscle fibers are stimulated by nerve impulses coming from the brain and the spinal

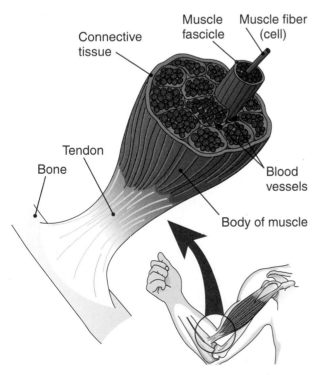

FIGURE **7•2** Structure of a skeletal muscle showing connective tissue coverings.

cord (see Chap. 8). Nerve cell fibers (axons) carry impulses to the muscles, each fiber branching to supply from a few to more than 100 individual muscle cells.

The Neuromuscular Junction

The point at which a nerve fiber contacts a muscle cell is called the *neuromuscular junction* (Fig. 7-3). It is here that a chemical classified as a *neurotransmitter* is released from the neuron to stimulate the muscle fiber. The specific neurotransmitter released here is *acetylcholine* (as-e-til-KO-lene), which is found elsewhere in the body as well. A great deal is known about the events that occur at this junction, and this information is important in understanding muscle action.

The neuromuscular junction is an example of a *synapse* (SIN-aps), a point of communication between cells. Between the cells there is a tiny space, the *synaptic cleft,* across which the neurotransmitter must travel. Until its release, the neurotransmitter is stored in tiny bubbles, called *vesicles,* in the endings of the nerve fiber. Once released, the neurotransmitter crosses the synaptic cleft and attaches to receptors, which are proteins imbedded in the muscle cell membrane. The membrane is folded at this point to increase surface area and hold a maximum number of receptors. The receiving membrane of the muscle cell is known as the *motor end plate.*

Muscle fibers, like nerve cells, show the property of *excitability;* that is, they are able to transmit electrical current along the cell membrane. When the muscle is stimulated at the neuromuscular junction, an electrical impulse is generated that spreads rapidly along the muscle cell membrane. This spreading wave of electrical current is called the *action potential* because it calls the muscle cell into action. Chapter 8 provides more information on synapses and the action potential.

✔ CHECKPOINT **3**:

Muscles are activated by the nervous system. What is the name of the special synapse where a nerve cell makes contact with a muscle cell?

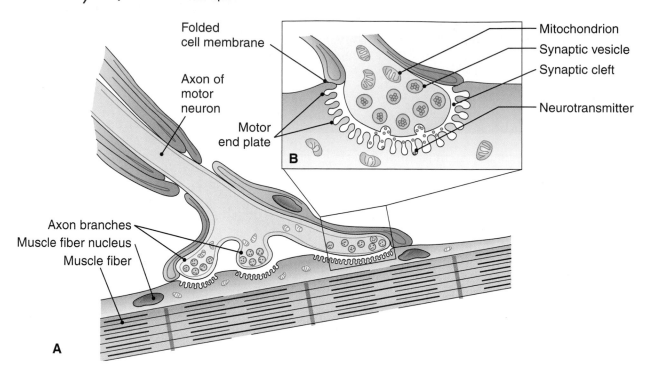

FIGURE **7•3**   Neuromuscular junction. **(A)** The branched end of a motor neuron makes contact with the membrane of a muscle fiber (cell). **(B)** Enlarged view.

Contraction

Another important property of muscle tissue is **contractility.** This is the capacity of a muscle fiber to undergo shortening and to change its shape, becoming thicker. Studies of muscle chemistry and observation of cells under the powerful electron microscope have given a concept of how muscle cells work.

These studies reveal that each skeletal muscle fiber contains many threads, or filaments, made of two kinds of proteins, called **actin** (AK-tin) and **myosin** (MI-o-sin). Filaments made of actin are thin and light; those made of myosin are heavy and dark. The filaments are present in alternating bundles within the muscle cell (Fig. 7-4). It is the alternating bands of light actin and heavy myosin filaments that give skeletal muscle its striated appearance. They also give a view of what occurs when muscles contract.

In movement, the myosin filaments "latch on" to the actin filaments by means of many paddle-like extensions. These attachments are described as *cross-bridges* between the two types of filaments. Using the energy of ATP for repeated movements, the cross-bridges, like the oars of a boat, pull all the actin strands closer together. As the overlapping filaments slide together, the muscle fiber contracts, becoming

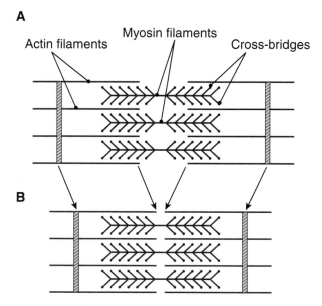

FIGURE **7•4**   The sliding filament mechanism of skeletal muscle contraction. **(A)** Muscle is in a relaxed state. **(B)** Muscle has contracted and the myosin cross bridges have moved to new sites to prepare for another "pull."

shorter and thicker. Figure 7-4 shows a section of muscle in the relaxed and contracted state. Note that the filaments overlap increasingly as the cell contracts. (In reality, not all the cross-bridges are moving at the same time. About one half are forward at any time, and the rest are preparing for another swing.)

✔ CHECKPOINT **4**:

What are two properties of muscle cells that are needed for response to a stimulus?

The Role of Calcium

It is well known that the mineral calcium is needed for muscle contraction. Calcium uncovers points on the actin where cross-bridges can form between the filaments so that the sliding action can begin. The calcium needed for contraction is stored within the endoplasmic reticulum (ER) of the muscle cell and is released into the cytoplasm when the cell is stimulated by a nerve fiber. Muscles relax when nerve stimulation stops and the calcium is pumped back into the ER (see Rigor Mortis).

Muscles and Energy

As noted earlier, all muscle contraction requires energy in the form of ATP. The source of this energy is the oxidation (commonly called "burning") of nutrients within the cells.

Rigor Mortis

After death, muscles enter a stage of rigidity known as **rigor mortis.** The calcium that triggers contraction escapes from its storage areas and causes the muscle filaments to slide together. Because all metabolism has ceased, however, there is no ATP to power further movement of the cross-bridges, and the filaments remain in a contracted position. This stiffness lasts for about 24 hours, then gradually fades as body tissues begin to decay. The rate at which these changes occur varies with the individual and the environment.

To produce ATP, muscle cells must have an adequate supply of oxygen and glucose or other usable nutrient. These substances are constantly brought to the cells by the circulation, but muscle cells also store a small reserve supply of each. Additional oxygen is stored in the form of a compound similar to the blood's hemoglobin but located specifically in muscle cells, as indicated by the prefix *myo-* in its name, **myoglobin** (mi-o-GLO-bin). Additional glucose is stored as a compound that is built from glucose molecules and is called **glycogen** (GLI-ko-jen). Glycogen can be broken down into glucose when needed by the muscle cells, for example, during vigorous exercise.

✔ CHECKPOINT **5**:

Muscle cells obtain energy for contraction from the oxidation of nutrients. What compound is formed in oxidation that supplies the energy for contraction?

Oxygen Debt

Oxygen plays an important role in preventing the accumulation of **lactic acid,** a waste product of metabolism that causes muscle fatigue. During strenuous activity, a person may not be able to breathe in oxygen rapidly enough to meet the needs of the hard-working muscles. The increased demands are met at first by the energy-rich compounds that are stored in the tissues. However, continual exercise depletes these stores.

For a short time, glucose may be used without the benefit of oxygen. In this case, lactic acid is formed in the cells by an alternate pathway of metabolism. This anaerobic process (occurring without oxygen) permits greater magnitude of activity than would otherwise be possible, as, for example, allowing sprinting instead of jogging.

Anaerobic metabolism can continue until buildup of lactic acid causes the muscle to fatigue. As lactic acid accumulates, the person is said to develop an **oxygen debt.** After stopping exercise, he or she must continue to take in more oxygen by continued rapid breathing (panting) until the debt is paid in full. That is, enough oxygen must be taken in to convert the lactic acid to other substances that can be metabolized further. In addition, the energy-rich compounds that are stored in the cells must be replenished.

✔ CHECKPOINT **6**:
_____

When muscles work without oxygen, a compound is produced that causes muscle fatigue. What is the name of this compound?

Effects of Exercise

Changes that occur as muscle metabolism increases during exercise cause *vasodilation* (vas-o-di-LA-shun)—an increase in the diameter of blood vessels—thereby allowing blood to flow more easily to these tissues. As muscles work, more blood is pumped back to the heart. The temporarily increased load on the heart acts to strengthen the heart muscle and to improve its circulation. The chambers of the heart gradually enlarge to accommodate more blood.

Regular exercise also improves breathing and respiratory efficiency. Circulation in the capillaries surrounding the alveoli (air sacs) is increased, and this brings about enhanced gas exchange. Athletic training leads to more efficient distribution and use of oxygen so that the onset of oxygen debt is delayed. Even moderate regular exercise has the additional benefits of weight control, strengthening of the bones, decreased blood pressure, and decreased risk of heart attacks. The effects of exercise on the body are studied in the fields of sports medicine and exercise physiology (see The Benefits of Regular Exercise).

Types of Muscle Contractions

Muscle *tone* refers to a partially contracted state of the muscles that is normal even when the muscles are not in use. The maintenance of this tone, or *tonus* (TO-nus), is due to the action of the nervous system in keeping the muscles in a constant state of readiness for action. Muscles that are little used soon become flabby, weak, and lacking in tone.

The Benefits of Regular Exercise

A well-balanced program of regular exercise can produce benefits to the muscular, cardiovascular, respiratory systems, and other systems, helping to build and maintain overall good health. Exercise can not only help you feel good, but look good as well. In order for an exercise program to produce maximum benefits, it must contain the following three components: stretching, aerobic exercise, and strength training.

Stretching helps to keep a muscle at its optimal length. Under the stress of repeated contractions, a muscle tends to shorten as each individual muscle fiber becomes stronger. Within groups of opposing or antagonistic muscles, one group of muscles or muscle fibers usually becomes stronger than the rest. This leads to muscle shortening on the side with the stronger fibers. Stretching promotes all fibers in the muscle relaxing to optimal length. A stretched muscle fiber is stronger because it contracts over a greater length. Stretching also helps to promote balance and keeps joints limber. Gentle stretching should be done both before and after a round of aerobic exercise or strength training.

Aerobic exercise is the heart of any program. Aerobic exercise should begin with a warm-up of about 5 minutes after stretching. The warm-up allows the cardiovascular and respiratory systems to gear up for increased oxygen demand. The aerobic cycle then involves a period of between 20 and 30 minutes of muscle work in which the muscles undergo a repetitive cycle of contraction and relaxation. This cycle increases the muscle stamina and, with consistency, can greatly increase endurance. Aerobic exercise prepares the muscle for the challenge of strength training.

Strength training uses resistance against active contraction to build muscle mass. This is known as the *primary principle;* all muscle tissue must work against a load to become stronger and larger. A muscle used repetitively against little or no load will not increase in strength, although some increase in size may occur. To increase strength, a muscle must be consistently contracted to at least 50% of its maximum length. This cycle should be repeated as 3 sets of 6 contractions, 3 times a week. At this level, the muscle achieves maximum strength while avoiding fatigue.

Any cycle of aerobic or strength training should be followed by a cooldown period. This involves reducing a muscle group's workload gradually over at least 10 minutes. A cooldown helps keep the blood from returning to the heart too quickly. It lets the heart and lungs readjust to a resting level and allows the circulatory system adequate time to flush out waste products built up during exercise.

A consistent regimen of appropriate exercise 3 times a week increases muscle size and strength and strengthens the cardiovascular and respiratory systems. The immune system is also stimulated by exercise. The road to good health is indeed best walked or biked instead of driven.

In addition to the partial contractions that are responsible for muscle tone, there are two other types of contractions on which the body depends:

- **Isotonic** (i-so-TON-ik) **contractions** are those in which the tone or tension within the muscle remains the same but the muscle as a whole shortens, producing movement; that is, work is accomplished. Lifting weights, walking, running, or any other activity in which the muscles become shorter and thicker (forming bulges) are isotonic contractions.
- **Isometric** (i-so-MET-rik) **contractions** are those in which there is no change in muscle length but there is a great increase in muscle tension. Pushing against an immovable force produces an isometric contraction. For example, if you push the palms of your hands hard against each other, there is no movement, but you can feel the increased tension in your arm muscles.

Most movements of the body involve a combination of both isotonic and isometric contractions. When walking, for example, some muscles contract isotonically to propel the body forward, but at the same time, other muscles are contracting isometrically to keep your body in position.

THE MECHANICS OF MUSCLE MOVEMENT

Attachments of Skeletal Muscles

Most muscles have two or more points of attachment to the skeleton. The muscle is attached to a bone at each end by means of a cordlike extension called a **tendon** (Fig. 7-5). All of the connective tissue within and around the muscle merges to form the tendon, which then attaches directly to the periosteum of the bone (see Fig. 7-2). In some instances, a broad sheet called an **aponeurosis** (ap-o-nu-RO-sis) may attach muscles to bones or to other muscles, as in the abdomen (Fig. 7-7) or across the top of the skull (Fig. 7-9).

In moving the bones, one end of a muscle is attached to a more freely movable part of the skeleton, and the other end is attached to a relatively stable part. The less movable (more fixed) attachment is called the **origin;** the attachment to the part of the body that the muscle puts into action is called the **insertion.** When a muscle contracts, it pulls on both points of attachment, bringing the more movable insertion closer to the origin and thereby causing movement of the body part. Figure 7-5 shows the action of the biceps brachii (in the upper arm) in flexing the arm at the elbow. The insertion on the radius of the forearm is brought to-

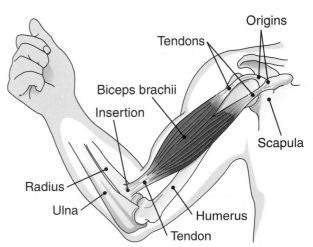

FIGURE **7•5** Diagram of a muscle showing three attachments to bones—two origins and one insertion.

A First-class lever

Scissors   Fulcrum

B Second-class lever

Fulcrum   Wheelbarrow   E

C Third-class lever   Fulcrum

Forceps   E   Fulcrum

FIGURE **7•6**   Levers. Three types of levers and tools that illustrate each. R = resistance (weight). E = effort (force).

ward the origin at the scapula of the shoulder girdle.

> ✔ CHECKPOINT **7**:
>
> Muscles are attached to bones by means of tendons: one attached to a less movable part of the skeleton, and one attached to a movable part. What are the names of these two attachment points?

Muscles Work Together

Many of the skeletal muscles function in pairs. A movement is performed by muscle called the ***prime mover;*** the muscle that produces an opposite movement is known as the ***antagonist.*** Clearly, for any given movement, the antagonist must relax when the prime mover contracts. For example, when the biceps brachii at the front of the arm contracts to flex the arm, the triceps brachii at the back must relax; when the triceps brachii contracts to extend the arm, the biceps brachii must relax. In addition to prime movers and antagonists, there are also muscles that serve to steady body parts or to assist prime movers.

As the muscles work together, body movements are coordinated, and a large number of complicated movements can be carried out. At first, however, the nervous system must learn to coordinate any new, complicated movement. Think of a child learning to walk or to write, and consider the number of muscles she or he uses unnecessarily or forgets to use when the situation calls for them.

> ✔ CHECKPOINT **8**:
>
> Muscles work together to produce movement. What is the name of the muscle that produces a movement as compared with the muscle that produces an opposite movement?

Levers and Body Mechanics

Proper body mechanics help conserve energy and ensure freedom from strain and fatigue; conversely, such ailments as lower back pain—a common complaint—can be traced to poor body

Orbicularis oculi

Masseter

Sternocleidomastoid

Deltoid

Pectoralis major

Serratus anterior

Biceps brachii

Brachioradialis

Flexor carpi

Extensor carpi

Abdominal aponeurosis

Adductors of thigh

Rectus femoris

Peroneus longus

Tibialis anterior

Temporalis

Orbicularis oris

Trapezius

External oblique

Intercostals

Internal oblique

Rectus abdominis

Sartorius

Vastus lateralis

Quadriceps femoris

Gastrocnemius

Soleus

7

FIGURE **7•7** Superficial muscles, anterior (front) view.

mechanics. Body mechanics have special significance to health workers, who are frequently called on to move patients and handle cumbersome equipment. Maintaining the body segments in correct relation to one another has a direct effect on the working capacity of the vital organs that are supported by the skeleton.

If you have had a course in physics, recall your study of levers. A lever is simply a rigid bar that moves about a fixed pivot point, the fulcrum. There are three classes of levers, which differ only in the location of the fulcrum,

the effort (force), and the resistance (weight) (see Fig. 7-6). In a first-class lever, the fulcrum is located between the resistance and the effort; a see-saw or a scissors is an example of this class. The second-class lever has the resistance located between the fulcrum and the effort; a wheelbarrow or a mattress lifted at one end is an illustration of this class. In the third-class lever, the effort is between the resistance and the fulcrum. A forceps or a tweezers is an example of this type of lever. The effort is applied in the center of the tool, between the fulcrum where the pieces join and the resistance at the tip.

The musculoskeletal system can be considered a system of levers, in which the bone is the lever, the joint is the fulcrum, and the force is applied by a muscle. Most lever systems in the body are of the third-class type. A muscle usually inserts over a joint and exerts force between the fulcrum and the resistance. That is, the fulcrum is behind both the point of effort and the weight. In Figure 7-5, the resistance is in the forearm and hand, the force is exerted at the muscle insertion on the forearm, and the fulcrum is the elbow joint.

✔ CHECKPOINT **9**:
_____

Muscles and bones work together as lever systems. Of the three classes of levers, which one represents the action of most muscles?

SKELETAL MUSCLE GROUPS

The study of muscles is made simpler by grouping them according to body regions. Knowing how muscles are named can also help in remembering them.

Naming of Muscles

A number of different characteristics are used in naming muscles, including the following:

- Location, named for a nearby bone, for example, or for position, such as lateral, medial, internal, or external
- Size, using terms such as maximus, major, minor, longus, brevis
- Shape, such as circular (orbicularis), triangular (deltoid), trapezoid (trapezius)
- Direction of fibers, including straight (rectus) or angled (oblique)
- Number of heads (attachment points) as indicated by the suffix *-ceps*, as in biceps, triceps, quadriceps
- Action, as in flexor, extensor, adductor, abductor, levator

Often, more than one feature is used in naming. Refer to Figures 7-7 and 7-8 as you study the locations and functions of some of the skeletal muscles and try to figure out why each has the name that it does. Although they are described in the singular, most of the muscles are present on both sides of the body. The information is summarized in Table 7-2.

Muscles of the Head

The principal muscles of the head are those of facial expression and of mastication (chewing) (see Fig. 7-9).

The muscles of facial expression include ring-shaped ones around the eyes and the lips, called the **orbicularis** (or-bik-u-LAH-ris) **muscles** because of their shape (think of "orbit"). The muscle surrounding each eye is called the **orbicularis oculi** (OK-u-li), whereas the muscle of the lips is the **orbicularis oris.** These muscles, of course, all have antagonists. For example, the **levator palpebrae** (PAL-pe-bre) **superioris,** or lifter of the upper eyelid, is the antagonist for the orbicularis oculi.

One of the largest muscles of expression forms the fleshy part of the cheek and is called the **buccinator** (BUK-se-na-tor). Used in whistling or blowing, it is sometimes referred to as the *trumpeter's muscle.* You can readily think of other muscles of facial expression: for instance, the antagonists of the orbicularis oris can produce a smile, a sneer, or a grimace. There are a number of scalp muscles by means of which the eyebrows are lifted or drawn together into a frown.

There are four pairs of muscles of mastication, all of which insert on the mandible and move it. The largest are the **temporal** (TEM-po-ral), located above and near the ear, and the **masseter** (mas-SE-ter) at the angle of the jaw.

The tongue has two groups of muscles. The first group, called the **intrinsic muscles,** is located entirely within the tongue. The second group, the **extrinsic muscles,** originate outside the tongue. It is because of these many muscles that the tongue has such remarkable flexibility and can perform so many different functions. Consider the intricate tongue motions involved in speaking, chewing, and swallowing.

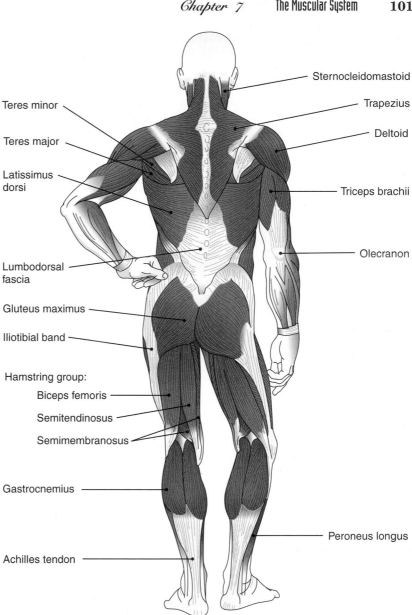

Sternocleidomastoid

Trapezius

Deltoid

Triceps brachii

Olecranon

Teres minor

Teres major

Latissimus dorsi

Lumbodorsal fascia

Gluteus maximus

Iliotibial band

Hamstring group:

Biceps femoris

Semitendinosus

Semimembranosus

Gastrocnemius

Peroneus longus

Achilles tendon

FIGURE **7•8** Superficial muscles, poste-

Muscles of the Neck

The neck muscles tend to be ribbonlike and extend up and down or obliquely in several layers and in a complex manner. The one you will hear of most frequently is the ***sternocleidomastoid*** (ster-no-kli-do-MAS-toyd), sometimes referred to simply as the *sternomastoid*. There are two of these strong muscles, which extend from the sternum upward, across either side of the neck, to the mastoid process. Working together, they bring the head forward on the chest (flexion).

Working alone, each muscle tilts and rotates the head so as to orient the face toward the side opposite that muscle. If the head is abnormally fixed in this position, the person is said to have ***torticollis*** (tor-tih-KOL-is), or *wryneck;* this condition may be due to injury or spasm of the muscle.

A portion of the trapezius muscle (described later) is located in the back of the neck, where it helps hold the head up (extension). Other larger deep muscles are the chief extensors of the head and neck.

Table 7•2   Review of Muscles

NAME	LOCATION	FUNCTION
Muscles of the Head and Neck		
Orbicularis oculi	Encircles eyelid	Closes eye
Levator palpebrae superioris	Back of orbit to upper eyelid	Opens eye
Orbicularis oris	Encircles mouth	Closes lips
Buccinator	Fleshy part of cheek	Flattens cheek; helps in eating, whistling, and blowing wind instruments
Temporal	Above and near ear	Closes jaw
Masseter	At angle of jaw	Closes jaw
Sternocleidomastoid	Along side of neck, to mastoid process	Flexes head; rotates head toward opposite side from muscle
Muscles of the Upper Extremities		
Trapezius	Back of neck and upper back, to clavicle and scapula	Raises shoulder and pulls it back; extends head
Latissimus dorsi	Middle and lower back, to humerus	Extends and adducts arm behind back
Pectoralis major	Upper, anterior chest, to humerus	Flexes and adducts arm across chest; pulls shoulder forward and downward
Serratus anterior	Below axilla on side of chest to scapula	Moves scapula forward; aids in raising arm
Deltoid	Covers shoulder joint, to lateral humerus	Abducts arm
Biceps brachii	Anterior arm, to radius	Flexes forearm and supinates hand
Triceps brachii	Posterior arm, to ulna	Extends forearm
Flexor and extensor carpi groups	Anterior and posterior forearm, to hand	Flex and extend hand
Flexor and extensor digitorum groups	Anterior and posterior forearm, to fingers	Flex and extend fingers
Muscles of the Trunk		
Diaphragm	Dome-shaped partition between thoracic and abdominal cavities	Dome descends to enlarge thoracic cavity from top to bottom
Intercostals	Between ribs	Elevate ribs and enlarge thoracic cavity
External and internal oblique; transversus and rectus abdominis	Anterolateral abdominal wall	Compress abdominal cavity and expel substances from body; flex spinal column
Levator ani	Pelvic floor	Aids defecation
Sacrospinalis	Deep in back, vertical mass	Extends vertebral column to produce erect posture
Muscles of the Lower Extremities		
Gluteus maximus	Superficial buttock, to femur	Extends thigh
Gluteus medius	Deep buttock, to femur	Abducts thigh
Iliopsoas	Crosses front of hip joint, to femur	Flexes thigh
Adductor group	Medial thigh, to femur	Adduct thigh
Sartorius	Winds down thigh, ilium to tibia	Flexes thigh and leg (to sit cross-legged)
Quadriceps femoris	Anterior thigh, to tibia	Extends leg
Hamstring group	Posterior thigh, to tibia and fibula	Flexes leg
Gastrocnemius	Calf of leg, to calcaneus	Extends foot (as in tiptoeing)
Tibialis anterior	Anterior and lateral shin, to foot	Dorsiflexes foot (as in walking on heels); inverts foot (sole inward)
Peroneus longus	Lateral leg, to foot	Everts foot (sole outward)
Flexor and extensor digitorum groups	Posterior and anterior leg, to toes	Flex and extend toes

Muscles of the Upper Extremities

Movement of the Shoulder and Arm

The Posterior Muscles

The position of the shoulder depends to a large extent on the degree of contraction of the ***trapez-*** *ius* (trah-PE-ze-us), a triangular muscle that covers the back of the neck and extends across the back of the shoulder to insert on the clavicle and scapula. The trapezius muscles enable one to raise the shoulders and pull them back. The upper portion of each trapezius can also extend the head and turn it from side to side.

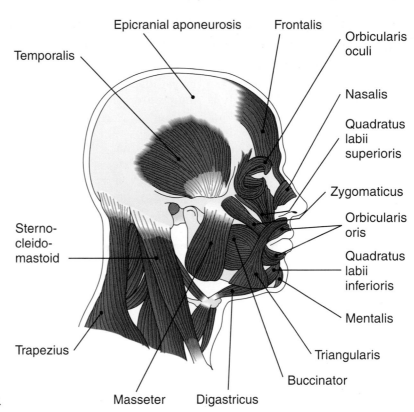

FIGURE **7•9**   Muscles of the head.

The *latissimus* (lah-TIS-ih-mus) *dorsi* originates from the vertebral spine in the middle and lower back and covers the lower half of the thoracic region. The fibers of each muscle converge to a tendon that inserts on the humerus. The latissimus dorsi powerfully extends the arm, bringing it down forcibly as, for example, in swimming.

The Anterior Muscles

A large *pectoralis* (pek-to-RAL-is) *major* is located on either side of the upper part of the chest at the front of the body. This muscle arises from the sternum, the upper ribs, and the clavicle and forms the anterior "wall" of the armpit, or axilla; it inserts on the upper part of the humerus. The pectoralis major flexes and adducts the arm, pulling it across the chest.

Below the axilla, on the side of the chest, is the *serratus* (ser-RA-tus) *anterior.* It originates on the upper eight or nine ribs on the side and the front of the thorax and inserts in the scapula on the side toward the vertebrae. The serratus anterior moves the scapula forward when, for example, one is pushing something. It also aids in raising the arm above the horizontal level.

The Shoulder Muscles

The *deltoid* covers the shoulder joint and is responsible for the roundness of the upper part of the arm just below the shoulder. Arising from the shoulder girdle (clavicle and scapula), the deltoid fibers converge to insert on the lateral side of the humerus. Contraction of this muscle abducts the arm, raising it laterally to the horizontal position.

The shoulder joint allows for a very wide range of movement. This freedom of movement is possible because the humerus fits into a shallow socket, the glenoid cavity of the scapula. This joint requires the support of four deep muscles and their tendons. In certain activities, such as swinging a golf club, playing tennis, or pitching a baseball, these four muscles, which compose the *rotator cuff,* may be injured, and even torn. Surgery is often required for repair of the rotator cuff.

Movement of the Forearm and Hand

The **biceps brachii** (BRA-ke-i), located on the front of the arm, is the muscle you usually display when you want to "flex your muscles" to show your strength. It inserts on the radius and serves to flex the forearm. It is a supinator of the hand (see Fig. 7-5).

The **triceps brachii**, located on the back of the arm, inserts on the olecranon of the ulna. The triceps has been called the *boxer's muscle* because it straightens the elbow when a blow is delivered. It is also important in pushing because it converts the arm and forearm into a sturdy rod.

Muscles That Move the Hand

Most of the muscles that move the hand and fingers originate from the radius and the ulna. Some of them insert on the carpal bones of the wrist, whereas others have long tendons that cross the wrist and insert on bones of the hand and the fingers.

The **flexor carpi** and the **extensor carpi muscles** are responsible for many movements of the hand. Muscles that produce finger movements are the several **flexor digitorum** (dij-e-TO-rum) and the **extensor digitorum muscles.**

Special groups of muscles in the fleshy parts of the hand are responsible for the intricate movements that can be performed with the thumb and the fingers. The freedom of movement of the thumb has been one of the most useful capacities of humans.

Muscles of the Trunk

Muscles of Respiration

The most important muscle involved in the act of breathing is the **diaphragm.** This dome-shaped muscle forms the partition between the thoracic cavity above and the abdominal cavity below (Fig. 7-10). When the diaphragm contracts, the central dome-shaped portion is pulled downward, thus enlarging the thoracic cavity from top to bottom.

The **intercostal muscles** are attached to and fill the spaces between the ribs. The external and internal intercostals run at angles in opposite directions. Contraction of the intercostal muscles serves to elevate the ribs, thus enlarging the thoracic cavity from side to side and from front to back. The mechanics of breathing are described in Chapter 16.

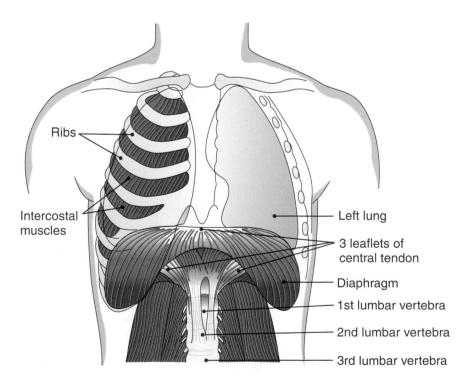

Ribs

Intercostal muscles

Left lung

3 leaflets of central tendon

Diaphragm

1st lumbar vertebra

2nd lumbar vertebra

3rd lumbar vertebra

FIGURE **7•10**   The diaphragm forms the partition between the thoracic cavity and the abdominal cavity.

Muscles of the Abdomen and Pelvis

The wall of the abdomen has three layers of muscle that extend from the back (dorsally) and around the sides (laterally) to the front (ventrally). They are the ***external abdominal oblique*** on the outside, the ***internal abdominal oblique*** in the middle, and the ***transversus abdominis,*** the innermost. The connective tissue from these muscles extends forward and encloses the vertical ***rectus abdominis*** of the anterior abdominal wall. The fibers of these muscles, as well as their connective tissue extensions (aponeuroses), run in different directions, resembling the layers in plywood and resulting in a strong abdominal wall. The midline meeting of the aponeuroses forms a whitish area called the ***linea alba*** (LIN-e-ah Al-ba), which is an important landmark on the abdomen. It extends from the tip of the sternum to the pubic joint (see Fig. 7-7).

These four pairs of abdominal muscles act together to protect the internal organs and compress the abdominal cavity, as in coughing, emptying the bladder (urination) and bowel (defecation), sneezing, vomiting, and childbirth (labor). The two oblique muscles and the rectus abdominis help bend the trunk forward and sideways.

The pelvic floor, or ***perineum*** (per-ih-NE-um), has its own form of diaphragm, shaped somewhat like a shallow dish. One of the principal muscles of this pelvic diaphragm is the ***levator ani*** (le-VA-tor A-ni), which acts on the rectum and thus aids in defecation. The superficial and deep muscles of the female perineum are shown in Figure 7-11.

Deep Muscles of the Back

The deep muscles of the back, which act on the vertebral column itself, are thick vertical masses that lie under the trapezius and latis-

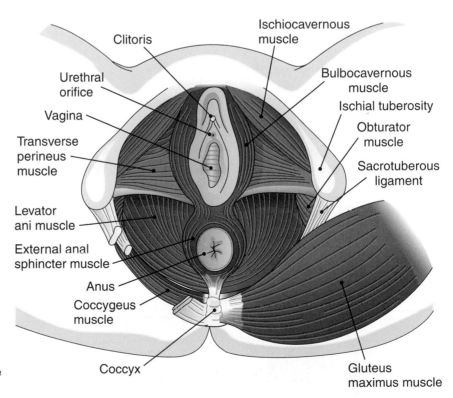

FIGURE **7•11**   Muscles of the female perineum (pelvic floor).

simus dorsi. The longest muscle is the **sacrospinalis** (sa-kro-spin-A-lis), which helps maintain the vertebral column in an erect posture.

Muscles of the Lower Extremities

The muscles in the lower extremities, among the longest and strongest muscles in the body, are specialized for locomotion and balance.

Movement of the Thigh and Leg

The **gluteus maximus** (GLU-te-us MAK-sim-us), which forms much of the fleshy part of the buttock, is relatively large in humans because of its support function when a person is standing in the erect position. This muscle extends the thigh and is important in walking and running. The **gluteus medius,** which is partially covered by the gluteus maximus, serves to abduct the thigh.

The **iliopsoas** (il-e-o-SO-as) arises from the ilium and the bodies of the lumbar vertebrae; it crosses the front of the hip joint to insert on the femur. It is a powerful flexor of the thigh and helps keep the trunk from falling backward when one is standing erect.

The **adductor muscles** are located on the medial part of the thigh. They arise from the pubis and ischium and insert on the femur. These strong muscles press the thighs together, as in grasping a saddle between the knees when riding a horse.

The **sartorius** (sar-TO-re-us) is a long, narrow muscle that begins at the iliac spine, winds downward and inward across the entire thigh, and ends on the upper medial surface of the tibia. It is called the *tailor's muscle* because it is used in crossing the legs in the manner of tailors, who in days gone by sat cross-legged on the floor.

The front and sides of the femur are covered by the **quadriceps femoris** (KWOD-re-seps FEM-or-is), a large muscle that has four heads of origin. The individual parts are as follows: in the center, covering the anterior thigh, the **rectus femoris**; on either side, the **vastus medialis** and **vastus lateralis;** deeper in the center, the **vastus intermedius.** One of these muscles (rectus femoris) originates from the ilium, and the other three are from the femur, but all four have a common tendon of insertion on the tibia.

You may remember that this is the tendon that encloses the knee cap, or patella. This muscle extends the leg, as in kicking a ball.

The **hamstring muscles** are located in the posterior part of the thigh. Their tendons can be felt behind the knee as they descend to insert on the tibia and fibula. The hamstrings flex the leg on the thigh, as in kneeling. Individually, moving from lateral to medial position, they are the **biceps femoris,** the **semimembranosus,** and the **semitendinosus.**

Movement of the Foot

The **gastrocnemius** (gas-trok-NE-me-us) is the chief muscle of the calf of the leg. It has been called the *toe dancer's muscle* because it is used in standing on tiptoe. It ends near the heel in a prominent cord called the **Achilles tendon,** which attaches to the calcaneus (heel bone). The Achilles tendon is the largest tendon in the body.

Another leg muscle that acts on the foot is the **tibialis** (tib-e-A-lis) **anterior,** located on the front of the leg. This muscle performs the opposite function of the gastrocnemius. Walking on the heels uses the tibialis anterior to raise the rest of the foot off the ground (dorsiflexion). This muscle is also responsible for inversion of the foot. The muscle for eversion of the foot is the **peroneus** (per-o-NE-us) **longus,** located on the side of the leg. The long tendon of this muscle crosses under the foot, forming a sling that supports the transverse (metatarsal) arch.

The toes, like the fingers, are provided with flexor and extensor muscles. The tendons of the extensor muscles are located in the top of the foot and insert on the superior surface of the toe bones (phalanges). The flexor digitorum tendons cross the sole of the foot and insert on the undersurface of the toe bones.

EFFECTS OF AGING ON MUSCLES

Beginning at about 40 years of age, there is a gradual loss of muscle cells with a resulting decrease in the size of each individual muscle. There is also a loss of power, notably in the extensor muscles, such as the large sacrospinalis near the vertebral column. This causes the "bent over" appearance of a hunchback (kyphosis), which in women is often referred to as the *dowager's hump.* Sometimes, there is a tendency to bend (flex) the hips and knees. In addition to causing the previously noted changes in the vertebral column (see Chap. 6), these effects on the extensor muscles result in a further decrease in the elderly person's height. Activity and exercise throughout life delay and decrease these undesirable effects of aging. Even among the elderly, resistance exercise, such as weight lifting, increases muscle strength and function.

Summary

I. Types of muscle
- **A.** Smooth muscle
  1. In walls of hollow organs, vessels, and respiratory passageways
  2. Cells tapered, single nucleus, nonstriated
  3. Involuntary; produces peristalsis; contracts and relaxes slowly
- **B.** Cardiac muscle
  1. Muscle of heart wall
  2. Cells branch; single nucleus; lightly striated
  3. Involuntary; self-excitatory
- **C.** Skeletal muscle
  1. Attached to bones and moves skeleton
  2. Cells long, cylindrical; multiple nuclei; heavily striated
  3. Voluntary; contracts and relaxes rapidly

II. Muscular system
- **A.** Functions
  1. Movement of skeleton
  2. Maintenance of posture
  3. Generation of heat
- **B.** Structure of a muscle
  1. Held by connective tissue around individual fibers, fascicles (bundles), whole muscle
- **C.** Muscle cells in action
  1. Neuromuscular junction—point where nerve fiber stimulates muscle cell
  2. Contraction—sliding together of filaments to shorten muscle
    a. Actin—thin and light
    b. Myosin—heavy and dark
  3. Calcium—allows cross-bridges to form between actin and myosin
- **D.** Muscles and energy
  1. ATP—supplies energy
  2. Myoglobin—stores energy
  3. Glycogen—stores glucose
  4. Oxygen debt—develops during strenuous exercise
    a. Anaerobic metabolism
    b. Yields lactic acid
- **E.** Effects of exercise
  1. Vasodilation to bring blood to tissues
  2. Improved breathing
- **F.** Types of muscle contractions
  1. Tonus—partially contracted state
  2. Isotonic contractions—muscle shortens to produce movement
  3. Isometric contractions—tension increases, but muscle does not shorten

III. Mechanics of muscle movement
- **A.** Attachments of skeletal muscles
  1. Tendon—cord of connective tissue that attaches muscle to bone
    a. Origin—attached to more fixed part
    b. Insertion—attached to moving part
  2. Aponeurosis—broad band of connective tissue that attaches muscle to bone or other muscle
- **B.** Muscles work together
  1. Prime mover—performs movement
  2. Antagonist—produces opposite movement
  3. Others—steady body parts and assist prime mover

C. Levers and body mechanics—muscles function with skeleton as lever systems
   1. Lever—bone
   2. Fulcrum—joint
   3. Force—muscle contraction

IV. Skeletal muscle groups
   A. Naming of muscles—location, size, shape, direction of fibers, number of heads, action

B. Muscles of the head
C. Muscles of the neck
D. Muscles of the upper extremities
E. Muscles of the trunk
F. Muscles of the lower extremities

V. Effects of aging on muscles
   1. Decrease in size of muscles
   2. Weakening of muscles, especially extensors

Questions for Study and Review

1. Compare smooth, cardiac, and skeletal muscle with respect to location, structure, and function.
2. List the functions of skeletal muscle.
3. Describe the structure of muscles from fiber to deep fascia.
4. Explain the role of each of the following in muscle contraction: actin and myosin, calcium, ATP, myoglobin, glycogen.
5. When does oxygen debt occur? What is the role of lactic acid in oxygen debt? How is oxygen debt eliminated?
6. What are some valuable effects of exercise?
7. Differentiate between the terms in each of the following pairs:
   a. *isotonic contraction* and *isometric contraction*
   b. *tendon* and *aponeurosis*
   c. *muscle origin* and *muscle insertion*
   d. *prime mover* and *antagonist*
8. What are levers and how do they work? The forceps is an example of which class of lever? When muscles and bones act as lever systems, what part of the body is the fulcrum?
9. List six characteristics by which muscles are named.
10. Name and describe the functions of the principal muscles of the head and neck, upper extremities, trunk, and lower extremities.
11. What effect does aging have on muscles?

✔ ANSWERS TO CHECKPOINTS

1. The three types of muscle are smooth muscle, cardiac muscle, and skeletal muscle.
2. The three main functions of skeletal muscle are movement of the skeleton, maintenance of posture, and generation of heat.
3. The special synapse where a nerve cell makes contact with a muscle cell is the neuromuscular junction.
4. Two properties of muscle cells that are needed for response to a stimulus are excitability and contractility.
5. ATP is the form of energy produced by the oxidation of nutrients that supplies the energy for contraction of muscle cells.
6. Lactic acid is produced when muscles work without oxygen, causing muscle fatigue.
7. The attachment of a muscle to a less movable part of the skeleton is the origin; the attachment of a muscle to a movable part of the skeleton is the insertion.
8. The muscle that produces a movement is called the prime mover; the muscle that produces an opposite movement is the antagonist.
9. The action of most muscles is represented by a third-class lever in which the fulcrum is behind the point of effort and the weight.
10. The diaphragm is the muscle most important in breathing.
11. The muscles of the abdominal wall are strengthened by having the fibers of these muscles run in different directions.

Of the four chapters in this unit, two describe the nervous system and some of its many parts and complex functions. The organs of special sense and other sensory receptors are allotted an additional separate chapter. The fourth chapter in this unit discusses hormones and the organs that produce them. Working with the nervous system, these hormones play an important role in coordination and control.

Unit III

COORDINATION AND CONTROL

The Nervous System: The Spinal Cord and Spinal Nerves

Chapter

SELECTED KEY TERMS

The following terms are defined in the Glossary:

acetylcholine
action potential
afferent
autonomic nervous system
axon
dendrite
effector
efferent
epinephrine
ganglion
interneuron
motor
nerve
nerve impulse
neuroglia
neurotransmitter
plexus
receptor
reflex
sensory
somatic nervous system
synapse
tract

BEHAVIORAL OBJECTIVES

After careful study of this chapter, you should be able to:

1. Describe the organization of the nervous system according to structure and function
2. Explain the purpose of neuroglia
3. Describe the structure of a neuron
4. Briefly describe the transmission of a nerve impulse
5. Explain the role of myelin in nerve conduction
6. Briefly describe transmission at a synapse
7. Define *neurotransmitter* and give several examples of neurotransmitters
8. Name three types of nerves and explain how they differ from each other
9. List the components of a reflex arc
10. Describe the spinal cord and name several of its functions
11. Define a reflex and give several examples
12. Describe and name the spinal nerves and three of their main plexuses
13. Compare the location and functions of the sympathetic and parasympathetic nervous systems

None of the body systems is capable of functioning alone. All are interdependent and work together as one unit to maintain normal conditions, termed *homeostasis*. The nervous system serves as the chief coordinating agency for all systems. Conditions both within and outside the body are constantly changing. The nervous system must detect and respond to these changes (known as *stimuli*) so that the body can adapt itself to new conditions. The nervous system has been compared to a telephone exchange, in that the brain and the spinal cord act as switching centers and the nerves act as cables for carrying messages to and from these centers.

THE NERVOUS SYSTEM AS A WHOLE

Structural Divisions

The parts of the nervous system may be grouped according to structure or function. The anatomic, or structural, divisions of the nervous system are as follows (Fig. 8-1):

- The ***central nervous system*** (CNS) includes the brain and spinal cord.
- The ***peripheral*** (per-IF-er-al) ***nervous system*** (PNS) is made up of all the nerves outside the CNS. It includes all the ***cranial nerves*** that carry impulses to and from the brain and all the ***spinal nerves*** that carry messages to and from the spinal cord.

The CNS and PNS together include all of the nervous tissue in the body.

Functional Divisions

Functionally, the nervous system is divided according to whether control is voluntary or involuntary and according to what type of tissue is stimulated (Table 8-1). Any tissue or organ that carries out a command from the nervous system is called an ***effector***, all of which are muscles or glands.

The ***somatic nervous system*** is controlled voluntarily (by conscious will), and all the effectors are skeletal muscles (described in Chap. 7). The involuntary division of the nervous system is called the ***autonomic nervous system*** (ANS), with reference to its automatic activity, or the ***visceral nervous system,*** because it controls smooth muscle, cardiac muscle, and glands, much of which make up the soft body organs, the viscera.

The ANS is further subdivided into a ***sympathetic nervous system*** and a ***parasympathetic nervous system*** based on organization and how each affects specific organs. The ANS is described later in this chapter.

Although these divisions are helpful for study

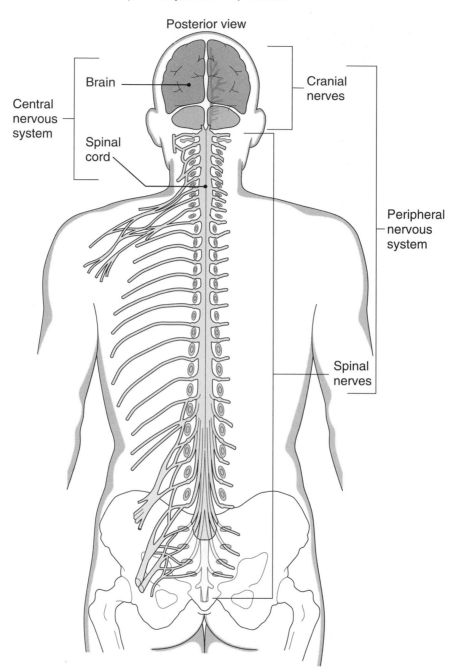

FIGURE **8•1**   Anatomic divisions of the nervous system.

purposes, the lines that divide the nervous system according to function are not as distinct as those that classify the system structurally. For example, the diaphragm, a skeletal muscle, typically functions in breathing without conscious thought. In addition, we have certain rapid reflex responses involving skeletal muscles—drawing the hand away from a hot stove, for example—that do not involve the brain. In contrast, people can be trained to consciously control involuntary functions, such as blood pressure, heart rate, and breathing rate, by techniques known as *biofeedback*.

To learn more about some of the effects of the

Table 8•1	Functional Divisions of the Nervous System	
DIVISION	**SOMATIC NERVOUS SYSTEM**	**AUTONOMIC NERVOUS SYSTEM**
Control	Voluntary	Involuntary
Effectors	Skeletal muscle	Smooth muscle, cardiac muscle, and glands
Subdivisions		Sympathetic and parasympathetic systems

nervous system on the rest of the body, see Mind Over Body: Your Own Healing Powers.

✔ CHECKPOINT **1**:

What are the two divisions of the nervous system based on structure?

✔ CHECKPOINT **2**:

The nervous system can be divided functionally into two divisions based on type of control and effectors. What division is voluntary and controls skeletal muscle, and what division is involuntary and controls involuntary muscles and glands?

Mind Over Body: Your Own Healing Powers

For more than 1000 years Eastern medicine has taught that the health of the body is entirely dependent upon the health of the mind. Western medicine has traditionally rejected this idea, preferring to rely upon well-documented studies of scientific fact. However, since the middle 1980s, western medical practitioners have put forth many well-founded studies to prove that our eastern colleagues have been right all along.

The earliest studies to indicate that the brain was indeed a very powerful physiological organ were undertaken in the early and middle 1960s. These studies set out to document that many "mental" illnesses such as schizophrenia and manic depression were indeed physiological disorders. In the years since, studies have continued to show that many physical symptoms are tied to what would have previously been thought of as "it's all just in your head."

"Bad" emotional stress, including feelings of depression, inability to cope, or anger, fear, loss, or rejection, causes distinct changes in the biochemistry of the brain, which may appear as physical ailments. When the body is experiencing "bad stress," the cardiovascular system works harder and less efficiently. The respiratory system has a harder time keeping up with demands for oxygen and the immune system has a more difficult time fighting off invading pathogens. The body's metabolism has trouble supplying the increased demand for energy needed to cope with the negative stress. In essence, the systems are geared more toward fighting the effects of stress than taking care of the body. As a result, people tend to get sick when they are under significant stress.

Conversely, positive or "good stress" leads to a general increase in a person's overall health. Feelings of happiness, joy, contentment, fulfillment, love, and companionship lead to positive changes in the biochemistry of the brain. The heart pumps more slowly and more efficiently, the lungs work more easily, the immune system is boosted to fight off disease.

Studies have now shown that:

- Men and women in solid, long-lasting relationships live longer than their single counterparts and experience less significant illness throughout their adult lives.
- Those who experience a significant stress are seven times more likely to become ill than the average person.
- Faith, prayer, and meditation, regardless of religious affiliation, may lead to shorter hospital stays, lower blood pressure, increased circulation, and extension of life-span by an average of 7.26 years.
- Laughter really is the best medicine, having been shown to directly stimulate the immune system.

Limiting our exposure to negative stress and exploiting the benefits of positive stress has a definite impact on our lives.

Neuroglia

In addition to conducting tissue, the nervous system contains cells that serve for support and protection. Collectively, these connective tissue cells are called ***neuroglia*** (nu-ROG-le-ah) or ***glial*** (GLI-al) ***cells.*** There are different types of neuroglia, each with specialized functions, some of which are the following:

* To protect nervous tissue
* To support nervous tissue and bind it to other structures
* To aid in repair of cells
* To act as phagocytes to remove pathogens and impurities
* To regulate the composition of fluids around and between cells

Unlike nerve cells, neuroglia continue to multiply throughout life. Because of their capacity to reproduce, most tumors of the nervous system are tumors of neuroglial tissue.

✔ CHECKPOINT **3**:

The nonconducting cells of the nervous system serve in protection and support. What are these cells called?

NEURONS AND THEIR FUNCTIONS

Structure of a Neuron

The functional cells of the nervous system are highly specialized cells called ***neurons*** (Fig. 8-2). The main portion of each neuron, the cell body, contains the nucleus and other organelles typically found in cells. A distinguishing feature of the neurons, however, are the long, threadlike fibers that extend out from the cell body and carry impulses across the cell. There are two kinds of fibers: dendrites and axons.

* ***Dendrites*** are neuron fibers that conduct impulses *to* the cell body. Most dendrites have a highly branched, treelike appearance (see Fig. 8-2). In fact, the name comes

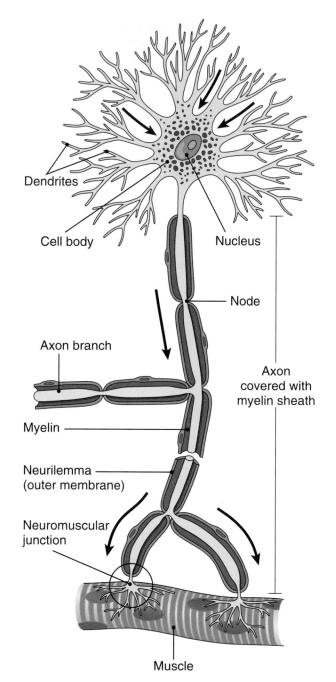

FIGURE **8•2**   Diagram of a motor neuron. The break in the axon denotes length. The arrows show the direction of the nerve impulse.

from a Greek word meaning "tree." Dendrites function as ***receptors*** in the nervous system. That is, they receive the stimulus that begins a neural pathway. In Chapter 10, we describe how the dendrites of the sensory system may be modified to respond to a specific type of stimulus.

- ***Axons*** (AK-sons) are neuron fibers that conduct impulses *away from* the cell body. These impulses may be delivered to another neuron, to a muscle, or to a gland. An axon is a single fiber, which may be quite long and which branches at its end.

The Myelin Sheath

Some axons are covered with a fatty material called ***myelin*** that insulates and protects the fiber (Fig. 8-3). In the PNS, this covering is produced by special neuroglia called ***Schwann*** (shvahn) ***cells,*** that wrap around the axon like a jelly roll depositing layers of myelin. When the sheath is complete, small spaces remain between the individual cells. These tiny gaps, called ***nodes,*** are important in speeding the conduction of nerve impulses.

The outermost membranes of the Schwann cells form a thin coating known as the ***neurilemma*** (nu-rih-LEM-mah). This covering is a part of the mechanism by which some peripheral nerves repair themselves when injured. Under some circumstances, damaged nerve cell fibers may regenerate by growing into the sleeve formed by the neurilemma. Cells of the brain and the spinal cord are myelinated, not by Schwann cells, but by other neuroglia. As a result, they have no neurilemma. If they are injured, the damage is permanent. Even in the peripheral nerves, however, repair is a slow and uncertain process.

Myelinated axons, because of the color of the myelin, are called ***white fibers*** and are found in the ***white matter*** of the brain and spinal cord as well as in the nerve trunks in all parts of the body. The fibers and cell bodies of the ***gray matter*** are not covered with myelin.

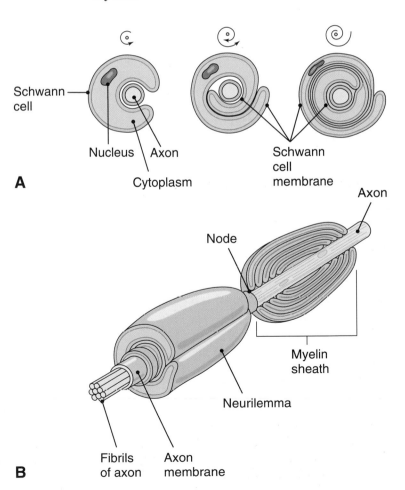

FIGURE **8•3** Formation of the myelin sheath. **(A)** Schwann cells wrap around the axon creating a myelin coating. **(B)** Outermost layer of the Schwann cell forms the neurilemma. Spaces between the cells are the nodes.

8

> ✔ CHECKPOINT **4**:
>
> The neuron, the functional unit of the nervous system, has long fibers extending from the cell body. What is the name of the fiber that carries impulses toward the cell body and what is the fiber that carries impulses away from the cell body?

> ✔ CHECKPOINT **5**:
>
> Myelin is a substance that covers and protects some axons. What color describes myelinated fibers, and what term describes unmyelinated tissue of the nervous system?

Types of Neurons

The job of neurons in the PNS is to relay information constantly either to or from the CNS. Neurons that conduct impulses *to* the spinal cord and brain are described as **sensory neurons,** also **afferent neurons.** Those cells that carry impulses *from* the CNS out to muscles and glands are **motor neurons,** also **efferent neurons.** Neurons that relay information within the CNS are **interneurons,** also called *central* or *association neurons.*

Nerves and Tracts

Everywhere in the nervous system, neuron fibers are collected into bundles of varying size. A bundle of fibers located within the PNS is a **nerve.** A bundle of fibers within the CNS is a **tract.**

Tracts are located in the brain and also in the spinal cord, where they conduct impulses to and from the brain. A nerve or tract can be compared to an electric cable made up of many wires. As with muscles, the "wires," or nerve cell fibers, in a nerve or tract are bound together with connective tissue.

A few of the cranial nerves contain only sensory fibers for conducting impulses toward the brain. These are described as **sensory (afferent) nerves.** A few of the cranial nerves contain only motor fibers for conducting impulses away from the brain and are classified as **motor (efferent) nerves.** Most of the cranial nerves and *all* of the

spinal nerves contain both sensory *and* motor fibers and are referred to as **mixed nerves.** Note that in a mixed nerve, impulses may be traveling in two directions (toward or away from the CNS), but each individual fiber in the nerve is carrying impulses in one direction only. Think of the nerve as a large highway. Traffic may be going north and south, for example, but each car is going forward in only one direction.

> ✔ CHECKPOINT **6**:
>
> Nerves are bundles of neuron fibers in the PNS. These nerves may be carrying impulses either toward or away from the CNS. What name is given to nerves that convey impulses toward the CNS, and what name is given to nerves that transport away from the CNS?

THE NERVOUS SYSTEM AT WORK

The Nerve Impulse

The mechanics of nerve impulse conduction are complex but can be compared to the spread of an electric current along a wire. What follows is a brief description of the electric changes that occur as a resting neuron is stimulated and transmits a nerve impulse.

The cell membrane of an unstimulated (resting) neuron carries an electric charge. This charge is maintained by ions (charged particles) concentrated on either side of the membrane. At rest, the inside of the membrane is negative as compared with the outside. In this state, the membrane is said to be *polarized.*

A **nerve impulse** starts with a local reversal in this charge, which then spreads along the membrane like a current (Fig. 8-4). This sudden electric change in the membrane is called an **action potential,** as described in Chapter 7 on the muscles. When this reversal occurs, the membrane is said to *depolarize.* The reversal occurs rapidly (in less than one thousandth of a second) and is followed at each point along the membrane by an immediate return to the original state so that the membrane can be stimulated again. When the membrane returns to its resting state, it is said to *repolarize.* Depolarization and repolarization are brought about by

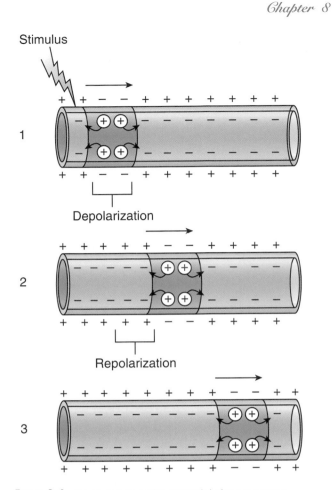

Stimulus

1

Depolarization

2

Repolarization

3

FIGURE **8•4** Spread of an action potential along a neuron.

✔ CHECKPOINT **7**:

An action potential occurs in two stages. In the first stage, the charge on the membrane reverses, and in the second stage, it returns to the resting state. What terms are used to describe the membrane in these two stages?

The Synapse

Neurons do not work alone; impulses must be transferred between neurons to convey information within the nervous system. The point of junction for transmission of the nerve impulse is the *synapse* (SIN-aps), a term that comes from a Greek word meaning "to clasp" (Fig. 8-5).

As described in Chapter 7, information must be passed from one cell to another across a tiny gap between the cells, the synaptic cleft. Within the branched endings of the axon are small vesicles (bubbles) containing a type of chemical known as a *neurotransmitter.* When a nerve impulse traveling along a neuron reaches the end of the axon, the axon releases its neurotransmitter into the narrow gap, the *synaptic cleft*, between the cells. The neurotransmitter then acts as a chemical signal to stimulate the next cell, described as the *postsynaptic cell.* The cell that releases the neurotransmitter is the *presynaptic cell.*

On the receiving membrane, usually that of a dendrite, but sometimes another part of the cell, there are special sites, or *receptors,* ready to pick up and respond to specific neurotransmitters. Receptors in the postsynaptic cell membrane influence how or if that cell will respond to a given neurotransmitter.

Neurotransmitters

Although there are many known neurotransmitters, the main ones are *epinephrine* (ep-ih-NEF-rin), also called *adrenaline;* a related compound, *norepinephrine* (nor-ep-ih-NEF-rin), or *noradrenaline;* and *acetylcholine* (as-e-til-KO-lene). Acetylcholine (ACh) is the neurotransmitter released at the neuromuscular junction, the synapse between a neuron and a muscle cell. All three of the above neurotransmitters function in the ANS. It is common

rapid shifts in sodium and potassium ions across the cell membrane. A stimulus can be defined as any force (*e.g.,* electric, chemical, or mechanical) that can start an action potential, which then spreads along the membrane as a nerve impulse.

The Role of Myelin in Conduction

In an unmyelinated fiber, the action potential spreads continuously along the membrane of the cell (see Fig. 8-4). When myelin is present on an axon, however, it insulates the fiber against the spread of current. This would appear to slow or stop conduction along these fibers, but in fact, the myelin sheath speeds conduction. In this case, the action potential must "jump" like a spark from node (space) to node along the sheath (see Fig. 8-3), and this type of conduction is actually faster than continuous conduction.

FIGURE **8•5** **(A)** A synapse. The axon ending has vesicles containing neurotransmitter, which is released across the synaptic cleft to the membrane of the next cell. **(B)** Close-up of a synapse. Showing receptors for neurotransmitter in the postsynaptic cell membrane.

to think of neurotransmitters as stimulating the cells they reach; in fact, they have been described as such in this discussion. Note, however, that some of these chemicals act to inhibit the postsynaptic cell and keep it from reacting.

The connections between neurons can be quite complex. One cell can branch to stimulate many receiving cells, or a single cell may be stimulated by a number of different axons (Fig. 8-6). The cell's response is based on the total effects of all the neurotransmitters it receives at any one time.

After its release into the synaptic cleft, the neurotransmitter may follow several paths for removal:

- It may slowly diffuse away from the synapse.
- It may be destroyed rapidly by enzymes in the synaptic cleft.
- It may be taken back into the presynaptic cell to be used again.

The method of removal is a factor in determining how long a neurotransmitter will act.

Dendrite

Axon

Cell body

Axon endings from other neurons

Nerve fibers from other neurons

FIGURE **8•6**   A single neuron is stimulated by axons of many other neurons.

✔ CHECKPOINT **8**:

Chemicals are needed to carry information across the synaptic cleft at a synapse. As group, what are all these chemicals called?

The Reflex Arc

As the nervous system functions, both external and internal stimuli are received, interpreted, and acted on. A complete pathway through the nervous system from stimulus to response is termed a ***reflex arc*** (Fig. 8-7). This is the basic functional pathway of the nervous system. The basic parts of a reflex arc are the following:

- ***Receptor***—the end of a dendrite or some specialized receptor cell, as in a special sense organ, that detects a stimulus
- ***Sensory neuron,*** or afferent neuron—a cell that transmits impulses *toward* the CNS
- ***Central nervous system***—where impulses

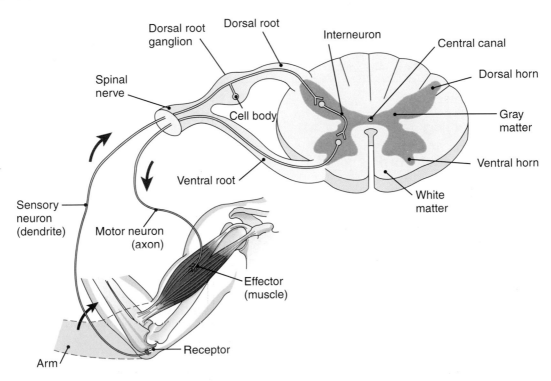

Dorsal root ganglion

Dorsal root

Interneuron

Central canal

Dorsal horn

Gray matter

Ventral horn

White matter

Spinal nerve

Cell body

Ventral root

Sensory neuron (dendrite)

Motor neuron (axon)

Effector (muscle)

Receptor

Arm

FIGURE **8•7**   Reflex arc showing the pathway of impulses and a cross section of the spinal cord.

are coordinated and a response is organized. One or more interneurons may carry impulses to and from the brain, may function within the brain, or may distribute impulses to different regions of the spinal cord. Almost every response involves connecting neurons in the CNS.

- *Motor neuron,* or efferent neuron—a cell that carries impulses *away from* the CNS
- *Effector*—a muscle or a gland outside the CNS that carries out a response

At its simplest, a reflex arc can involve just two neurons, one sensory and one motor, with a synapse in the CNS. There are few reflex arcs that require only this minimal number of neurons. The knee-jerk reflex described later is one of the few examples in humans. Most reflex arcs involve many more, even hundreds, of connecting neurons within the CNS. The many intricate patterns that make the nervous system so responsive and adaptable also make it difficult to study, and investigation of the nervous system is one of the most active areas of research today.

✔ CHECKPOINT **9**:

What name is given to a pathway through the nervous system from a stimulus to an effector?

THE SPINAL CORD

Location of the Spinal Cord

The spinal cord is contained in and protected by the vertebrae, which fit together to form a continuous tube extending from the occipital bone to the coccyx (Fig. 8-8). In the embryo, the spinal cord occupies the entire spinal canal, extending down into the tail portion of the vertebral column. The column of bone grows much more rapidly than the nerve tissue of the cord, however, and eventually, the end of the cord no longer reaches the lower part of the spinal canal. This disparity in growth continues to increase, so that in adults, the cord ends in the region just below the area to which the last rib attaches (between the first and second lumbar vertebrae).

Structure of the Spinal Cord

The spinal cord (see Fig. 8-7) has a small, irregularly shaped internal section that consists of gray matter (nerve cell bodies) and a larger area surrounding this gray part that consists of white matter (nerve cell fibers). The gray matter is so arranged that a column of cells extends up and down dorsally, one on each side; another column is found in the ventral region on each side. These two pairs of columns, called the **dorsal** and **ventral horns,** give the gray matter an H-shaped appearance in cross-section. In the center of the gray matter is a small channel, the **central canal**, that contains cerebrospinal fluid, the liquid that circulates around the brain and spinal cord. The white matter consists of thousands of myelinated axons arranged in three areas external to the gray matter on each side.

✔ CHECKPOINT **10**:

The spinal cord contains both gray and white matter. How is this tissue arranged in the spinal cord?

Functions of the Spinal Cord

Linking the Spinal Nerves to the Brain
The white matter of the spinal cord is divided into tracts that convey impulses to and from the brain. As shown in Figure 8-7, sensory impulses from peripheral receptors enter the dorsal horn of the spinal cord. They are then transmitted upward toward the brain in *ascending tracts* of the white matter.

Motor impulses traveling down from the brain are carried in *descending tracts* until they exit through the ventral horn of the gray matter to reach an effector.

Reflex Activities
A **reflex** is a rapid, simple, and automatic response involving very few neurons. Reflexes are

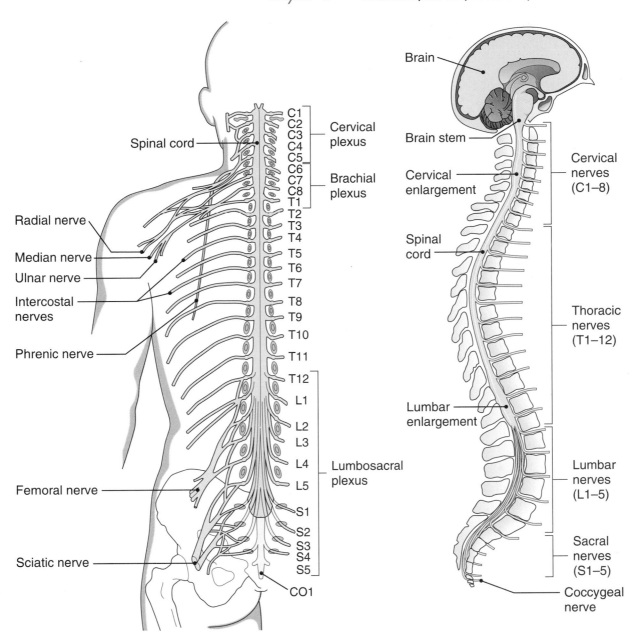

FIGURE **8•8**　Spinal cord and spinal nerves showing plexuses. **(A)** Interior view. **(B)** Lateral view.

specific; a given stimulus always produces the same response.

When you fling out an arm or leg to catch your balance, withdraw from a painful stimulus, or blink to avoid an object approaching your eyes, you are experiencing reflex behavior. A simple reflex arc that passes through the spinal cord alone and does not involve the brain is termed a ***spinal reflex.***

The ***stretch reflex,*** in which a muscle is stretched and responds by contracting, is one example. If you tap the tendon below the kneecap (the patellar tendon), the muscle of the anterior thigh (quadriceps femoris) contracts, eliciting the knee-jerk reflex (Fig. 8-9).

Such stretch reflexes may be evoked by appropriate tapping of most large muscles (such as the triceps brachii in the arm and the gas-

8

FIGURE **8•9**   The patellar (knee-jerk) reflex.

any collection of nerve cell bodies located outside the CNS. Fibers from sensory receptors throughout the body lead to these dorsal root ganglia.

The ventral roots of the spinal nerves are a combination of motor (efferent) fibers that supply muscles and glands (effectors). The cell bodies of these neurons are located in the ventral gray matter (ventral horns) of the cord. Because the dorsal (sensory) and ventral (motor) roots are combined to form the spinal nerve, all spinal nerves are mixed nerves.

Branches of the Spinal Nerves

Each spinal nerve continues only a short distance away from the spinal cord and then branches into small posterior divisions and larger anterior divisions. The larger anterior branches interlace to form networks called ***plexuses*** (PLEK-sus-eze), which then distribute branches to the body parts (see Fig. 8-8). The three main plexuses are described as follows:

- The ***cervical plexus*** supplies motor impulses to the muscles of the neck and receives sensory impulses from the neck and the back of the head. The phrenic nerve, which activates the diaphragm, arises from this plexus.
- The ***brachial*** (BRA-ke-al) ***plexus*** sends numerous branches to the shoulder, arm, forearm, wrist, and hand. The radial nerve emerges from the brachial plexus.
- The ***lumbosacral*** (lum-bo-SA-kral) ***plexus*** supplies nerves to the pelvis and legs. The largest branch in this plexus is the ***sciatic*** (si-AT-ik) ***nerve,*** which leaves the dorsal part of the pelvis, passes beneath the gluteus maximus muscle, and extends down the back of the thigh. At its beginning, it is nearly 1 inch thick, but it soon branches to the thigh muscles; near the knee, it forms two subdivisions that supply the leg and the foot.

trocnemius in the calf of the leg). Because reflexes are simple and predictable, they are used in physical examinations to test the condition of the nervous system.

> ✔ CHECKPOINT **11**:
>
> What are the two main functions of the spinal cord?

SPINAL NERVES

Location and Structure of the Spinal Nerves

There are 31 pairs of spinal nerves, each pair numbered according to the level of the spinal cord from which it arises (see Fig. 8-8). Each nerve is attached to the spinal cord by two roots: the ***dorsal root*** and the ***ventral root*** (see Fig. 8-7). On each dorsal root is a marked swelling of gray matter called the ***dorsal root ganglion,*** which contains the cell bodies of the sensory neurons. A ***ganglion*** (GANG-le-on) is

To learn about how the organization of the spinal nerves affects skin sensations, see Dermatomes.

✔ CHECKPOINT **12**:

How many pairs of spinal nerves are there?

THE AUTONOMIC NERVOUS SYSTEM

Characteristics of the Autonomic Nervous System

The autonomic (visceral) nervous system regulates the action of the glands, the smooth muscles of hollow organs and vessels, and the heart muscle. These actions are carried on automatically; whenever a change occurs that calls for a regulatory adjustment, it is made without conscious awareness.

Dermatomes

Sensory neurons from all over the skin, except for the skin of the face and scalp, feed information into the spinal cord through the spinal nerves. The skin surface can be mapped into distinct regions that are supplied by a single spinal nerve. Each of these regions is called a *dermatome* (DER-mah-tome) (see illustration below).

Stimulation of the skin within a given dermatome is carried over the corresponding spinal nerve. This information can be used to identify the spinal nerve or spinal segment that is involved in an injury. In some areas, the dermatomes are not absolutely distinct. Some dermatomes may share a nerve supply with neighboring regions. For this reason, it is necessary to numb several adjacent dermatomes to achieve successful anesthesia.

Dermatomes

8

SYMPATHETIC SYSTEM

PARASYMPATHETIC SYSTEM

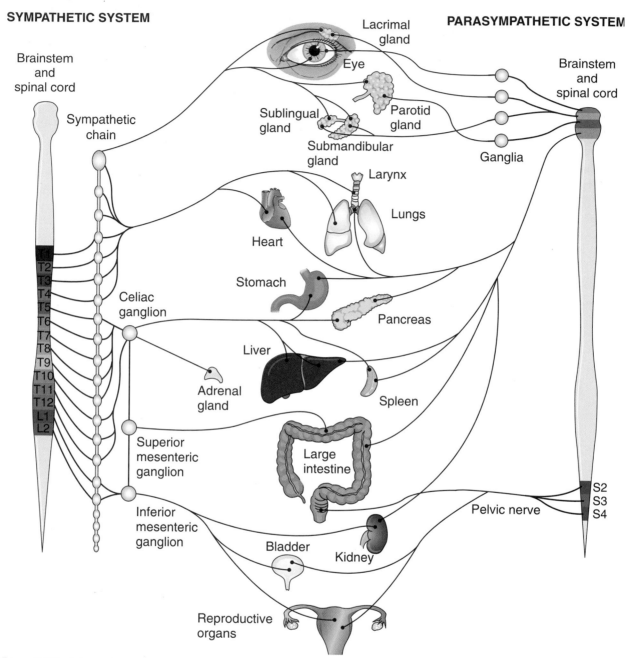

FIGURE **8•10**   Autonomic nervous system (only one side is shown for each division).

The sensory neurons in this system are grouped with those that come from the skin and voluntary muscles. In contrast, the *efferent* neurons, which supply the glands and the involuntary muscles, are arranged in a distinct pattern, which has led to their separation for study purposes into *sympathetic* and *parasympathetic* divisions (Fig. 8-10).

All autonomic pathways contain two motor neurons connecting the spinal cord with the effector organ. The two neurons synapse in ganglia that serve as relay stations along the way. The first neuron, the ***preganglionic neuron,*** extends from the spinal cord to the ganglion. The second neuron, the ***postganglionic neuron,*** travels from the ganglion to the effector. This differs from the voluntary (somatic) nervous system, in which each motor nerve fiber extends all the way from the spinal cord to the skeletal muscle with no intervening synapse. Some of the autonomic fibers are within the spinal nerves; some are within the cranial nerves (see Chap. 9).

✔ CHECKPOINT **13**:

How many neurons are there in each motor pathway of the ANS?

Divisions of the Autonomic Nervous System

The characteristics of the two divisions of the ANS are described below. The information is summarized in Table 8-2.

Sympathetic Nervous System
The sympathetic motor neurons originate in the spinal cord with cell bodies in the thoracic and lumbar regions, the ***thoracolumbar*** (tho-rah-ko-LUM-bar) area. These fibers arise from the spinal cord at the level of the first thoracic nerve down to the level of the second lumbar spinal nerve. From this part of the cord, nerve fibers extend to ganglia where they synapse with second neurons, the fibers of which extend to the glands and involuntary muscle tissues.

Many of the sympathetic ganglia form the ***sympathetic chains,*** two cordlike strands of ganglia that extend along either side of the spinal column from the lower neck to the upper abdominal region.

In addition, the nerves that supply the organs of the abdominal and pelvic cavities synapse in three single ***collateral ganglia*** farther from the spinal cord.

The postganglionic neurons of the sympathetic system, with few exceptions, act on their effectors by releasing the neurotransmitter epinephrine (adrenaline) and the related compound norepinephrine (noradrenaline). This system is therefore described as ***adrenergic,*** which means "activated by adrenaline."

Parasympathetic Nervous System
The parasympathetic motor pathways begin in the ***craniosacral*** (kra-ne-o-SAK-ral) areas, with fibers arising from cell bodies in the brainstem (midbrain and medulla) and the lower (sacral) part of the spinal cord. From these centers, the first fibers extend to autonomic ganglia that are usually located near or within the walls of the effector organs and are called ***terminal ganglia.*** The pathways then continue along postganglionic neurons that stimulate the involuntary tissues.

The neurons of the parasympathetic system release the neurotransmitter acetylcholine, leading to the description of this system as ***cholinergic*** (activated by acetylcholine).

Functions of the Autonomic Nervous System

Most organs are supplied by both sympathetic and parasympathetic fibers, and the two systems generally have opposite effects. The sympathetic part of the ANS tends to act as an accelerator for those organs needed to meet a stressful situation. It promotes what is called the ***fight-or-flight response*** because in the most primitive terms, the person must decide to

Table 8•2 Divisions of the Autonomic Nervous System		
DIVISION	SYMPATHETIC NERVOUS SYSTEM	PARASYMPATHETIC NERVOUS SYSTEM
Origin of fibers	Thoracic and lumbar regions of the spinal cord; thoracolumbar	Brain stem and sacral regions of the spinal cord; craniosacral
Location of ganglia	Sympathetic chain and three single collateral ganglia	Terminal ganglia in or near the effector organ
Neurotransmitter	Adrenaline and noradrenaline; adrenergic	Acetylcholine; cholinergic
Effects (see Table 8-3)	Response to stress; fight-or-flight response	Reverses stress response; stimulates some activities

8

Table 8•3 Effects of the Sympathetic and Parasympathetic Systems on Selected Drugs		
EFFECTOR	SYMPATHETIC SYSTEM	PARASYMPATHETIC SYSTEM
Pupils of eye	Dilation	Constriction
Sweat glands	Stimulation	None
Digestive glands	Inhibition	Stimulation
Heart	Increased rate and strength of beat	Decreased rate and strength of beat
Bronchi of lungs	Dilation	Constriction
Muscles of digestive system	Decreased contraction (peristalsis)	Increased contraction
Kidneys	Decreased activity	None
Urinary bladder	Relaxation	Contraction and emptying
Liver	Increased release of glucose	None
Penis	Ejaculation	Erection
Adrenal medulla	Stimulation	None
Blood vessels to		
Skeletal muscles	Dilation	Constriction
Skin	Constriction	None
Respiratory system	Dilation	Constriction
Digestive organs	Constriction	Dilation

stay and "fight it out" with the enemy or to run away from danger. If you think of what happens to a person who is frightened or angry, you can easily remember the effects of impulses from the sympathetic nervous system:

- Increase in the rate and force of heart contractions
- Increase in blood pressure due partly to the more effective heartbeat and partly to constriction of small arteries in the skin and the internal organs
- Dilation of blood vessels to skeletal muscles, bringing more blood to these tissues
- Dilation of the bronchial tubes to allow more oxygen to enter
- Stimulation of the central portion of the adrenal gland. This produces hormones, including epinephrine, that prepare the body to meet emergency situations in many ways (see Chap. 11). The sympathetic nerves and hormones from the adrenal gland reinforce each other
- Increase in metabolism
- Dilation of the pupil and decrease in focusing ability (for near objects)

The sympathetic system also acts as a brake on those systems not directly involved in the re-

sponse to stress, such as the urinary and digestive systems. If you try to eat while you are angry, you may note that your saliva is thick and so small in amount that you can swallow only with difficulty. Under these circumstances, when food does reach the stomach, it seems to stay there longer than usual.

The parasympathetic part of the ANS normally acts as a balance for the sympathetic system once a crisis has passed. The parasympathetic system brings about constriction of the pupils, slowing of the heart rate, and constriction of the bronchial tubes. It also stimulates the formation and release of urine and activity of the digestive tract. Saliva, for example, flows more easily and profusely, and its quantity and fluidity increase.

Most organs of the body receive both sympathetic and parasympathetic stimulation, the effects of the two systems on a given organ generally being opposite. Table 8-3 shows some of the actions of these two systems.

✔ CHECKPOINT **14**:

Which division of the ANS stimulates a stress response, and which division reverses the stress response?

Summary

I. The nervous system as a whole
A. Structural divisions—anatomic
1. Central nervous system (CNS)—brain and spinal cord
2. Peripheral nervous system (PNS)—spinal and cranial nerves
B. Functional divisions—physiologic
1. Somatic nervous system—voluntary; supplies skeletal muscles
2. Autonomic (visceral) nervous system—involuntary; supplies smooth muscle, cardiac muscle, glands
C. Neuroglia
1. Nonconducting cells
2. Protect and support nervous tissue

II. Neurons and their functions
A. Structure of a neuron
1. Cell body
2. Cell fibers
a. Dendrite—carries impulses to cell body
b. Axon—carries impulses away from cell body
3. Myelin sheath
a. Covers and protects some axons
b. Speeds conduction
c. Made by Schwann cells in PNS; neuroglia in CNS
d. Neurilemma—outermost layer of Schwann cell; aids axon repair
e. White matter—myelinated tissue; gray matter—unmyelinated tissue
B. Types of neurons
1. Sensory (afferent)—carry impulses toward CNS
2. Motor (efferent)—carry impulses away from CNS
C. Nerves and tracts—bundles of neuron fibers
1. Nerve—in peripheral nervous system
a. Sensory (afferent) nerve—con-tains only fibers that carry impulses toward the CNS (from a receptor)
b. Motor (efferent) nerve—contains only fibers that carry impulses away from the CNS (to an effector)
c. Mixed nerve—contains both sensory and motor fibers
2. Tract—in central nervous system

III. The nervous system at work
A. Nerve impulse (action potential)—electric current that spreads along nerve fiber
B. Synapse—junction between neurons where a nerve impulse is transmitted from one neuron to the next
1. Neurotransmitter—carries impulse across synapse
2. Receptors—in postsynaptic membrane; pick up neurotransmitters
3. Neurotransmitter removed by diffusion, enzyme destruction, return to presynaptic cell
C. Reflex arc—pathway through the nervous system
1. Receptor—detects stimulus
2. Sensory neuron—receptor to CNS
3. Central neuron—in CNS
4. Motor neuron—CNS to effector
5. Effector—muscle or gland that responds

IV. Spinal cord
A. Location of the spinal cord—in vertebral column; ends between first and second lumbar vertebrae
B. Structure of the spinal cord—H-shaped area of gray matter surrounded by white matter
C. Functions of the spinal cord
1. Links spinal nerves to brain
2. Reflex activities
a. Reflex—simple, rapid, automatic response using few neurons
b. Examples—stretch reflex, eye blink, withdrawal reflex
c. Spinal reflex—coordinated in spinal cord

V. Spinal nerves—31 pairs
  A. Location and structure of the spinal nerves
    1. Roots
      a. Sensory (dorsal)
      b. Motor (ventral)
  B. Branches of the spinal nerves—plexuses: networks formed by anterior branches
    1. Cervical plexus
    2. Brachial plexus
    3. Lumbosacral plexus

VI. Autonomic nervous system—motor (efferent) division of the visceral (involuntary) nervous system
  A. Characteristics of the autonomic nervous system
    1. Involuntary
    2. Controls glands, smooth muscle, heart (cardiac) muscle
  B. Divisions of the autonomic nervous system
    1. Sympathetic nervous system
      a. Thoracolumbar
      b. Adrenergic—uses adrenaline
    2. Parasympathetic system
      a. Craniosacral
      b. Cholinergic—uses acetylcholine
  C. Functions of the autonomic nervous system
    1. Sympathetic—stimulates fight-or-flight (stress) response
    2. Parasympathetic—returns body to normal
    3. Usually have opposite effects on an organ

Questions for Study and Review

1. What is the main function of the nervous system?
2. Name the two structural divisions of the nervous system.
3. Name the organs or structures controlled by the somatic nervous system; by the visceral nervous system.
4. Define the following terms: *neuron, myelin, synapse, ganglion, Schwann cell.*
5. What are neuroglia? Give some examples of their functions.
6. Differentiate between the terms in each of the following pairs:
   a. *axon* and *dendrite*
   b. *gray matter* and *white matter*
   c. *receptor* and *effector*
   d. *afferent* and *efferent*
   e. *sensory* and *motor*
   f. *nerve* and *tract*
7. Without the label, how would you know that the neuron in Figure 8-2 is a motor neuron? Is this neuron a part of the somatic or visceral nervous system?
8. What is a mixed nerve? Give several examples.
9. Describe a nerve impulse. How does conduction along a myelinated fiber differ from conduction along an unmyelinated fiber?
10. What is a synapse? Briefly describe what occurs at a synapse.
11. What are neurotransmitters? Give several examples of neurotransmitters.
12. Name the components of a reflex arc.
13. Locate and describe the spinal cord. Name two of its functions.
14. Describe a reflex. Give several examples of reflexes.
15. Define a spinal nerve. How many pairs of spinal nerves are there?
16. Differentiate between the dorsal and ventral roots of a spinal nerve.
17. Define a *plexus.* Name the three main plexuses of the spinal nerves.

18. What are the functions of the sympathetic part of the ANS, and how do these compare with those of the parasympathetic nervous system?

✔ Answers to Checkpoints

1. Structurally, the nervous system can be divided into a central and a peripheral nervous system.
2. The somatic nervous system is voluntary and controls skeletal muscle; the autonomic (visceral) nervous system is involuntary and controls involuntary muscles and glands.
3. The nonconducting cells of the nervous system that serve in protection and support are the neuroglia (glial cells).
4. The fiber of the neuron that carries impulses toward the cell body is the dendrite; the fiber that carries impulses away from the cell body is the axon.
5. Myelinated fibers are white, and unmyelinated tissues are gray.
6. Nerves that convey impulses toward the CNS are sensory (afferent) nerves; nerves that convey impulses away from the CNS are motor (efferent) nerves.
7. In the first stage of an action potential, the charge on the membrane reverses and the membrane is described as being depolarized. In the second stage of an action potential, the membrane returns to the resting state and is described as repolarized.
8. All the chemicals used to carry information across the synaptic cleft are neurotransmitters.
9. A reflex arc is a pathway through the nervous system from a stimulus to an effector.
10. In the spinal cord, an H-shaped section of gray matter is located internally, and the white matter is located around it. The gray matter extends in two pairs of columns called dorsal and ventral horns.
11. The spinal cord links the spinal nerves to the brain and coordinates reflexes.
12. There are 31 pairs of spinal nerves.
13. There are two neurons in each motor pathway of the autonomic nervous system.
14. The sympathetic system stimulates a stress response, and the parasympathetic system reverses it.

8

The Nervous System: The Brain and Cranial Nerves

SELECTED KEY TERMS

The following terms are defined in the Glossary:

brain stem
cerebellum
cerebral cortex
cerebrospinal fluid
cerebrum
diencephalon
hypothalamus
medulla oblongata
meninges
midbrain
pons
thalamus
ventricle

BEHAVIORAL OBJECTIVES

After careful study of this chapter, you should be able to:

1. Give the location and functions of the four main divisions of the brain
2. Name and locate the three subdivisions of the brain stem
3. Name and describe the three meninges
4. Cite the function of cerebrospinal fluid and describe where and how this fluid is formed
5. Cite one function of the cerebral cortex in each lobe of the cerebrum
6. Cite the names and functions of the 12 cranial nerves
7. Describe several methods used to image the brain

THE BRAIN AND ITS PROTECTIVE STRUCTURES

Main Parts of the Brain

The brain occupies the cranial cavity and is covered by membranes, fluid, and the bones of the skull. Although the various regions of the brain are in communication and function together, the brain may be divided into distinct areas for ease of study (Fig. 9-1):

- The *cerebrum* (SER-e-brum) is the largest part of the brain. It is divided into right and left *cerebral* (SER-e-bral) *hemispheres* by a deep groove called the *longitudinal fissure*.
- The *diencephalon* (di-en-SEF-ah-lon) is the area between the cerebral hemispheres and the brain stem. It includes the thalamus and the hypothalamus.
- The *brain stem* connects the cerebrum and diencephalon with the spinal cord. The upper portion of the brain stem is the *midbrain*. Below that, and plainly visible from the inferior view of the brain, are the *pons* (ponz) and the *medulla oblongata* (meh-DUL-lah ob-long-GAH-tah). The pons connects the midbrain with the medulla, whereas the medulla connects the brain with the spinal cord through a large opening in the base of the skull (foramen magnum).
- The *cerebellum* (ser-eh-BEL-um) is located immediately below the back part of the cerebral hemispheres and is connected with the cerebrum, brain stem, and spinal cord by means of the pons. The word *cerebellum* means "little brain."

Each of these divisions is described in greater detail later in this chapter.

✔ CHECKPOINT **1**:

What are the main divisions of the brain?

Coverings of the Brain and Spinal Cord

The *meninges* (men-IN-jez) are three layers of connective tissue that surround both the brain and spinal cord to form a complete enclosure. The outermost of these membranes, the *dura mater* (DU-rah MA-ter), is the thickest and toughest of the meninges. (*Mater* is from the Latin meaning "mother," referring to the protective function of the meninges; *dura* means "hard"). Inside the skull, the dura mater splits in certain places to provide venous channels,

9

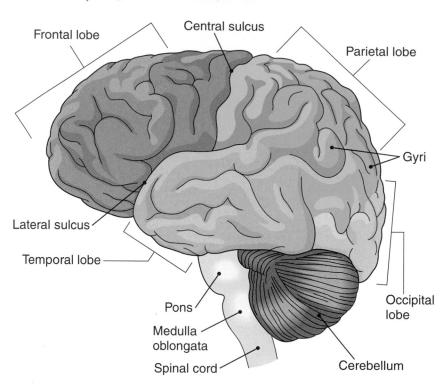

Frontal lobe

Central sulcus

Parietal lobe

Gyri

Lateral sulcus

Temporal lobe

Pons

Medulla oblongata

Spinal cord

Occipital lobe

Cerebellum

FIGURE **9•1** External surface of the brain showing the main parts and some of the lobes and sulci of the cerebrum.

called **dural sinuses,** for the drainage of blood coming from the brain tissue.

The middle layer of the meninges is the **arachnoid** (ah-RAK-noyd). This membrane is loosely attached to the deepest of the meninges by weblike fibers, allowing a space for the movement of cerebrospinal fluid (CSF) between the two membranes. (*Arachnoid* is from the Latin word for spider because of its weblike appearance).

The innermost layer around the brain, the **pia mater** (PI-ah MA-ter), is attached to the nervous tissue of the brain and spinal cord and follows all the contours of these structures (Fig. 9-2). It is made of a delicate connective tissue in which there are many blood vessels (*pia* meaning "tender" or "soft"). The blood supply to the brain is carried, to a large extent, by the pia mater.

> ✔ CHECKPOINT **2**:
>
> The meninges are protective membranes around the brain and spinal cord. What are the names of the three layers of the meninges from the outermost to the innermost?

Cerebrospinal Fluid

Cerebrospinal (ser-e-bro-SPI-nal) **fluid** is a clear liquid that circulates in and around the brain and spinal cord (Fig. 9-3). The function of the CSF is to support nervous tissue and to cushion shocks that would otherwise injure these delicate structures. This fluid also carries nutrients to the cells and transports waste products from the cells.

CSF flows freely through the brain and spinal cord and finally flows out into the subarachnoid space of the meninges. Much of the fluid is then returned to the blood through projections called *arachnoid villi* in the dural sinuses.

Ventricles

CSF is formed in four spaces within the brain called **ventricles** (VEN-trih-klz) (Fig. 9-4). A vascular network in each ventricle, the **choroid** (KOR-oyd) **plexus,** forms CSF by filtration of the blood and by cellular secretion.

The four ventricles that produce CSF extend somewhat irregularly into the various parts of the brain. The largest are the lateral ventricles in the two cerebral hemispheres. Their exten-

Figure **9•2** Frontal (coronal) section of the top of the head showing meninges and related parts.

sions into the lobes of the cerebrum are called *horns.* These paired ventricles communicate with a midline space, the third ventricle, by means of openings called *foramina* (fo-RAM-in-ah). The third ventricle is surrounded by the diencephalon. Continuing down from the third ventricle, a small canal, called the *cerebral aqueduct,* extends through the midbrain into the fourth ventricle, which is located between the brain stem and the cerebellum. This ventricle is continuous with the central canal of the spinal cord. In the roof of the fourth ventricle are three openings that allow the escape of CSF to the area that surrounds the brain and spinal cord.

✔ CHECKPOINT **3:**

In addition to the meninges, CSF helps to support and protect the brain and spinal cord. Where is CSF produced?

DIVISIONS OF THE BRAIN
Cerebral Hemispheres

Each cerebral hemisphere is divided into four visible *lobes* named for the overlying cranial bones. These are the frontal, parietal, temporal, and occipital lobes (see Fig. 9-1). In addition, there is a small fifth lobe deep within each hemisphere that cannot be seen from the surface. Not much is known about this lobe, which is called the *insula.*

The outer nervous tissue of the cerebral hemispheres is gray matter that makes up the *cerebral cortex.* This thin layer of gray matter is the most highly evolved portion of the brain and is responsible for conscious thought, reasoning, and abstract mental functions. Specific functions are localized in the cortex of the different lobes, as described in greater detail later.

The cortex is arranged in folds forming elevated portions known as *gyri* (JI-ri), which are

9

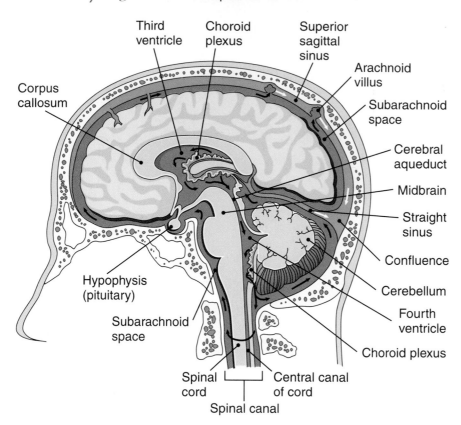

FIGURE **9•3** Flow of CSF from choroid plexuses back to the blood in dural sinuses is shown by the black arrows; flow of blood is shown by the white arrows.

separated by shallow grooves called *sulci* (SUL-si) (see Fig. 9-1). Although there are many sulci, the following two are especially important landmarks:

- The *central sulcus,* which lies between the frontal and parietal lobes of each hemisphere at right angles to the longitudinal fissure
- The *lateral sulcus,* which curves along the side of each hemisphere and separates the temporal lobe from the frontal and parietal lobes (see Fig. 9-1)

Internally, the cerebral hemispheres are made largely of white matter and a few islands of gray matter. The white matter consists of myelinated fibers that connect the cortical areas with each other and with other parts of the nervous system.

An important band of white matter is the *corpus callosum* located at the bottom of the longitudinal fissure (see Fig. 9-3). This band acts as a bridge between the right and left hemispheres, permitting impulses to cross from one side of the brain to the other.

The *internal capsule* is a crowded strip of white matter composed of many myelinated fibers (forming tracts).

Basal ganglia are masses of gray matter located deep within each cerebral hemisphere. These groups of neurons help regulate body movement and facial expressions communicated from the cerebral cortex. The neurotransmitter *dopamine* (DO-pah-mene) is secreted by the neurons of the basal ganglia.

Functions of the Cerebral Cortex

It is within the cerebral cortex, the layer of gray matter that forms the surface of each cerebral hemisphere, that impulses are received and analyzed. These activities form the basis of knowledge. The brain "stores" information, much of which can be recalled on demand by means of the phenomenon called *memory*. It is in the cerebral cortex that thought processes such as association, judgment, and discrimination take

A

B

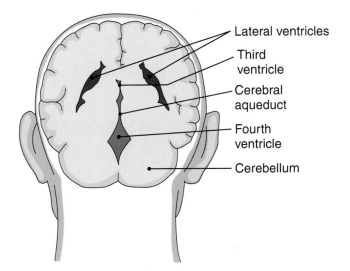

FIGURE **9•4** Ventricles of the brain seen from three views. **(A)** superior. **(B)** Lateral. **(C)** Posterior.

C

place. Conscious deliberation and voluntary actions also arise from the cerebral cortex.

Although the various areas of the brain act in coordination to produce behavior, particular functions are localized in the cortex of each lobe. Some of these are described below:

- The *frontal lobe,* which is relatively larger in humans than in any other organism, lies in front of the central sulcus. This lobe contains the motor area, which directs movement (Fig. 9-5). Because of the way in which motor fibers cross to opposite sides in the central nervous system, the left side of the brain governs the right side of the body, and the right side of the brain governs the left side of the body. The frontal lobe also contains two areas important in speech (the speech centers are discussed later).
- The *parietal lobe* occupies the upper part of each hemisphere and lies just behind the central sulcus. This lobe contains the *sensory area,* in which impulses from the skin, such as touch, pain, and temperature, are interpreted. The estimation of distances, sizes, and shapes also take place here.
- The *temporal lobe* lies below the lateral sulcus and folds under the hemisphere on each side. This lobe contains the *auditory area* for receiving and interpreting impulses from the ear. The *olfactory area,* concerned with the sense of smell, is located in the medial part of the temporal lobe; it is stimulated by impulses arising from receptors in the nose.
- The *occipital lobe* lies behind the parietal lobe and extends over the cerebellum. This lobe contains the *visual area* for interpreting impulses arising from the retina of the eye.

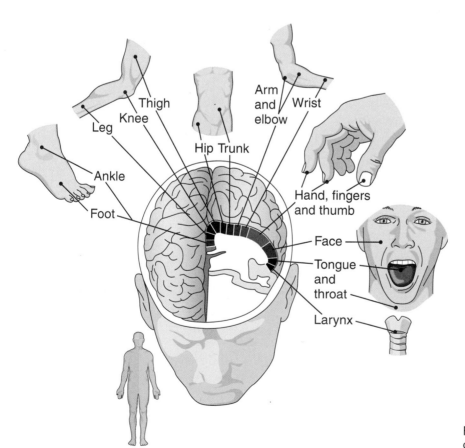

FIGURE **9•5** Motor areas of the cerebral cortex (frontal lobe).

> ✔ CHECKPOINT **4**:
>
> Higher functions of the brain occur in a thin layer of gray matter on the surface of the cerebral hemispheres. What is the name of this outer layer of gray matter?

Communication Areas

The ability to communicate by written and verbal means is an interesting example of the way in which areas of the cerebral cortex are interrelated (Fig. 9-6). The development and use of these areas are closely connected with the process of learning.

- The ***auditory areas*** are located in the temporal lobe. In one of these areas, sound impulses transmitted from the environment are detected, whereas in the surrounding area (auditory association area), the sounds are interpreted and understood. The beginnings of language are learned by auditory means; thus, the auditory area for understanding sounds is near the auditory

receiving area of the cortex. Babies often appear to understand what is being said long before they do any talking themselves. It is usually several years before children learn to read or write words.

- The ***motor areas*** for communication by speech and writing are located in front of the lowest part of the motor cortex in the frontal lobe. Because the lower part of the motor cortex controls the muscles of the head and neck, it seems logical to think of the motor speech center as an extension forward in this area. The muscles of speech (in the tongue, the soft palate, and the larynx) are controlled here, in a region named ***Broca's*** (bro-KAHZ) ***area***, after its discoverer. A person who suffers damage to this area, as by a stroke, may have difficulty in producing speech (motor aphasia). Similarly, the written speech center is located in front of the cortical area that controls the muscles of the arm and hand. The ability to write words is usually one of the last phases in the development of learning words and their meanings.

- The ***visual areas*** of the cortex in the oc-

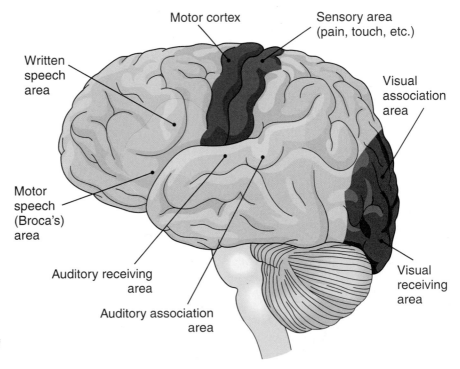

FIGURE **9•6** Functional areas of the cerebral cortex.

Motor cortex
Sensory area (pain, touch, etc.)
Written speech area
Visual association area
Motor speech (Broca's) area
Auditory receiving area
Auditory association area
Visual receiving area

cipital lobe are also involved in communication. Here, visual images of language are received. These visual impulses are then interpreted as words in the visual area that lies in front of the receiving cortex. The ability to read with understanding is also developed in this area. You might *see* writing in the Japanese language, for example, but this would involve only the visual receiving area in the occipital lobe unless you could also *read* the words.

There is a functional relation among areas of the brain. Many neurons must work together to enable a person to receive, interpret, and respond to verbal and written messages as well as to touch (tactile stimulus) and other sensory stimuli.

Memory and the Learning Process

Memory is the mental faculty for recalling ideas. In the initial stage of the memory process, sensory signals (*e.g.,* visual, auditory) are retained for a very short time, perhaps only fractions of a second. Nevertheless, they can be used for further processing. **Short-term memory** refers to the retention of bits of information for a few seconds or perhaps a few minutes, after which the information is lost unless reinforced. **Long-term memory** refers to the storage of information that can be recalled at a later time. There is a tendency for a memory to become more fixed the more often a person repeats the remembered experience; thus, short-term memory signals can lead to long-term memories. Furthermore, the more often a memory is recalled, the more indelible it becomes; such a memory can be so deeply fixed in the brain that it can be recalled immediately.

Careful anatomic studies have shown that tiny extensions called *fibrils* form at the synapses in the cerebral cortex, so that impulses can travel more easily from one neuron to another. The number of these fibrils increases with age. Physiologic studies show that rehearsal (repetition) of the same information again and again accelerates and potentiates the degree of transfer of short-term memory into long-term memory. A person who is wide awake memorizes far better than does a person who is in a state of mental fatigue. It has also been noted that the brain is able to organize information so that new ideas are stored in the same areas in which similar ones had been stored before.

To learn about preventing damage to the brain and loss of memory, read about preventing concussion in Watch Your Head!

Watch Your Head!

Closed head injury (CHI) is the leading cause of death due to neurologic illness or injury for people under 50 years of age. Damage to brain tissues occurs either from penetrating trauma of the head or from acceleration–deceleration events where a head in motion suddenly comes to a stop. Nervous tissue, blood vessels, and possibly the meninges may be bruised, torn, lacerated, or ruptured. Depending upon the degree and type of tissue damage, the patient may be said to have suffered a concussion, cerebral contusion, or cerebral laceration along with edema. Recovery from a concussion is usually complete, with no long-standing effects. However, recovery from a significant contusion or a laceration with edema is a serious challenge. Mortality rates in these more severe injuries approach 50%; treatment is usually supportive in nature and may do little to change the outcome. The most unfortunate fact regarding CHIs is that they are largely preventable.

Any head injury may be lessened, if not prevented, by taking a few precautions.

- Whenever riding in a moving vehicle, wear both the lap and shoulder belts, and adjust the headrest to sit directly behind the back of your skull.
- Whenever you participate in outside sports or activities, wear a safety helmet. Young children are especially vulnerable since their skulls may not be completely fused and calcified at the time of injury.
- Children should never be swung around to play "airplane" nor should they ever be vigorously bounced or shaken.

Although treatment of CHIs has advanced in recent years, prevention is still the best weapon we have against these potentially serious and fatal injuries.

The Diencephalon

The *diencephalon,* or interbrain, is located between the cerebral hemispheres and the brain stem. It can be seen by cutting into the central section of the brain. The *thalamus* (THAL-ah-mus) and the *hypothalamus* are included in the diencephalon (Fig. 9-7).

The two parts of the thalamus form the lateral walls of the third ventricle. Nearly all sensory impulses travel through the masses of gray matter that form the thalamus. The role of the thalamus is to sort out the impulses and direct them to particular areas of the cerebral cortex.

The hypothalamus is located in the midline area below the thalamus and forms the floor of the third ventricle. It helps to maintain homeostasis by controlling body temperature, water balance, sleep, appetite, and some emotions, such as fear and pleasure. Both the sympathetic and parasympathetic divisions of the autonomic nervous system are under the control of the hypothalamus, as is the pituitary gland. The hypothalamus thus influences the heartbeat, the contraction and relaxation of the walls of blood vessels, hormone secretion, and other vital body functions.

✔ CHECKPOINT **5**:

What are the two main portions of the diencephalon and what do they do?

To learn more about the function of sleep, see Sleep.

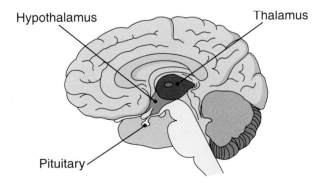

FIGURE **9•7** Diagram showing the relationship among the thalamus, hypothalamus, and pituitary (hypophysis).

Sleep

Although everybody does it, there are still many mysteries about how, why, and when we sleep. Study of brain waves with the electroencephalograph has shown that sleep occurs in two phases. One of these, rapid-eye-movement (REM) sleep, is associated with dreaming.

As we descend from drowsiness into deep sleep, we progress through a non–rapid-eye-movement (NREM) phase. Although all the triggers for falling asleep are not known, a major factor is the amount of light received through the eyes. This signals the hypothalamus to regulate sleep–wake cycles. About 1 to 1½ hours after falling asleep, short periods of REM sleep with dreaming occur. These then alternate with NREM sleep at intervals of about 90 minutes. Extreme fatigue and sedatives decrease the amount of REM sleep in favor of deep NREM sleep. Also, infants have a much greater percentage of REM sleep; this declines with age.

Sleep rests the body, improves learning, and strengthens the immune system. There is also evidence that REM sleep helps the brain to sort memories.

The Limbic System

Along the border between the cerebrum and the diencephalon is a region known as the *limbic system.* This system is involved in emotional states and behavior. It includes the *hippocampus* (shaped like a sea horse), located under the lateral ventricles, which functions in learning and the formation of long-term memory. It also includes regions that stimulate the *reticular formation,* a network that extends along the brain stem and governs wakefulness and sleep. The limbic system thus links the conscious functions of the cerebral cortex and the automatic functions of the brain stem.

The Brain Stem

The brain stem is composed of the midbrain, the pons, and the medulla oblongata. These structures connect the cerebrum and diencephalon with the spinal cord.

The Midbrain

The **midbrain,** located below the center of the cerebrum, forms the forward part of the brain stem. Four rounded masses of gray matter that are hidden by the cerebral hemispheres form the upper part of the midbrain; these four bodies act as relay centers for certain eye and ear reflexes. The white matter at the front of the midbrain conducts impulses between the higher centers of the cerebrum and the lower centers of the pons, medulla, cerebellum, and spinal cord. Cranial nerves III and IV originate from the midbrain.

The Pons

The **pons** lies between the midbrain and the medulla, in front of the cerebellum (see Fig. 9-1). It is composed largely of myelinated nerve fibers, which serve to connect the two halves of the cerebellum with the brain stem as well as with the cerebrum above and the spinal cord below.

The pons is an important connecting link between the cerebellum and the rest of the nervous system, and it contains nerve fibers that carry impulses to and from the centers located above and below it. Certain reflex (involuntary) actions, such as some of those regulating respiration, are integrated in the pons. Cranial nerves V through VIII originate from the pons.

The Medulla Oblongata

The **medulla oblongata** of the brain is located between the pons and the spinal cord (see Fig. 9-1). It appears white externally because, like the pons, it contains many myelinated nerve fibers. Internally, it contains collections of cell bodies (gray matter) called **nuclei,** or *centers.* Among these are vital centers, such as the following:

- The **respiratory center** controls the muscles of respiration in response to chemical and other stimuli.
- The **cardiac center** helps regulate the rate and force of the heartbeat.
- The **vasomotor** (vas-o-MO-tor) **center** regulates the contraction of smooth muscle in the blood vessel walls and thus controls blood flow and blood pressure.

The ascending sensory fibers that carry messages through the spinal cord up to the brain travel through the medulla, as do descending motor fibers. These groups of fibers form tracts (bundles) and are grouped together according to function.

The motor fibers from the motor cortex of the cerebral hemispheres extend down through the medulla, and most of them cross from one side to the other (decussate) while going through this part of the brain. It is the crossing of motor fibers in the medulla that causes the right cerebral hemisphere to control muscles in the left side of the body and the left cerebral hemisphere to control muscles in the right side of the body, a characteristic termed *contralateral* (opposite side) *control.*

The medulla is an important reflex center; here, certain neurons end, and impulses are relayed to other neurons. The last four pairs of cranial nerves (IX through XII) are connected with the medulla.

> ✔ CHECKPOINT **6**:
>
> What are the three subdivisions of the brain stem?

The Cerebellum

The **cerebellum** is made up of three parts: the middle portion (vermis) and two lateral hemispheres. Like the cerebral hemispheres, the cerebellum has an outer area of gray matter and an inner portion that is largely white matter. The functions of the cerebellum are as follows:

- To aid in the **coordination of voluntary muscles** so that they will function smoothly and in an orderly fashion. Disease of the cerebellum causes muscular jerkiness and tremors.
- To aid in the **maintenance of balance** in standing, walking, and sitting as well as during more strenuous activities. Messages from the internal ear and from sensory receptors in tendons and muscles aid the cerebellum.

- To aid in the ***maintenance of muscle tone*** so that all muscle fibers are slightly tensed and ready to produce necessary changes in position as quickly as may be necessary.

✔ CHECKPOINT **7**:

What are some functions of the cerebellum?

BRAIN STUDIES

Imaging the Brain

A major tool for clinical study of the brain is the ***CT*** (computed tomography) ***scan,*** which provides multiple x-ray pictures taken from different angles simultaneously. By means of a computer, the information is organized and displayed as photographs of the bone, soft tissue, and cavities of the brain (Fig. 9-8). Anatomic lesions, such as tumors or scar tissue accumulations, are readily seen.

MRI (magnetic resonance imaging) gives even clearer pictures of the brain without the use of dyes or x-rays. The method is based on computerized interpretation of the movements of atomic nuclei following their exposure to radio waves within a powerful magnetic field. Although MRI is more expensive and takes longer than CT imaging, it gives more views of the brain and may reveal tumors, scar tissue, and hemorrhaging not shown by CT.

With ***PET*** (positron emission tomography) one can actually visualize the brain in action. With this method, a radioactively labeled substance (*e.g.,* glucose) is followed as it moves through the brain. As tasks are performed, regions of the cortex that are involved become "hot."

The Electroencephalograph

The interactions of the billions of nerve cells in the brain give rise to measurable electric currents. These may be recorded by an instrument called the ***electroencephalograph*** (e-lek-tro-en-SEF-ah-lo-graf). The recorded tracings or brain waves produce an electroencephalogram (EEG).

FIGURE **9•8** CT scanner. (Photograph courtesy of Philips Medical Systems)

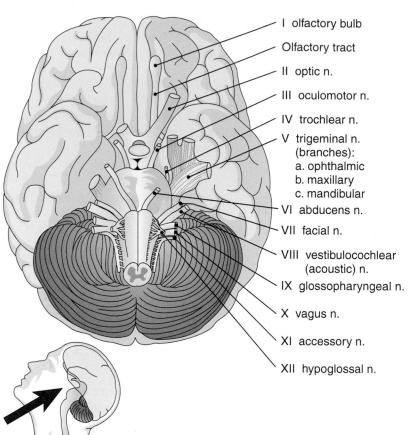

I olfactory bulb

Olfactory tract

II optic n.

III oculomotor n.

IV trochlear n.

V trigeminal n.
(branches):
a. ophthalmic
b. maxillary
c. mandibular

VI abducens n.

VII facial n.

VIII vestibulocochlear
(acoustic) n.

IX glossopharyngeal n.

X vagus n.

XI accessory n.

XII hypoglossal n.

FIGURE **9•9** Base of the brain showing cranial nerves.

CRANIAL NERVES

Location of the Cranial Nerves

There are 12 pairs of cranial nerves (in this discussion, when a cranial nerve is identified, a pair is meant). They are numbered, usually in Roman numerals, according to their connection with the brain, beginning at the front and proceeding back (Fig. 9-9). Except for the first two pairs, all the cranial nerves arise from the brain stem. The first 9 pairs and the 12th pair supply structures in the head.

General Functions of the Cranial Nerves

From a functional point of view, we may think of the kinds of messages the cranial nerves handle as belonging to one of four categories:

- ***Special sensory impulses,*** such as those for smell, taste, vision, and hearing
- ***General sensory impulses,*** such as those for pain, touch, temperature, deep muscle sense, pressure, and vibrations
- ***Somatic motor impulses*** resulting in voluntary control of skeletal muscles
- ***Visceral motor impulses*** producing involuntary control of glands and involuntary muscles (cardiac muscle and smooth muscle). These motor pathways are part of the autonomic nervous system, parasympathetic division.

Names and Functions of the Cranial Nerves

A few of the cranial nerves (I, II, and VIII) contain only sensory fibers; some (III, IV, VI, XI, and XII) contain all or mostly motor fibers. The remainder (V, VII, IX, and X) contain both sensory and motor fibers; they are known as *mixed nerves*. All 12 nerves are listed below:

I. The *olfactory nerve* carries smell impulses from receptors in the nasal mucosa to the brain.

II. The *optic nerve* carries visual impulses from the eye to the brain.

III. The *oculomotor nerve* is concerned with the contraction of most of the eye muscles.

IV. The *trochlear* (TROK-le-ar) *nerve* supplies one eyeball muscle.

V. The *trigeminal* (tri-JEM-in-al) *nerve* is the great sensory nerve of the face and head. It has three branches that transport general sense impulses (*e.g.,* pain, touch, temperature) from the eye, the upper jaw, and the lower jaw. The third branch is joined by motor fibers to the muscles of mastication (chewing).

VI. The *abducens* (ab-DU-senz) *nerve* is another nerve sending controlling impulses to an eyeball muscle.

VII. The *facial nerve* is largely motor. The muscles of facial expression are all supplied by branches from the facial nerve. This nerve also includes special sensory fibers for taste (anterior two thirds of the tongue), and it contains secretory fibers to the smaller salivary glands (the submandibular and sublingual) and to the lacrimal (tear) gland.

VIII. The *vestibulocochlear* (ves-tib-u-lo-KOK-le-ar) *nerve* carries sensory impulses for hearing and for equilibrium from the inner ear. This nerve was formerly called the *auditory* or *acoustic nerve.*

IX. The *glossopharyngeal* (glos-o-fah-RIN-ge-al) *nerve* contains general sensory fibers from the back of the tongue and the pharynx (throat). This nerve also contains sensory fibers for taste from the posterior third of the tongue, secretory fibers that supply the largest salivary gland (parotid), and motor nerve fibers to control the swallowing muscles in the pharynx.

X. The *vagus* (VA-gus) *nerve* is the longest cranial nerve. (Its name means "wanderer.") It supplies most of the organs in the thoracic and abdominal cavities. This nerve also contains motor fibers to the larynx (voice box) and pharynx and to glands that produce digestive juices and other secretions.

XI. The *accessory nerve* (formerly called the *spinal accessory nerve*) is a motor nerve with two branches. One branch controls two muscles of the neck, the trapezius and sternocleidomastoid; the other supplies muscles of the larynx.

XII. The *hypoglossal nerve,* the last of the 12 cranial nerves, carries impulses controlling the muscles of the tongue.

✔ CHECKPOINT **8**: _____

How many pairs of cranial nerves are there?

✔ CHECKPOINT **9**: _____

The cranial nerves are classified as being sensory, motor, or mixed. What is a mixed nerve?

AGING OF THE NERVOUS SYSTEM

The nervous system is one of the first systems to develop in the embryo. By the beginning of the third week of development, the rudiments of the central nervous system have appeared.

Beginning with maturity, the nervous system begins to undergo changes. The brain begins to decrease in size and weight due to a loss of cells, especially in the cerebral cortex. These losses are accompanied by a decrease in synapses and in neurotransmitters. The speed of processing information decreases, and movements are slowed. Memory diminishes, especially for recent events. Changes in the vascular system throughout the body with a narrowing of the arteries (atherosclerosis) reduce blood flow to the brain. Degeneration of vessels increases the likelihood of stroke.

Despite this depressing news, the nervous system, like other body systems, has vast reserves. Changes vary from person to person in location and severity, and most elderly people are able to cope with life's demands.

Summary

I. **The brain and its protective structures**
   A. Main parts of the brain—cerebrum, diencephalon, brain stem, cerebellum
   B. Coverings of the brain and spinal cord
      1. Meninges
         a. Dura mater—tough outermost layer
         b. Arachnoid—weblike middle layer
         c. Pia mater—vascular innermost layer
      2. Meningitis—inflammation of the meninges
   C. Cerebrospinal fluid (CSF)
      1. Circulates around and within brain and spinal cord
      2. Cushions and protects
      3. Ventricles—four spaces within brain where CSF is produced
         a. Choroid plexus—vascular network in ventricle that produces CSF

II. **Divisions of the brain**
   A. Cerebral hemispheres
      1. Lobes—frontal, parietal, temporal, occipital, insula
      2. Cortex—outer layer of gray matter
         (a) Functions—interpretation, memory, conscious thought, judgment, voluntary actions
      3. Corpus callosum—connecting band of white matter
   B. Diencephalon—area between cerebral hemispheres and brain stem
      1. Thalamus—directs sensory impulses to cortex

      2. Hypothalamus—maintains homeostasis, controls pituitary
      3. Limbic system
         a. Contains parts of cerebrum and diencephalon
         b. Controls emotion and behavior
   C. Brain stem
      1. Midbrain—involved in eye and ear reflexes
      2. Pons—connecting link for other divisions
      3. Medulla oblongata
         a. Connects with spinal cord
         b. Contains vital centers for respiration, heart rate, vasomotor activity
   D. The cerebellum—regulates coordination, balance, muscle tone

III. **Brain studies**
   A. Imaging the brain
      1. Computed tomography (CT)
      2. Magnetic resonance imaging (MRI)
      3. Positron emission tomography (PET)
   B. Electroencephalograph (EEG)

IV. **Cranial nerves**—12 pairs
   A. Location of the cranial nerves
   B. General functions of the cranial nerves
      1. Carry special and general sensory impulses
      2. Carry somatic and visceral motor impulses
   C. Names and functions of the cranial nerves
      1. Sensory (I, II, VIII)
      2. Motor (III, IV, VI, XI, XII)
      3. Mixed (V, VII, IX, X)

V. **Aging of the nervous system**

Questions for Study and Review

1. Name and locate the main parts of the brain and briefly describe the main functions of each.
2. Name the covering of the brain and the spinal cord. Name and describe its three layers. What is an infection of this covering called?
3. What is the purpose of the CSF? Where and how is CSF formed?
4. Name the four surface lobes of the cerebral hemispheres and describe functions of the cortex in each.
5. Name and describe the communication areas.
6. What are the differences between short-term and long-term memory, and how is each attained?
7. Describe the thalamus. Where is it located? What are its functions?
8. What activities does the hypothalamus regulate?
9. What is the limbic system and what are its functions?
10. Name and locate three divisions of the brain stem.
11. Name four general functions of the cranial nerves.
12. Name and describe the functions of the 12 cranial nerves. What are some disorders of the cranial nerves?

✔ ANSWERS TO CHECKPOINTS

1. The main divisions of the brain are the cerebrum, the diencephalon, the brain stem, and the cerebellum.
2. The three layers of the meninges are the dura mater, the arachnoid, and the pia mater.
3. CSF is produced in the ventricles of the brain. The two lateral ventricles are in the cerebral hemispheres, the third ventricle is in the diencephalon, and the fourth is between the brain stem and the cerebellum.
4. The outer layer of gray matter of the cerebral hemispheres where higher functions occur is the cerebral cortex.
5. The thalamus of the diencephalon directs sensory input to the cerebral cortex; the hypothalamus helps to maintain homeostasis.
6. The three subdivisions of the brain stem are the midbrain, the pons, and the medulla oblongata.
7. The cerebellum aids in coordination of voluntary muscles, maintenance of balance, and maintenance of muscle tone.
8. There are 12 pairs of cranial nerves.
9. A mixed nerve has both sensory and motor fibers.

The Sensory System

SELECTED KEY TERMS

The following terms are defined in the Glossary:

accommodation

choroid

cochlea

conjunctiva

convergence

cornea

lacrimal

lens (crystalline lens)

organ of Corti

ossicle

proprioceptor

refraction

retina

sclera

semicircular canal

tympanic membrane

vestibule

vitreous body

BEHAVIORAL OBJECTIVES

After careful study of this chapter, you should be able to:

1. Describe the function of the sensory system

2. Differentiate between the special and general senses and give examples of each

3. Describe the structure of the eye

4. Define *refraction* and list the refractive media of the eye

5. Differentiate between the rods and the cones of the eye

6. Compare the functions of the extrinsic and intrinsic muscles of the eye

7. Describe the nerve supply to the eye

8. Describe the three divisions of the ear

9. Describe the receptors for hearing and for equilibrium with respect to location and function

THE SENSES

The sensory system serves to protect the individual by detecting changes in the environment. An environmental change becomes a *stimulus* when it initiates a nerve impulse, which then travels to the central nervous system (CNS) by way of a sensory (afferent) neuron. Many stimuli arrive from the external environment and are detected at or near the surface of the body. Others, such as the stimuli from the viscera, originate internally and help to maintain homeostasis.

Receptors

The part of the nervous system that detects a stimulus is the **receptor,** which may be one of the following:

- The free dendrite of a sensory neuron, such as the receptors for pain
- A modified ending, or **end-organ,** on the dendrite of an afferent neuron, such as those for touch and temperature
- A special cell associated with an afferent neuron, such as the rods and cones of the retina of the eye and the receptors in the other special sense organs.

Regardless of the type of stimulus or the type of receptor involved, a stimulus becomes a sensation—something we experience—only when the nerve impulse it generates is interpreted by a specialized area of the cerebral cortex to which it travels.

Special and General Senses

One way of classifying the senses is according to the distribution of the receptors. A **special sense** is localized in a special sense organ; a **general sense** is widely distributed throughout the body.

- **Special senses**
  - **Vision** from receptors in the eye
  - **Hearing** from receptors in the internal ear
  - **Equilibrium** from receptors in the internal ear
  - **Taste** from the tongue receptors
  - **Smell** from receptors in the upper nasal cavities
- **General senses**
  - **Pressure,** *heat*, *cold*, *pain*, and *touch* from the skin and internal organs
  - Sense of **position** from the muscles, tendons, and joints

Mechanoreceptors

Sensory receptors can be classified according to the stimulus to which they respond. Thermoreceptors, such as those in the skin, detect change in temperature; photoreceptors in the retina of the eye respond to light; and chemoreceptors, such as those for taste and smell, detect chemicals.

Mechanoreceptors respond to movement, such as stretch, pressure, or vibration. The receptors that provide awareness of body position are examples, as are those that monitor stretch and tone of muscle fibers. Pressure and touch receptors in the skin are also mechanoreceptors.

In the ear, the receptors for hearing and equilibrium are mechanoreceptors. Both these receptors function by means of ciliated cells that respond to movement. In the vestibular apparatus, movements of the head trigger impulses that help to regulate balance. In the cochlea, sound waves cause movement of cilia and generate the impulses involved in hearing.

For more information, see Mechanoreceptors.

THE EYE AND VISION

Protection of the Eyeball

In the embryo, the eye develops as an outpocketing of the brain. The eye is a delicate organ, and nature has carefully protected it by means of the following structures:

- The skull bones form the walls of the eye orbit (cavity) and serve to protect more than half of the dorsal part of the eyeball.
- The eyelid aids in protecting the front of the eye. The eyelid can be closed to keep harmful materials out of the eye, and blinking helps to lubricate the eye. A muscle, the levator palpebrae, is attached to the upper eyelid. When this muscle contracts, it keeps the eye open. If the muscle becomes weaker with age, the eyelids may droop and interfere with vision, a condition called *ptosis*.
- The eyelashes and eyebrow help to keep foreign matter out of the eye.
- A thin membrane, the ***conjunctiva*** (kon-junk-TI-vah), lines the eyelid and covers the anterior portion of the eyeball.
- Tears, produced by the ***lacrimal*** (LAK-rih-mal) ***glands,*** lubricate the eye, wash away small foreign objects that enter the eye, and contain an enzyme that protects against infection.

The Conjunctiva

The conjunctiva is a thin membrane that lines the inner surface of the eyelid and covers the anterior part of the eyeball up to the edge of the cornea at the center. Cells within the conjunctiva produce mucus that aids in lubricating the eye. As the conjunctiva extends from the eyelid to the front of the eye, a sac is formed. The lower portion of the conjunctival sac can be used to instill drops of medication.

With age, there is often a thinning and drying of the conjunctiva, resulting in inflammation and enlarged blood vessels.

The Lacrimal Apparatus

Tears, produced by the ***lacrimal*** (LAK-rih-mal) ***gland*** (Fig. 10-1), serve to keep the conjunctiva moist. As tears flow across the eye from the lacrimal gland, located in the upper lateral part of the orbit, the fluid carries

FIGURE **10•1** Lacrimal apparatus.

away small particles that have entered the conjunctival sacs. The tears are then carried into ducts near the nasal corner of the eye where they drain into the nose by way of the *nasolacrimal* (na-zo-LAK-rih-mal) *duct* (see Fig. 10-1). Any excess of tears causes a "runny nose"; a greater overproduction of them results in the spilling of tears onto the cheeks.

With age, the lacrimal gland produces less secretion, but those tears that are produced may overflow to the cheek because of plugging of the nasolacrimal ducts, which would normally carry the tears away from the eye.

See Protecting the Eye.

✔ CHECKPOINT **1**:

What are some structures that protect the eye?

Coats of the Eyeball

The eyeball has three separate coats, or tunics (Fig. 10-2). The outermost tunic, called the *sclera* (SKLE-rah), is made of tough connective tissue. It is commonly referred to as the *white of the eye.*

The second tunic of the eyeball is the *choroid* (KO-royd). Composed of a delicate network of connective tissue interlaced with many blood vessels, this coat contains much dark brown pigment. The choroid may be compared to the dull black lining of a camera in that it prevents incoming light rays from scattering and reflecting off the inner surface of the eye. The blood vessels at the back of the eye can reveal signs of disease, and visualization of these vessels with an *ophthalmoscope* (of-THAL-mo-skope) is an important part of a medical examination.

The innermost tunic, the *retina* (RET-ih-nah), is the actual receptor layer of the eye. It contains the light-sensitive cells known as *rods* and *cones,* which generate the nerve impulses associated with the sense of vision.

✔ CHECKPOINT **2**:

What are the names of the tunics of the eyeball?

Protecting the Eye

Keeping the eyes out of harm's way is a daily task that should become habit. Vision represents a significant portion of the total sensory input that our brains depend on to decipher our situation and surroundings. Although the visual process is quite complex, there are three basic areas in which a person may take steps to protect the eyes.

Everyone should have a routine complete eye exam by an optometrist or ophthalmologist at least every 2 years, every year after age 40. This exam should include:

- A direct visualization of the patient's retinas to check for damage to the retina or to the many blood vessels that supply it
- A pressure test to determine whether or not a patient is at risk of developing glaucoma

Each of us should protect our eyes from the environment and potential hazards:

- Wear sunglasses to block some of the harmful light that enters the eye from the front
- Wear a hat to shield against light coming from above
- To protect the eye from the wind and airborne particles, wear sunglasses and hats.
- Whenever working with chemicals or operating machinery that has moving parts, wear protective eyewear.

Make sure that any acute injury to the eye is treated promptly. Even what seems like a simple scratch can have significant complications. Have a doctor evaluate any signs of infection in the eye immediately.

Pathway of Light Rays and Refraction

As light rays pass through the eye toward the retina, they travel through a series of transparent, colorless parts (see Fig. 10-2). On the way, they undergo a process known as *refraction,* which is the bending of light rays as they pass from one substance to another substance of different density. This refraction of the light rays makes it possible for light from a very large area to be focused on a very small surface, the retina, where the receptors are located. The following are, in order from the outside to the in-

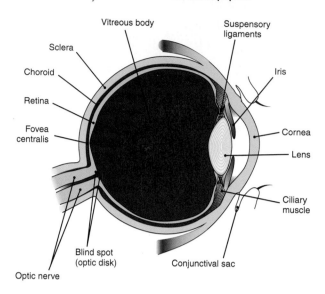

FIGURE **10•2** The eye.

side, the transparent refracting parts, or **media,** of the eye:

- The **cornea** (KOR-ne-ah) is a forward continuation of the sclera, but it is transparent and colorless, whereas the rest of the sclera is opaque and white. The cornea is referred to frequently as the *window* of the eye. It bulges forward slightly and is the main refracting structure of the eye. The cornea has no blood vessels; it is nourished by the fluids that constantly wash over it.
- The **aqueous** (A-kwe-us) **humor,** a watery fluid that fills much of the eyeball in front of the lens, helps maintain the slight forward curve of the cornea.
- The **lens,** technically called the *crystalline lens*, is a clear, circular structure made of a firm, elastic material. The lens has two bulging surfaces and is thus described as biconvex. The lens is important in light refraction because it is elastic and its thickness can be adjusted to focus light for near or distance vision.
- The **vitreous** (VIT-re-us) **body** is a soft jellylike substance that fills the entire space behind the lens. Like the aqueous humor, it is important in maintaining the shape of the eyeball as well as in aiding in refraction.

Note that the light rays passing through the eye are actually overrefracted so that an image falls on the retina upside down and backward. It is the job of the visual centers of the brain to reverse the images.

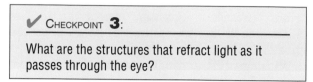

✔ CHECKPOINT **3**:

What are the structures that refract light as it passes through the eye?

Function of the Retina

The retina has a complex structure with multiple layers of cells (Fig. 10-3). The deepest layer is a pigmented layer just anterior to the choroid. Next are the rods and cones, the receptor cells of the eye, named for their shape. Details on how these two types of cells differ are presented Table 10-1.

The rods are highly sensitive to light and thus function in dim light, but they do not provide a sharp image. They are more numerous than the cones and are distributed more toward the front of the retina. When you enter into dim light, such as a darkened movie theater, you cannot see for a short period. It is during this time that the rods are beginning to function, a change that is described as **dark adaptation.** When you are able to see again, images are blurred and appear only in shades of gray because the rods are unable to differentiate colors.

The cones function in bright light, are sensitive to color, and give sharp images. The cones are localized at the center of the retina, especially at a point near the optic nerve called the **fovea centralis** (FO-ve-ah sen-TRA-lis). There are three types of cones, each sensitive to either red, green, or blue light. Color blindness results from a lack of cones in the retina. People who completely lack cones are totally color blind; those who lack one type of cone are partially color blind. This disorder, because of its pattern of inheritance, occurs almost exclusively in males.

The rods and cones function by means of pigments that are sensitive to light. The rod pigment is **rhodopsin** (ro-DOP-sin) or visual purple. Manufacture of these pigments requires

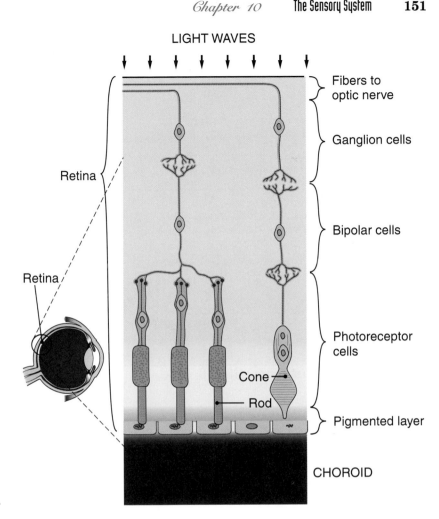

FIGURE **10•3**   Structure of the retina.

Table 10•1	**Comparison of the Rods and Cones of the Retina**	
CHARACTERISTIC	RODS	CONES
Shape	Cylindrical	Flask shaped
Number	About 120 million in each retina	About 6 million in each retina
Distribution	Toward the periphery (front) of the retina	Concentrated at the center of the retina
Stimulus	Dim light	Bright light
Visual acuity (sharpness)	Low	High
Pigments	Rhodopsin (visual purple)	Pigments sensitive to red, green, or blue
Color perception	None; shades of gray	Respond to color

vitamin A. If vitamin A is lacking in the diet, a person may have difficulty seeing in dim light because there is too little light to activate the rods, a condition termed ***night blindness.***

Nerve impulses from the rods and cones flow into sensory neurons that eventually merge to form the optic nerve (cranial nerve II), which connects with the retina at the back of the eye (see Fig. 10-2). The impulses travel to the visual center in the occipital cortex of the brain.

The coordinated actions needed for vision are summarized in Table 10-2.

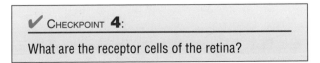

✔ CHECKPOINT **4**:

What are the receptor cells of the retina?

Table 10•2 **Events Needed for Vision**
Refraction of light
Adjustment of the pupil by muscles of the iris
Adjustment of the lens by the ciliary muscle (accommodation)
Convergence of the eyes by extrinsic eye muscles
Stimulation of receptor cells (rods and cones) in retina
Transmission of impulses to the brain by means of the optic nerve
Interpretation of impulses in cortex of occipital lobe

Muscles of the Eye

There are two groups of muscles associated with the eye:

- The voluntary muscles attached to the outer surface of the eyeball are the ***extrinsic*** (eks-TRIN-sik) ***muscles***.
- The involuntary muscles located within the eyeball are the ***intrinsic*** (in-TRIN-sik) ***muscles***.

The Extrinsic Muscles

The six ribbonlike extrinsic muscles connected with each eye originate on the bones of the orbit and insert on the surface of the sclera (Fig. 10-4). They are named for their location and the direction of the muscle fibers. These muscles

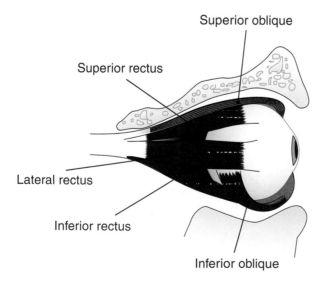

FIGURE **10•4** Extrinsic muscles of the eye (medial rectus not shown)

pull on the eyeball in a coordinated fashion so that both eyes center on one visual field. This process of ***convergence*** is necessary to formation of a clear image on the retina. Having the image come from a slightly different angle from each retina is believed to be important for three-dimensional (stereoscopic) vision, a characteristic of primates.

> ✔ CHECKPOINT **5**:
>
> What is the function of the extrinsic muscles of the eye?

The Intrinsic Muscles

The intrinsic muscles are found in two circular structures within the eye (see Fig. 10-2):

- The ***iris,*** the colored or pigmented part of the eye, is composed of two types of muscles. The size of the central opening of the iris, called the ***pupil,*** is governed by the action of these two sets of muscles, one of which is arranged in a circular fashion, and the other of which extends in a radial manner like the spokes of a wheel.
- The ***ciliary muscle*** is shaped somewhat like a flattened ring with a hole the size of the outer edge of the iris. This muscle alters the shape of the lens during the process of accommodation (described later).

The purpose of the iris is to regulate the amount of light entering the eye. In the presence of bright light, the circular muscle fibers of the iris contract, reducing the size of the pupil. This narrowing is termed *constriction.* In contrast, if the light is dim, the radial muscles contract, and the opening is pulled outward and enlarged. This enlargement of the pupil is known as *dilation.*

The pupil changes size, too, according to whether one is looking at a near object or a distant one. Viewing a near object causes the pupil to become smaller; viewing a distant object causes it to enlarge.

The muscle of the ciliary body is similar in direction and method of action to the radial muscle of the iris. When the ciliary muscle contracts, it draws forward and removes the tension on the **suspensory ligaments,** which hold the lens in place (see Fig. 10-2). The elastic lens then recoils and becomes thicker in much the same way that a rubber band thickens when the pull on it is released. When the ciliary body relaxes, the lens becomes flattened. These actions change the refractive ability of the lens.

The process of **accommodation** involves coordinated eye changes to enable a person to focus on near objects. The ciliary body contracts, thereby thickening the lens, and the circular muscle fibers of the iris contract to decrease the size of the opening of the pupil. In young people, the lens is elastic, and therefore its thickness can be readily adjusted according to the need for near or distance vision. With aging, the lens loses its elasticity and therefore its ability to adjust to near vision by thickening, making it difficult to focus clearly on close objects. This condition is called **presbyopia** (pres-be-O-pe-ah), which literally means "old eye."

✔ CHECKPOINT **6**:

What is the function of the iris?

✔ CHECKPOINT **7**:

What is the function of the ciliary muscle?

Nerve Supply to the Eye

Two sensory nerves supply the eye (Fig. 10-5):

* The **optic nerve** (cranial nerve II) carries visual impulses from the retinal rods and cones to the brain.
* The **ophthalmic** (of-THAL-mik) **branch of the trigeminal nerve** (cranial nerve V) carries impulses of pain, touch, and temperature from the eye and surrounding parts to the brain.

The optic nerve arises from the retina a little toward the medial or nasal side of the eye. There are no retinal rods and cones in the area of the optic nerve. Consequently, no image can form on the retina at this point, which is known as the blind spot or **optic disk.**

Near the optic disk is the tiny depressed area in the retina known as the fovea centralis, which contains the highest concentration of cones and is the point of sharpest vision (see

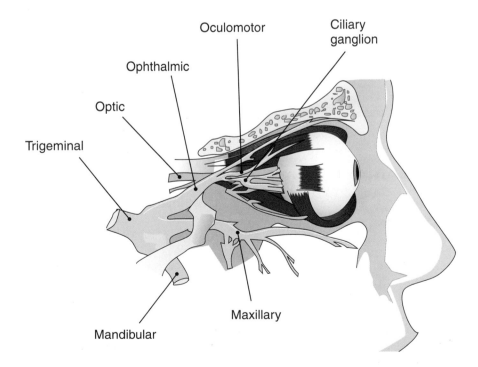

FIGURE **10•5**   Nerves of the eye.

Fig. 10-2). The fovea is contained within a yellowish spot, the macula. This area may show degenerative changes with age.

There are three nerves that carry motor impulses to the muscles of the eyeball. The largest is the oculomotor nerve (cranial nerve III), which supplies voluntary and involuntary motor impulses to all the muscles but two. The other two nerves, the trochlear (cranial nerve IV) and the abducens (cranial nerve VI), each supply one voluntary muscle.

✔ CHECKPOINT **8**:

What is cranial nerve II and what does it do?

THE EAR

The ear is the sense organ for both hearing and equilibrium (Fig. 10-6). It may be divided into three main sections:

- The *outer ear* includes an outer projection and a canal.
- The *middle ear* is an air space containing three small bones.
- The *inner ear* is the most complex and contains the sensory receptors for hearing and equilibrium.

The Outer Ear

The external portion of the ear consists of a visible projecting portion, the *pinna* (PIN-nah), or the *auricle* (AW-rih-kl), and a canal that leads into the deeper parts of the ear. The purpose of the pinna is to direct sound waves into the ear, but it is probably of little importance in humans. Leading in from the pinna is an opening, the *external auditory canal,* or *meatus* (me-A-tus), which extends medially for about 2.5 cm or more, depending on which wall of the canal is measured. The skin lining this tube is thin and, in the first part of the canal, contains many *ceruminous* (seh-RU-mih-nus) *glands.* The *cerumen* (seh-RU-men), or wax, may become dried and impacted in the canal and must then be removed. The same kinds of disorders that

involve the skin elsewhere—atopic dermatitis, boils, and other infections—may also affect the skin of the external auditory canal.

At the end of the auditory canal is the *tympanic* (tim-PAN-ik) *membrane,* or eardrum, which serves as a boundary between the external auditory canal and the middle ear cavity. It vibrates freely as sound waves enter the ear.

The Middle Ear

The Ossicles

The middle ear cavity is a small, flattened space that contains three small bones, or *ossicles* (OS-ih-klz). The three ossicles are joined in such a way that they amplify the sound waves received by the tympanic membrane and then transmit the sounds to the fluid in the inner ear. The handlelike part of the first bone, or *malleus* (MAL-e-us), is attached to the tympanic membrane, whereas the headlike portion is connected with the second bone, called the *incus* (ING-kus). The innermost of the ossicles is shaped somewhat like a stirrup and is called the *stapes* (STA-peze). The base of the stapes is in contact with a membrane covering the *oval window* of the inner ear. This membrane in turn vibrates and transmits the sound waves to the fluid of the inner ear.

✔ CHECKPOINT **9**:

What are the ossicles of the ear and what do they do?

The Eustachian Tube

The *eustachian* (u-STA-shun) *tube* (auditory tube) connects the middle ear cavity with the throat, or *pharynx* (FAR-inks) (see Fig. 10-6). This tube opens to allow pressure to equalize on the two sides of the tympanic membrane. The valve that closes the tube can be forced open by swallowing hard, yawning, or blowing with the nose and mouth sealed, as is done when one is experiencing pain from pressure changes in an airplane.

The mucous membrane of the pharynx is continuous through the eustachian tube into the

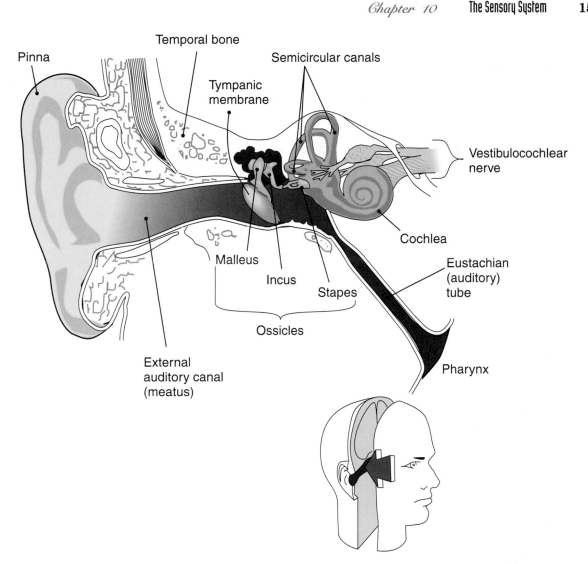

FIGURE **10•6**   The ear, showing the outer, middle, and inner divisions.

middle ear cavity, and organisms may travel along the membrane, causing infection of the middle ear.

At the back of the middle ear cavity is an opening into the mastoid air cells, which are spaces inside the mastoid process of the temporal bone.

The Inner Ear

The most complicated and important part of the ear is the internal portion, which is described as a *labyrinth* (LAB-ih-rinth) because it has a complex mazelike construction. It consists of three separate areas hollowed out inside the temporal bone (see Fig. 10-6). The skeleton of the inner ear is called the **bony labyrinth.** Its three divisions are as follows:

* The **vestibule,** which is next to the oval window and is composed of two chambers (the utricle and saccule)
* The **semicircular canals,** three projecting bony tubes located toward the back
* The **cochlea** (KOK-le-ah), coiled like a snail shell and located toward the front

All three divisions of the bony labyrinth contain a fluid called **perilymph** (PER-e-limf).

Within the bony labyrinth is an exact replica of this bony shell made of membrane, much like an inner tube within a tire. The tubes and chambers of this ***membranous labyrinth*** are filled with a fluid called ***endolymph*** (EN-do-limf). The endolymph is within the membranous labyrinth, and the perilymph is all around it. These fluids are important to the sensory functions of the inner ear.

Hearing

The organ of hearing, called the ***organ of Corti*** (KOR-te), consists of ciliated receptor cells located inside the membranous cochlea, or ***cochlear duct*** (Fig. 10-7). Sound waves enter the external auditory canal and cause the tympanic membrane to vibrate. These vibrations are amplified by the ossicles and transmitted by them to the perilymph of the inner

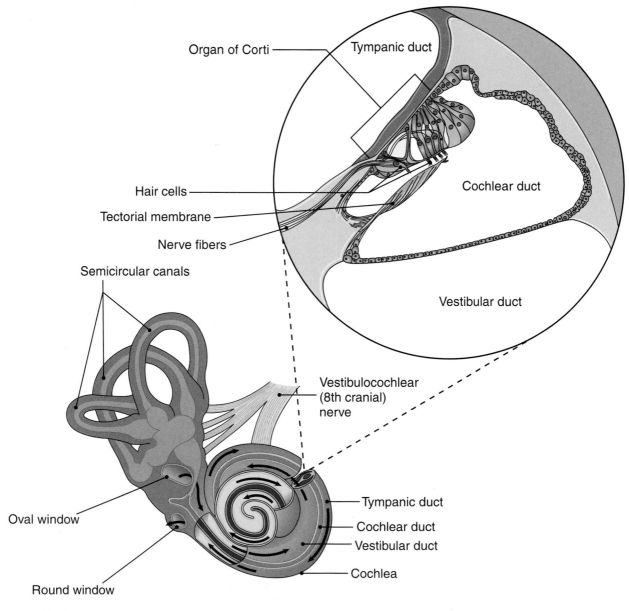

FIGURE **10•7** Cochlea and organ of Corti. The arrows show the direction of sound waves in the cochlea.

ear. The sound waves enter the upper chamber of the cochlea (the vestibular duct), travel to the top of the cochlea, and then continue through the lower chamber of the cochlea (the tympanic duct). As the sound waves move through the fluids in these chambers, they set up vibrations in the endolymph of the cochlear duct. These vibrations stimulate the tiny, hairlike cilia on the receptor cells, setting up nerve impulses that travel to the brain in the **cochlear nerve,** a branch of the eighth cranial nerve (formerly called the *auditory* or *acoustic nerve*).

Sound waves ultimately leave the ear through another membrane-covered space in the bony labyrinth, the **round window.**

✔ CHECKPOINT **10**:

What is the name of the organ of hearing and where is it located?

Equilibrium

The other sensory receptors in the inner ear are those related to equilibrium (Fig. 10-8). They are located in the vestibule and the semicircular canals, which together make up the **vestibular apparatus.**

Receptors located in the two small sacs of the vestibule function to sense the position of the head or the position of the body when moving in a straight line, as in a moving vehicle. This aspect of equilibrium is termed **static equilibrium.**

The receptors for **dynamic equilibrium,** which function when the body is spinning or moving in a different direction, are located at the bases of the semicircular canals.

Receptors for the sense of equilibrium are also ciliated cells. As the head moves, a shift in the position of the cilia within their surrounding fluid generates a nerve impulse. Nerve fibers from the vestibule and from the semicircular canals form the **vestibular** (ves-TIB-u-lar) **nerve,** which joins the cochlear nerve to form the vestibulocochlear nerve, the eighth cranial nerve.

✔ CHECKPOINT **11**:

Where are the receptors for equilibrium located?

OTHER SPECIAL SENSE ORGANS

The sense organs of taste and smell are designed to respond to chemical stimuli.

Sense of Taste

The sense of taste involves receptors in the tongue and two different nerves that carry taste impulses to the brain (Fig. 10-9). The taste receptors, known as **taste buds,** are located along the edges of small, depressed areas called **fissures.** Taste buds are stimulated only if the substance to be tasted is in solution or dissolves in the fluids of the mouth. Receptors for four basic tastes are localized in different regions, forming a "taste map" of the tongue:

- **Sweet** tastes are most acutely experienced at the tip of the tongue (hence the popularity of lollipops and ice cream cones).
- **Sour** tastes are most effectively detected by the taste buds located at the sides of the tongue.
- **Salty** tastes are most acute at the anterior sides of the tongue.
- **Bitter** tastes are detected at the back part of the tongue.

The nerves of taste include the facial and the glossopharyngeal cranial nerves (VII and IX). The interpretation of taste impulses is probably accomplished by the lower front portion of the brain, although there may be no sharply separate taste, or **gustatory** (GUS-tah-to-re) **center**.

Sense of Smell

The importance of the sense of smell is often underestimated. This sense helps to detect gases and other harmful substances in the environment and helps to warn of spoiled food. Smells can trigger memories and other psychological responses. Smell is also important in sexual behavior.

The receptors for smell are located in the **olfactory** (ol-FAK-to-re) **epithelium** of the upper

FIGURE **10•8** Inner ear showing action of receptors for dynamic equilibrium.

part of the nasal cavity (see Fig. 10-9). Again, the chemicals detected must be in solution in the fluids that line the nose. Because these receptors are high in the nasal cavity, one must "sniff" to bring odors upward in the nose.

The impulses from the receptors for smell are carried by the olfactory nerve (I), which leads directly to the olfactory center in the temporal cortex of the brain. The interpretation of smell is closely related to the sense of taste, but a greater variety of dissolved chemicals can be detected by smell than by taste. The smell of foods is just as important in stimulating appetite and

the flow of digestive juices as is the sense of taste.

The olfactory receptors deteriorate with age, with the result that food becomes less appealing. It is important when presenting food to elderly people that the food look inviting so as to stimulate their appetites.

✔ CHECKPOINT **12**:

What are the special senses that respond to chemical stimuli?

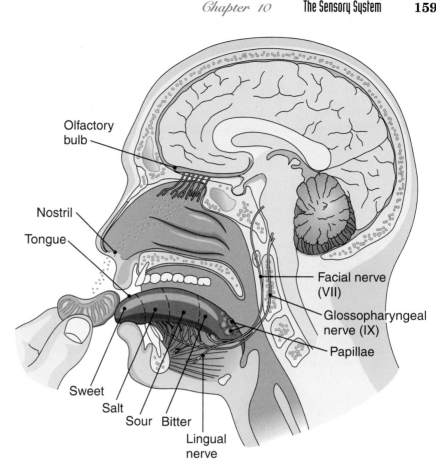

Olfactory bulb

Nostril

Tongue

Facial nerve (VII)

Glossopharyngeal nerve (IX)

Papillae

Sweet

Salt

Sour   Bitter

Lingual nerve

FIGURE **10•9**   Organs of taste and smell.

THE GENERAL SENSES

Unlike the *special* sensory receptors, which are localized within specific sense organs, limited to a relatively small area, the *general* sensory receptors are scattered throughout the body. These include receptors for touch, pressure, heat, cold, position, and pain (Fig. 10-10).

Sense of Touch

The touch receptors, **tactile** (TAK-til) **corpuscles,** are found mostly in the dermis of the skin and around hair follicles. Sensitivity to touch varies with the number of touch receptors in different areas. They are especially numerous and close together in the tips of the fingers and the toes. The lips and the tip of the tongue also contain many of these receptors and are very sensitive to touch. Other areas, such as

the back of the hand and the back of the neck, have fewer receptors and are less sensitive to touch.

Sense of Pressure

It has been found that even when the skin is anesthetized, there is still consciousness of pressure. These sensory end-organs for deep sensibility are located in the subcutaneous tissues beneath the skin and also near joints, muscles, and other deep tissues. They are sometimes referred to as *receptors for deep touch.*

Sense of Temperature

The temperature receptors are free nerve endings. They are widely distributed in the skin. There are separate receptors for heat and cold, and they vary in distribution. A warm object

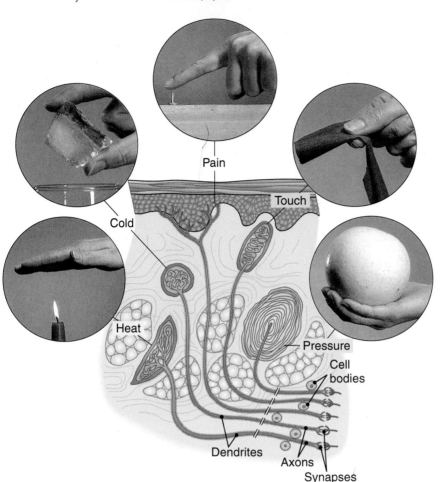

Pain

Touch

Cold

Heat

Pressure

Cell bodies

Dendrites

Axons

Synapses

FIGURE **10•10** Sensory receptors in the skin. Synapses are in the spinal cord.

stimulates only the heat receptors, and a cool object affects only the cold receptors. Internally, there are temperature receptors in the hypothalamus of the brain, which help to adjust body temperature according to the temperature of the blood passing through.

Sense of Position

Receptors located in muscles, tendons, and joints relay impulses that aid in judging one's position and changes in the locations of body parts in relation to each other. They also inform the brain of the amount of muscle contraction and tendon tension. These rather widespread receptors, known as ***proprioceptors*** (pro-pre-o-SEP-tors), are aided in this function by the equilibrium receptors of the internal ear.

Information received by these receptors is needed for the coordination of muscles and is important in such activities as walking, running, and many more complicated skills, such as playing a musical instrument. These muscle receptors also play an important part in maintaining muscle tone and good posture as well as allowing for the adjustment of the muscles for the particular kind of work to be done. The nerve fibers that carry impulses from these receptors enter the spinal cord and ascend to the brain in the posterior part of the cord. The cerebellum is a main coordinating center for these impulses.

✔ CHECKPOINT **13**:

What are proprioceptors and where are they located?

Sense of Pain

Pain is the most important protective sense. The receptors for pain are widely distributed. They are found in the skin, muscles, and joints and to a lesser extent in most internal organs (including the blood vessels and viscera). Pain receptors are not enclosed in capsules as are the sensory end-organs; rather, they are merely branchings of the nerve fiber, called *free nerve endings.*

There are two pathways for the transmission of pain to the CNS, one for acute, sharp pain, and the other for slow, chronic pain. Thus, a single strong stimulus produces the immediate sharp pain, followed in a second or so by the slow, diffuse, burning pain that increases in severity with the passage of time.

SENSORY ADAPTATION

When sensory receptors are exposed to a continuous stimulus, receptors often adjust themselves so that the sensation becomes less acute. The term for this phenomenon is *sensory adaptation.* For example, if you immerse your hand in very warm water, it may be uncomfortable; however, if you leave your hand there, soon the water will feel less hot (even if it has not cooled appreciably).

Receptors adapt at different rates. Those for warmth, cold, and light pressure adapt rapidly. In contrast, those for pain do not adapt. In fact, the sensations from the slow pain fibers tend to increase over time. This variation in receptors allows us to save energy by not responding to unimportant stimuli while always heeding the warnings of pain.

Summary

I. **The senses**—protect by detecting changes (stimuli) in the environment
   A. **Special and general senses**
      1. Special senses—vision, hearing, equilibrium, taste, smell
      2. General senses—pain, touch, temperature, pressure, position

II. **The eye and vision**
   A. Protection of the eyeball—bony orbit, eyelid, eyelashes, conjunctiva, tears (lacrimal apparatus)
   B. Coats of the eyeball
      1. Sclera—white of the eye
         a. Cornea—anterior
      2. Choroid—pigmented; contains blood vessels
      3. Retina—receptor layer
   C. Pathway of light rays and refraction
      1. Refraction—bending of light rays as they pass through substances of different density
      2. Refracting parts (media)—cornea, aqueous humor, lens, vitreous body
   D. Function of retina
      1. Cells
         a. Rods—cannot detect color; function in dim light
         b. Cones—detect color; function in bright light
      2. Pigments—sensitive to light; rod pigment is rhodopsin
   E. Muscles of the eye
      1. Extrinsic muscles—six move each eyeball
      2. Intrinsic muscles
         a. Iris—colored ring around pupil; regulates the amount of light entering the eye
         b. Ciliary body—regulates the thickness of the lens for accommodation
   F. Nerve supply to the eye
      1. Sensory nerves
         a. Optic nerve (II)—carries impulses from retina to brain

b. Ophthalmic branch of trigeminal (V)
2. Motor nerves—move eyeball
a. Oculomotor (III), trochlear (IV), abducens (VI)

III. The ear
A. Outer ear—pinna, auditory canal (meatus), tympanic membrane (eardrum)
B. Middle ear
1. Ossicles—malleus, incus, stapes
2. Eustachian tube—connects middle ear with pharynx to equalize pressure
C. The inner ear—bony labyrinth and membranous labyrinth
1. Vestibule—contains receptors for static equilibrium
2. Semicircular canals—contain receptors for dynamic equilibrium
3. Cochlea—contains receptors for hearing (organ of Corti)
4. Nerve—vestibulocochlear (auditory) nerve (VIII)

IV. Other special sense organs
A. Sense of taste—gustatory sense
1. Receptors—taste buds
2. Tastes—sweet, sour, salty, bitter
3. Nerves—facial (VII) and glossopharyngeal (IX)
B. Sense of smell—olfactory sense
1. Receptors—in upper part of nasal cavity
2. Nerve—olfactory nerve (I)

V. General senses
A. Sense of touch
B. Sense of pressure
C. Sense of temperature
D. Sense of position—receptors are proprioceptors in muscles, tendons, joints
E. Sense of pain—receptors are free nerve endings

VI. Sensory adaptation—adjustment of receptors so that sensation becomes less acute

Questions for Study and Review

1. What is the function of the senses?
2. Define *sensory receptor* and give several examples.
3. List the five special senses.
4. List six general senses.
5. List five protective devices for the eye.
6. Name the three coats (tunics) of the eye.
7. Trace the path of a light ray from the outside of the eye to the retina.
8. What happens to light when it is refracted and what causes refraction?
9. How does the retina function in vision?
10. List the extrinsic muscles of the eye. What is their function?
11. List the intrinsic muscles of the eye. What is their function?
12. What is near accommodation? What structures of the eye are necessary for near accommodation?
13. List five cranial nerves associated with the eye and give the function of each.
14. Describe the structures that sound waves pass through in traveling through the ear to the receptors for hearing.
15. What parts of the ear function in equilibrium?
16. What cranial nerve carries impulses from the ear? Name the two branches.
17. Name the four basic tastes. Where are the taste receptors?
18. Describe the olfactory apparatus.

19. Where are the receptors for the sense of position located?
20. What does *adaptation* mean with respect to the senses? How does sensory adaptation differ among the senses?
21. Differentiate between the terms in each of the following pairs:
    a. *special sense* and *general sense*
    b. *rods* and *cones*
    c. *static* and *dynamic equilibrium*
    d. *endolymph* and *perilymph*
    d. *gustatory* and *olfactory*

✔ ANSWERS TO CHECKPOINTS

1. Structures that protect the eye include the skull bones, eyelid, eyelashes, eyebrow, conjunctiva, and lacrimal gland.
2. The tunics (coats) of the eyeball are the sclera, choroid, and retina.
3. The structures that refract light as it passes through the eye to the retina are the cornea, aqueous humor, lens, and vitreous body.
4. The receptor cells of the retina are the rods and cones.
5. The extrinsic eye muscles pull on the eyeball so that both eyes center on one visual field, a process known as convergence.
6. The iris adjusts the size of the pupil to regulate the amount of light that enters the eye.
7. The ciliary muscle adjusts the thickness of the lens to allow for accommodation for near vision.
8. Cranial nerve II is the optic nerve. It carries impulses from the retinal rods and cones to the brain.
9. The ossicles of the middle ear are three small bones, the malleus, incus, and stapes, that transmit sound waves from the tympanic membrane to the inner ear.
10. The organ of hearing is the organ of Corti located in the cochlear duct within the cochlea.
11. The receptors for equilibrium are located in the vestibular apparatus, which consists of the vestibule and the semicircular canals.
12. The senses of taste and smell are the special senses that respond to chemical stimuli.
13. Proprioceptors are the receptors that respond to change in position. They are located in muscles, tendons, and joints.

10

Chapter 11

The Endocrine System: Glands and Hormones

SELECTED KEY TERMS

The following terms are defined in the Glossary:

endocrine

hormone

hypothalamus

pituitary (hypophysis)

prostaglandin

receptor

steroid

target tissue

BEHAVIORAL OBJECTIVES

After careful study of this chapter, you should be able to:

1. Compare the effects of the nervous system and the endocrine system in controlling the body

2. Describe the functions of hormones

3. Explain how hormones are regulated

4. Identify the glands of the endocrine system on a diagram

5. List the hormones produced by each endocrine gland and describe the effects of each on the body

6. Describe how the hypothalamus controls the anterior and posterior pituitary

7. List tissues other than the endocrine glands that produce hormones

8. Explain how the endocrine system responds to stress

The endocrine system consists of a group of glands that produces regulatory chemicals called *hormones.* The endocrine system and the nervous system work together to control and coordinate all other systems of the body. The nervous system and the endocrine system are the two main controlling and coordinating systems of the body. The nervous system controls such rapid activity as muscle movement and intestinal activity by means of electrical and chemical stimuli. The effects of the endocrine system occur more slowly and over a longer period and involve chemical stimuli only. The effects of these chemical messengers are widespread.

Although the nervous and endocrine systems differ in some respects, the two systems are closely related. The activity of the pituitary gland, which in turn regulates other glands, is controlled by a part of the brain. The connections between the nervous system and the endocrine system enable endocrine function to adjust to the demands of a changing environment.

HORMONES

Functions of Hormones

Hormones are chemical messengers that have specific regulatory effects on certain cells or organs in the body. Hormones are released directly into the bloodstream, by which they are carried to all parts of the body. They regulate growth, metabolism, reproduction, and behavior. Some hormones affect many tissues, for example, growth hormone, thyroid hormone, and insulin. Others affect only specific tissues. One pituitary hormone, thyroid-stimulating hormone (TSH), acts only on the thyroid gland; another (ACTH) stimulates only the outer portion of the adrenal gland.

The specific tissue acted on by each hormone is the *target tissue.* The cells that make up these tissues have *receptors* in the plasma membrane or within the cytoplasm to which the hormone attaches. Once attached to the cell, the hormone affects cell activities, regulating the manufacture of proteins, changing the permeability of the membrane, or affecting metabolic reactions.

Chemistry

Chemically, hormones fall into two main categories:

- *Amino acid compounds.* Most hormones are proteins or related compounds also made of amino acids. All hormones except those of the adrenal cortex and the sex glands fall into this category.
- *Steroids* are hormones derived from lipids.

They are produced by the adrenal cortex and the sex glands.

Regulation of Hormones

The amount of each hormone that is secreted is normally kept within a specific range. Negative feedback is the method used to regulate these levels. That is, the concentration of the hormone itself acts as a brake on further secretion of that hormone. Each endocrine gland tends to over-secrete its hormone, exerting more effect on the target tissue. When the target tissue becomes too active, there is a negative effect on the endocrine gland, which then decreases its secretory action.

The release of hormones may fall into a rhythmic pattern. Hormones of the adrenal cortex follow a 24-hour cycle related to a person's sleeping pattern, with the level of secretion greatest just before arising and least at bedtime. Hormones of the female menstrual cycle follow a monthly pattern.

The remainder of this chapter deals with hormones and the tissues that produce them. Refer to Figure 11-1 to locate each of the endocrine glands as you study. The information on the endocrine glands and their hormones is summarized in Table 11-1.

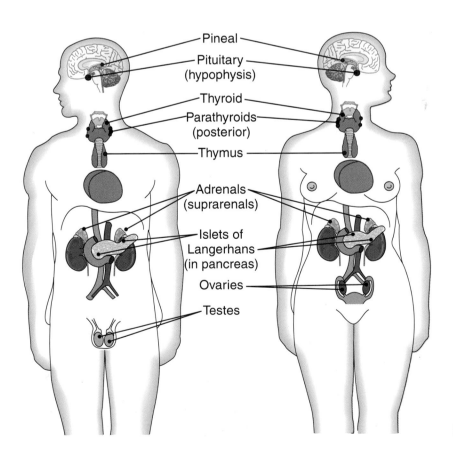

Pineal
Pituitary (hypophysis)
Thyroid
Parathyroids (posterior)
Thymus
Adrenals (suprarenals)
Islets of Langerhans (in pancreas)
Ovaries
Testes

FIGURE **11•1** The endocrine glands.

Table 11•1 The Endocrine Glands and Their Hormones

GLAND	HORMONE	PRINCIPAL FUNCTIONS
Anterior pituitary	GH (growth hormone)	Promotes growth of all body tissues
	TSH (thyroid-stimulating hormone)	Stimulates thyroid gland to produce thyroid hormones
	ACTH (adrenocorticotropic hormone)	Stimulates adrenal cortex to produce cortical hormones; aids in protecting body in stress situations (injury, pain)
	PRL (prolactin)	Stimulates secretion of milk by mammary glands
	FSH (follicle-stimulating hormone)	Stimulates growth and hromone activity of ovarian follicles; stimulates growth of testes; promotes development of sperm cells
	LH (luteinizing hormone); ICSH (interstitial cell–stimulating hormone) in males	Causes development of corpus luteum at site of ruptured ovarian follicle in female; stimulates secretion of testosterone in male
Posterior pituitary	ADH (antidiuretic hormone; vasopressin)	Promotes reabsorption of water in kidney tubules; stimulates smooth muscle tissue of blood vessels to constrict
	Oxytocin	Causes contraction of muscle of uterus; causes ejection of milk from mammary glands
Thyroid	Thyroxine (T_4) and triiodothyronine (T_3)	Increases metabolic rate, influencing both physical and mental activities; required for normal growth
	Calcitonin	Decreases calcium level in blood
Parathyroids	Parathyroid hormone	Regulates exchange of calcium between blood and bones; increases calcium level in blood
Adrenal medulla	Epinephrine and norephinephrine	Increases blood pressure and heart rate; activates cells influenced by sympathetic nervous system plus many not affected by sympathetic nerves
Adrenal cortex	Cortisol (95% of glucocorticoids)	Aids in metabolism of carbohydrates, proteins, and fats; active during stress
	Aldosterone (95% of mineralcorticoids)	Aids in regulating electrolytes and water balance
	Sex hormones	May influence secondary sexual characteristics
Pancreatic islets	Insulin	Aids transport of glucose into cells; required for cellular metabolism of foods, especially glucose; decreases blood sugar levels
	Glucagon	Stimulates liver to release glucose, thereby increasing blood sugar levels
Testes	Testosterone	Stimulates growth and development of sexual organs (testes, penis) plus development of secondary sexual characteristics, such as hair growth on body and face and deepening of voice; stimulates maturation of sperm cells
Ovaries	Estrogens (*e.g.,* estradiol)	Stimulates growth of primary sexual organs (uterus, tubes) and development of secondary sexual organs, such as breasts, plus changes in pelvis to ovoid, broader shape
	Progesterone	Stimulates development of secretory parts of mammary glands; prepares uterine lining for implantation of fertilized ovum; aids in maintaining pregnancy
Thymus	Thymosin	Promotes growth of T cells active in immunity
Pineal	Melatonin	Regulates mood, sexual development, and daily cycles in response to the amount of light in the environment

THE ENDOCRINE GLANDS AND THEIR HORMONES

The Pituitary

The *pituitary* (pih-TU-ih-tar-e), or *hypophysis* (hi-POF-ih-sis), is a small gland about the size of a cherry. It is located in a saddlelike depression of the sphenoid bone just behind the point at which the optic nerves cross. It is surrounded by bone except where it connects with the brain by a stalk called the *infundibulum* (in-fun-DIB-u-lum). The gland is divided into two parts, the *anterior lobe* and the *posterior lobe.* The hormones released from each lobe are shown in Figure 11-2.

The pituitary is often called the *master gland* because it releases hormones that affect the working of other glands, such as the thyroid, gonads (gonads), and adrenal glands. (Hormones

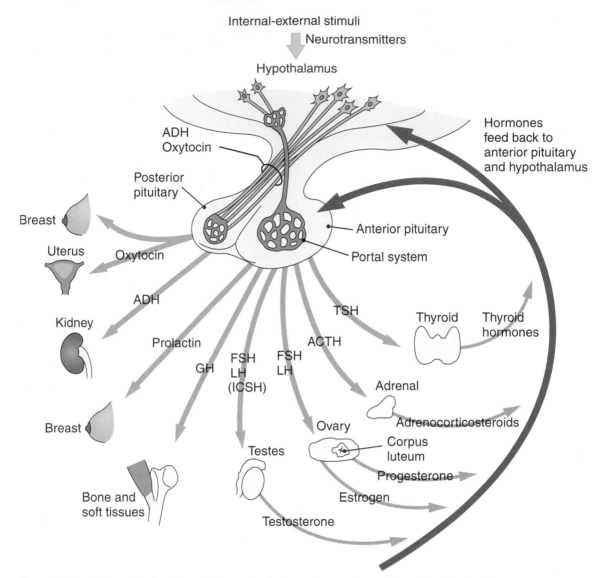

FIGURE **11•2** Pituitary gland and its relations to the brain and target tissues. Hypothalamic-releasing hormones influence the anterior pituitary through a portal system. Tropic hormones from the anterior pituitary affect the working of various other glands. The hypothalamus communicates with the posterior pituitary through tracts.

that stimulate other glands may be recognized by the ending *-tropin,* as in *thyrotropin,* which means "acting on the thyroid gland.") However, the pituitary itself is controlled by the ***hypothalamus*** of the brain, to which it is connected by the infundibulum (stalk) (see Fig. 11-2). The infundibulum carries secretions and nerve impulses from the hypothalamus to the pituitary.

The hormones produced in the anterior pituitary are not released from the gland until chemical messengers called ***releasing hormones*** arrive from the hypothalamus. These releasing hormones are sent to the anterior pituitary by way of a special type of circulatory pathway called a ***portal system.*** By this circulatory "detour," some of the blood that leaves the hypothalamus travels to capillaries in the anterior pituitary before returning to the heart.

As the blood circulates through the capillaries, it delivers the hormones that stimulate the release of anterior pituitary secretions.

The two hormones of the posterior pituitary (antidiuretic hormone, or ADH, and oxytocin) are actually produced in the hypothalamus and stored in the posterior pituitary. Their release is controlled by nerve impulses that travel over pathways (tracts) between the hypothalamus and the posterior pituitary.

✔ CHECKPOINT **3**:

What part of the brain controls the pituitary?

Hormones of the Anterior Lobe

- *Growth hormone (GH)*, or *somatotropin* (so-mah-to-TRO-pin), acts directly on most body tissues, promoting protein manufacture that is essential for growth. Produced throughout life, GH causes increase in size and height to occur in youth, before the closure of the epiphyses of long bones. A young person with a deficiency of GH will remain small, though well proportioned, unless treated with adequate hormone (see Growth Hormone).
- *Thyroid-stimulating hormone (TSH),* or *thyrotropin* (thi-ro-TRO-pin), stimulates the thyroid gland to produce thyroid hormones.
- *Adrenocorticotropic* (ad-re-no-kor-te-ko-TRO-pik) *hormone (ACTH)* stimulates the cortex of the adrenal glands.
- *Prolactin* (pro-LAK-tin) *(PRL)* stimulates the production of milk in the female.
- *Gonadotropins* (gon-ah-do-TRO-pinz), acting on the gonads, regulate the growth, development, and functioning of the reproductive systems in both males and females. The two gonadotropins are the following:
  - Follicle-stimulating hormone *(FSH)* stimulates the development of eggs in the ovaries and sperm cells in the testes.
  - Luteinizing (LU-te-in-i-zing) *hormone (LH)* causes ovulation in females and sex hormone secretion in both males and females; in males, the hormone is called

Growth Hormone

Growth hormone, also called *somatotropin,* is produced by the anterior pituitary gland. Its release is regulated by growth hormone–releasing hormone (GHRH) and growth hormone–inhibiting hormone (GHIH), also called *somatostatin,* from the hypothalamus.

Although growth hormone mainly affects the development of bones and muscles, it has a general effect on most other tissues as well, stimulating an increase in protein synthesis. It also stimulates the liver to release fatty acids for energy when the level of blood glucose drops. In this capacity, it is released during times of stress. The production of growth hormone is controlled by its concentration in the blood; by the level of other hormones, including those from the adrenal, thyroid, and sex glands; and by the level of nutrients in the blood.

Insufficient growth hormone results in pituitary dwarfism. This condition can be prevented by administering growth hormone to children who lack it. Growth hormone is now produced by genetic engineering. The gene for the hormone is introduced into harmless bacteria, which then produce large quantities in laboratory cultures.

interstitial cell–stimulating hormone (ICSH).

Hormones of the Posterior Lobe

- *Antidiuretic* (an-ti-di-u-RET-ik) *hormone (ADH)* promotes the reabsorption of water from the kidney tubules and thus decreases the excretion of water. Large amounts of this hormone cause contraction of the smooth muscle of blood vessels and raise blood pressure. Inadequate amounts of ADH cause excessive loss of water and result in a disorder called *diabetes insipidus*. This type of diabetes should not be confused with diabetes mellitus, which is due to inadequate amounts of insulin.
- *Oxytocin* (ok-se-TO-sin) causes contraction of the muscle of the uterus and milk ejec-

tion from the breasts. Under certain circumstances, commercial preparations of this hormone are administered during or after childbirth to cause the uterus to contract.

✔ CHECKPOINT **4**:

Some of the anterior pituitary hormones end with the suffix *-tropin*. What does this suffix mean?

The Thyroid Gland

The largest of the endocrine glands is the *thyroid,* which is located in the neck (Fig. 11-3). The thyroid has two oval parts called the *lateral lobes,* one on either side of the larynx (voice box). A narrow band called the *isthmus* (IS-mus) connects these two lobes. A connective tissue capsule encloses the entire gland.

Hormones of the Thyroid Gland

The thyroid produces two hormones that regulate metabolism. The principal hormone is *thyroxine* (thi-ROK-sin), which is symbolized as T_4, based on the iodine content. The other hormone, triiodothyronine (tri-i-o-do-THI-ro-nin), is T_3. These hormones function to increase the rate of metabolism in body cells. In particular, they increase energy metabolism and protein metabolism. Thyroid hormones are necessary along with growth hormones for normal growth to occur.

The thyroid gland needs an adequate supply of iodine in the blood to produce these hormones. Iodine deficiency is rare now due to widespread availability of this mineral in vegetables, seafood, dairy products, and processed foods.

Another hormone produced by the thyroid gland is *calcitonin* (kal-sih-TO-nin), which is active in calcium metabolism. This hormone is discussed later in connection with the parathyroid gland.

The Parathyroid Glands

Behind the thyroid gland, and embedded in its capsule, are four tiny *parathyroid glands* (Fig. 11-4). The secretion of these glands, *parathyroid hormone (PTH),* is one of three substances that regulate calcium metabolism. The other two hormones are *calcitonin* and *hydroxycholecalciferol* (hi-drok-se-ko-le-kal-SIF-eh-rol)

Calcium Metabolism

PTH promotes the release of calcium from bone tissue, thus increasing the amount of calcium circulating in the bloodstream. PTH also causes the kidney to retain calcium. Calcitonin, produced by the thyroid gland, lowers the amount of calcium circulating in the blood. Calcitonin does this by promoting the deposit of calcium in bone tissue. Hydroxycholecalciferol, the active form of vitamin D, is produced by modification of the vitamin in the liver and then the kidney. Hydroxycholecalciferol increases absorption of calcium by the intestine to raise blood calcium levels. These three substances work together to regulate the amount of calcium in the blood and provide calcium for bone maintenance and other functions.

✔ CHECKPOINT **5**:

What mineral is regulated by parathyroid hormone?

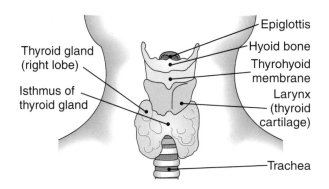

FIGURE **11•3** Thyroid gland (anterior view) in relation to the larynx and trachea.

Thyroid gland (right lobe)
Isthmus of thyroid gland
Epiglottis
Hyoid bone
Thyrohyoid membrane
Larynx (thyroid cartilage)
Trachea

The Adrenal Glands

The *adrenals,* or *suprarenals,* are two small glands located above the kidneys. Each adrenal gland has two parts that act as separate glands.

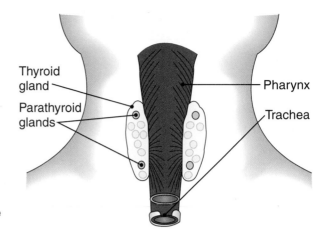

FIGURE **11•4** Posterior view of the thyroid gland showing the parathyroid glands embedded in its surface.

The inner area is called the **medulla,** and the outer portion is called the **cortex.**

Hormones From the Adrenal Medulla

The hormones of the adrenal medulla are released in response to stimulation by the sympathetic nervous system. The principal hormone produced by the medulla is **epinephrine,** also called **adrenaline.** Another hormone released from the adrenal medulla, **norepinephrine,** is closely related chemically and is similar in its actions to epinephrine. These two hormones are referred to as the *fight-or-flight hormones* because of their effects during emergency situations. We have already learned about these hormones in studying the autonomic nervous system. When released from nerve endings instead of being released directly into the bloodstream, they function as neurotransmitters.

Some of their effects are as follows:

* Stimulation of the involuntary muscle in the walls of the arterioles, causing these muscles to contract and blood pressure to rise accordingly
* Conversion of the glycogen stored in the liver into glucose. The glucose is poured into the blood and brought to the voluntary muscles, permitting them to do an extraordinary amount of work
* Increase in the heart rate
* Increase in the metabolic rate of body cells
* Dilation of the bronchioles, through relaxation of the smooth muscle of their walls

> ✔ CHECKPOINT **6**:
>
> The main hormone from the adrenal medulla also functions as a neurotransmitter in the sympathetic nervous system. What is the name of this hormone?

Hormones From the Adrenal Cortex

There are three main groups of hormones secreted by the adrenal cortex:

* **Glucocorticoids** (glu-ko-KOR-tih-koyds) maintain the carbohydrate reserve of the body by promoting the conversion of amino acids into glucose (sugar) instead of protein. The production of these hormones increases in times of stress to aid the body in responding to unfavorable conditions. Glucocorticoids also have the ability to suppress the inflammatory response and are often administered as medication for this purpose. The major hormone of this group is **cortisol,** which is also called *hydrocortisone.*
* **Mineralocorticoids** (min-er-al-o-KOR-tih-koyds) are important in the regulation of electrolyte balance. They control the reabsorption of sodium and the secretion of potassium by the kidney tubules. The major hormone of this group is **aldosterone** (al-DOS-ter-one).
* **Sex hormones** are normally secreted, but in small amounts; their effects in the body are slight.

✔ CHECKPOINT **7**:

What effect does cortisol have on glucose levels in the blood?

The Pancreas

Hormones of the Pancreas

Scattered throughout the **pancreas** are small groups of specialized cells called **islets** (I-lets), also known as the **islets of Langerhans** (LAHNG-er-hanz). A microscopic view of the pancreas showing the islet cells is presented in Figure 11-5. These cells make up the endocrine portion of the pancreas and function independently from the exocrine part of the pancreas, which produces digestive juices and releases them through ducts. The most important hormone secreted by these islets is **insulin.**

Insulin is active in the transport of glucose across plasma membranes. Once inside a cell, glucose is metabolized for energy. Insulin also increases the rate at which the liver changes excess glucose into fatty acids, which can then be converted to fats and stored in adipose tissue. Through these actions, insulin has the effect of lowering the level of sugar in the blood. Insulin has other metabolic effects as well. It promotes the uptake of amino acids into cells and improves the manufacture of these amino acids into proteins.

A second hormone produced by the islet cells is **glucagon** (GLU-kah-gon), which works with insulin to regulate blood sugar levels. Glucagon causes the liver to release stored glucose into the bloodstream. Glucagon also increases the rate at which glucose is made from proteins in the liver. In these two ways, glucagon increases blood sugar.

✔ CHECKPOINT **8**:

What two hormones produced by the islets of the pancreas act to regulate glucose levels in the blood?

The Sex Glands

The sex glands, the ovaries of the female and the testes of the male, not only produce the sex cells but also are important endocrine organs. The hormones produced by these organs are needed in the development of the sexual characteristics, which usually appear in the early teens, and for the maintenance of the reproductive organs once full development has been attained. Those features that typify a male or female other than the structures directly concerned with reproduction are termed **secondary sex characteristics.** They include a deep voice and facial and body hair in males, and wider hips and a greater ratio of fat to muscle in females.

acini (digestive cells)

pancreatic islet

blood vessel

FIGURE **11•5**   Microscopic view of pancreatic cells. Light staining islet cells are seen among the cell clusters (acini) that produce digestive juices. (Courtesy of Dana Morse Bittus and B. J. Cohen)

Hormones of the Sex Glands

The main male sex hormone or **androgen** (AN-dro-jen) produced by the male sex glands is **testosterone** (tes-TOS-ter-one).

In the female, the hormones that most nearly parallel testosterone in their actions are the **estrogens** (ES-tro-jens). Estrogens contribute to the development of the female secondary sex characteristics and stimulate the development of the mammary glands, the onset of menstruation, and the development and functioning of the reproductive organs.

The other hormone produced by the female sex glands, called **progesterone** (pro-JES-ter-one), assists in the normal development of pregnancy. All the sex hormones are discussed in more detail in Chapter 20.

 CHECKPOINT **9**:

In addition to controlling reproduction, sex hormones confer certain features associated with male and female gender. What are these features called as a group?

The Thymus Gland

The **thymus gland** is a mass of lymphoid tissue that lies in the upper part of the chest above the heart. This gland is important in the development of immunity. Its hormone, **thymosin** (THI-mo-sin), assists in the maturation of certain white blood cells known as T cells (T lymphocytes) after they have left the thymus gland and taken up residence in lymph nodes throughout the body.

The Pineal Gland

The **pineal** (PIN-e-al) **gland** is a small, flattened, cone-shaped structure located posterior to the midbrain and connected to the roof of the third ventricle. The pineal produces the hormone **melatonin** (mel-ah-TO-nin) during the dark period of each day. Little hormone is produced during daylight hours. This pattern of hormone secretion influences the regulation of sleep–wake cycles. Melatonin also appears to delay the onset of puberty.

OTHER HORMONE-PRODUCING TISSUES

Originally, the word *hormone* applied to the secretions of the endocrine glands only. The term now includes various substances produced in the body that have regulatory actions, either locally or at a distance from where they are produced. Many body tissues produce substances that have strong effects in regulating the local environment. Some of these other hormone-producing organs are the following:

- The stomach secretes a hormone that stimulates its digestive activity.
- The small intestine secretes hormones that stimulate the production of digestive juices and help regulate the process of digestion.
- The kidneys produce a hormone called **erythropoietin** (e-rith-ro-POY-eh-tin), which stimulates red blood cell production in the bone marrow. This hormone is produced when there is a decreased supply of oxygen in the blood.
- The atria of the heart produce a substance called **atrial natriuretic** (na-tre-u-RET-ik) **peptide (ANP)** in response to increased filling of the atria. ANP increases loss of sodium by the kidneys and lowers blood pressure.
- The **placenta** (plah-SEN-tah) produces several hormones during pregnancy. These cause changes in the uterine lining and, later in pregnancy, help to prepare the breasts for lactation. Pregnancy tests are based on the presence of placental hormones.

Prostaglandins

Prostaglandins (pros-tah-GLAN-dins) are a group of local hormones made by most body tissues. They are produced, act, and are rapidly inactivated in or close to the sites of origin. A bewildering array of functions has been ascribed to these substances. Some prostaglandins cause constriction of blood vessels, of bronchial tubes, and of the intestine, whereas others cause dilation of these same structures. Prostaglandins are active in promoting inflammation; certain anti-inflammatory drugs, such as aspirin, act by blocking the production of prostaglandins. Some of the prostaglandins have been used to induce labor or abortion and have been recommended as possible contraceptive agents.

Overproduction of prostaglandins by the uterine lining (endometrium) can cause painful cramps of the muscle of the uterus. Treatment with drugs that are prostaglandin inhibitors has been successful in some cases. Much has been written about these substances, and extensive research on them continues.

HORMONES AND STRESS

Stress in the form of physical injury, disease, emotional anxiety, and even pleasure calls forth a specific response from the body that involves both the nervous system and the endocrine system. The nervous system response, the "fight-or-flight" response, is mediated by parts of the brain, especially the hypothalamus, and by the autonomic nervous system. The hypothalamus also triggers the release of ACTH from the anterior pituitary. The hormones released from the adrenal cortex as a result of stimulation by ACTH raise the levels of glucose and other nutrients in the blood and inhibit inflammation. Growth hormone, thyroid hormones, sex hormones, and insulin may also be released.

These hormones help the body meet stressful situations. Unchecked, however, they are harmful to the body and may lead to such stress-related disorders as high blood pressure, heart disease, ulcers, back pain, and headaches. Cortisones decrease the immune response, leaving the body more open to infection.

Although no one would enjoy a life totally free of stress in the form of stimulation and challenge, unmanaged stress, or "distress," has negative effects on the body. For this reason, techniques such as biofeedback and meditation to control stress are useful. The simple measures of setting priorities, getting adequate periods of

Taking Control of the Stress in Your Life

In today's complicated world, everyday stress is a part of our normal routine. Every now and then the pressures build until we are "stressed out." Research has conclusively shown that this feeling is not simply in your mind but is a physiologic reaction to stress.

When we encounter a stressful event, our nervous system signals the adrenal medulla to secrete the hormones epinephrine and norepinephrine directly into the bloodstream. This results in similar effects as when these hormones are released from nerve endings upon stimulation of the sympathetic nervous system. The difference is, when the hormones are secreted directly into the bloodstream, their effects are as much as 3 to 5 times stronger, and last up to 10 times longer than when they are released from nerve endings. When we encounter excessive stress, both hormones build up in the bloodstream and cause adverse effects such as restlessness, feeling jittery, inability to concentrate, inability to eat or sleep, and ultimately significant fatigue and possibly depression. Most of these effects can be reduced or eliminated by techniques of stress reduction, for example:

- Biofeedback focuses on an unconscious process to bring it into conscious perception; with structured, focused thought, the process can often be changed.
- Transcendental meditation uses a repetition of a "mantra," a specific word closely associated with a process to control or change that process.
- Guided imagery uses pleasing music, natural sounds, and visual images to steal focus away from unpleasant stimuli.
- Repetitive physical modalities use a physical action (exercise) rather than a mantra to focus attention.
- Coordinated relaxation exercises such as slow, deep breathing or repetitive contraction and relaxation of muscles also focus the mind's control.

relaxation, and getting regular physical exercise are important in maintaining total health. See Taking Control of the Stress in Your Life.

✔ CHECKPOINT **10**:
_____

What are some hormones released in time of stress?

AGING AND THE ENDOCRINE SYSTEM

Some of the changes associated with aging, such as loss of muscle and bone tissue, can be linked to changes in the endocrine system. The main clinical conditions associated with the endocrine system involve the pancreas and the thyroid.

Many elderly people develop adult-onset diabetes mellitus as a result of decreased secretion of insulin, which is made worse by poor diet, inactivity, and increased body fat. Some elderly people also show the effects of decreased thyroid hormone secretion.

Decline in the sex hormones during the middle-aged years occurs in both males and females. These changes come from decreased activity of the gonads but also involve the more basic level of the pituitary gland and the secretion of gonadotropic hormones. Decrease in bone mass leading to osteoporosis is one result of these declines. With age, there is also a decrease in levels of growth hormone and diminished activity of the adrenal cortex.

Thus far, the only commonly applied treatment for endocrine failure associated with age has been sex hormone replacement therapy for women at menopause. This supplementation has shown beneficial effects on mucous membranes, the cardiovascular system, bone mass, and mental function.

Summary

I. Hormones
  A. Functions of hormones
   1. Affect other cells or organs—target tissue
   2. Widespread effects on growth, metabolism, reproduction
   3. Local effects
  B. Chemistry—chemical types
   1. Amino acid compounds—proteins and related compounds
   2. Steroids
      a. Derived from lipids
      b. Produced by adrenal cortex and sex glands
  C. Regulation of hormones—negative feedback

II. Endocrine glands and their hormones
  A. Pituitary
   1. Regulated by hypothalamus
      a. Anterior pituitary—releasing hormones sent through portal system
      b. Posterior pituitary—stores hormones; released by nervous stimulation
   2. Anterior lobe hormones
      a. Growth hormone (GH)
      b. Thyroid-stimulating hormone (TSH)
      c. Adrenocorticotropic hormone (ACTH)
      d. Prolactin (PRL)
      e. Follicle-stimulating hormone (FSH)
      f. Luteinizing hormone (LH)
   3. Posterior lobe hormones
      a. Antidiuretic hormone (ADH)
      b. Oxytocin
  B. Thyroid gland
   1. Hormones
      a. Thyroxine—influences cell metabolism
      b. Calcitonin—decreases blood calcium levels
  C. Parathyroid glands—secrete parathyroid hormone (PTH), which increases blood calcium levels

11

D. Adrenal glands
1. Hormones of adrenal medulla (inner region)
a. Epinephrine and norepinephrine—act as neurotransmitters
2. Hormones of adrenal cortex (outer region)
a. Glucocorticoids—released during stress; e.g., cortisol
b. Mineralocorticoids—regulate water and electrolyte balance; e.g., aldosterone
c. Sex hormones—produced in small amounts
E. Pancreas—islet cells of pancreas secrete hormones
1. Insulin
a. Lowers blood glucose
2. Glucagon
a. Raises blood glucose
F. Sex glands—needed for reproduction and development of secondary sex characteristics
1. Testes—secrete testosterone
2. Ovaries—secrete estrogen and progesterone
G. Thymus gland—secretes thymosin,

which aids in development of T lymphocytes
H. Pineal gland—secretes melatonin
1. Regulates sexual development and sleep–wake cycles
2. Controlled by environmental light

III. Other hormone-producing tissues
1. Stomach and small intestine—secrete hormones that regulate digestion
2. Kidneys—secrete erythropoietin, which increases production of red blood cells
3. Atria of heart—ANP causes loss of sodium by kidney and lowers blood pressure
4. Placenta—secretes hormones that maintain pregnancy and prepare breasts for lactation
A. Prostaglandins—other cells throughout body produce prostaglandins, which have varied effects

IV. Hormones and stress

V. Aging and the endocrine system

Questions for Study and Review

1. Compare the actions of the nervous system and the endocrine system.
2. Define *hormone.* Describe some general functions of hormones.
3. Give three examples of amino acid hormones; of steroid hormones.
4. Define *target tissue.*
5. Name the two divisions of the pituitary gland. Name the hormones released from each division and describe the effects of each.
6. What type of system connects the anterior pituitary with the hypothalamus? What is carried to the pituitary by this system?
7. Where is the thyroid gland located? What is its main hormone, and what does it do?
8. What is the main purpose of PTH?
9. Name the two divisions of the adrenal glands and describe the effects of the hormones from each.
10. What are the main purposes of insulin in the body? Name and describe the condition characterized by insufficient production of insulin.
11. Name the male and female sex hormones and briefly describe what each does.
12. Name the hormone produced by the thymus gland; by the pineal body. What are the effects of each?

13. Name five organs other than the endocrine glands that secrete hormones.
14. What are some of the various functions that have been ascribed to prostaglandins?
15. List several hormones that are released during stress.

✔ ANSWERS TO CHECKPOINTS

1. Hormones are chemicals that have specific regulatory effects on certain cells or organs in the body. Some of their effects are to regulate growth, metabolism, reproduction, and behavior.
2. Negative feedback is used to regulate the secretion of hormones.
3. The hypothalamus controls the pituitary.
4. The ending -*tropin* means a hormone that acts on another gland.
5. Thyroxine increases metabolism in cells.
6. The mineral calcium is regulated by PTH.
7. The main hormone from the adrenal medulla is epinephrine (adrenaline).
8. Cortisol raises the level of glucose in the blood.
9. The two hormones produced by the pancreatic islets that regulate glucose levels are insulin and glucagon.
10. Secondary sex characteristics are features associated with gender other than reproductive activity.
11. Some hormones released in time of stress are epinephrine, norepinephrine, ACTH, cortisol, growth hormone, thyroid hormones, sex hormones, and insulin.

11

The chapters of this unit discuss the blood, the heart, the blood vessels, and the lymphatic system as well as body defenses, immunity, and vaccines. It is the purpose of this unit to emphasize the importance of transportation and immune systems in maintaining normal body functions.

Unit IV

CIRCULATION AND BODY DEFENSE

The Blood

Chapter

12

SELECTED KEY TERMS

The following terms are defined in the Glossary:

agglutination

antiserum

coagulation

erythrocyte

fibrin

hematocrit

hemoglobin

hemostasis

leukocyte

plasma

platelet (thrombocyte)

serum

BEHAVIORAL OBJECTIVES

After careful study of this chapter, you should be able to:

1. List the functions of the blood
2. List the main ingredients in plasma
3. Name the three types of formed elements in the blood and give the function of each
4. Describe five types of leukocytes
5. Describe the formation of blood cells
6. Define hemostasis and cite three steps in hemostasis
7. Briefly describe the steps in blood clotting
8. Define *blood type* and explain the relation between blood type and transfusions
9. Describe the tests used to study blood

The circulating blood is of fundamental importance in maintaining homeostasis. This life-giving fluid brings nutrients and oxygen to the cells and carries away waste. Blood is pumped continuously by the heart through a closed system of vessels. The heart and blood vessels are described in Chapters 13 and 14.

Blood is classified as a connective tissue because nearly half of it is made up of cells. Blood cells share many characteristics of origination and development with other connective tissues. However, blood differs from other connective tissues in that its cells are not fixed in position; instead, they move freely in the liquid portion of the blood.

Blood is a viscous (thick) fluid that varies in color from bright scarlet to dark red, depending on how much oxygen it is carrying. The quantity of circulating blood differs with the size of the person; the average adult male, weighing 70 kg (154 pounds), has about 5 liters (5.2 quarts) of blood. This volume accounts for about 8% of total body weight.

FUNCTIONS OF THE BLOOD

The circulating blood serves the body in three ways: transportation, regulation, and protection.

Transportation

- Oxygen from inhaled air diffuses into the blood through the thin lung membranes and is carried to all the tissues of the body. Carbon dioxide, a waste product of cell metabolism, is carried from the tissues to the lungs, where it is breathed out.
- The blood transports nutrients and other needed substances, such as electrolytes (salts) and vitamins, to the cells. These materials may enter the blood from the digestive system or may be released into the blood from body stores.
- The blood transports the waste products from the cells to the sites from which they are released. For example, the kidney removes excess water, acid, electrolytes, and urea (a nitrogen-containing waste). The liver removes blood pigments, hormones, and drugs, and the lungs eliminate carbon dioxide.
- The blood carries hormones from their sites of origin to the organs they affect.

Regulation

- Buffers in the blood help keep the pH of body fluids at about 7.4. (The pH is a measure of the acidity of a solution.)

- The blood serves to regulate the amount of fluid in the tissues by means of substances (mainly proteins) that maintain the proper osmotic pressure.
- The blood transports heat that is generated in the muscles to other parts of the body, thus aiding in the regulation of body temperature.

Protection

- The blood is important in defense against disease. It carries the cells and antibodies of the immune system that protect against pathogens.
- The blood contains factors that protect against blood loss from the site of an injury.

CHECKPOINT 1:

What are some substances transported in the blood?

BLOOD CONSTITUENTS

The blood is divided into two main components. The liquid portion is the *plasma.* The *formed elements,* which include cells and cell fragments, fall into three categories, as follows:

- *Erythrocytes* (eh-RITH-ro-sites), from *erythro,* meaning "red," are the red blood cells, which transport oxygen.
- *Leukocytes* (LU-ko-sites), from *leuko,* meaning "white," are the several types of white blood cells, which protect against infection.
- *Platelets,* also called *thrombocytes* (THROM-bo-sites), are cell fragments that participate in blood clotting.

CHECKPOINT 2:

What are the two main components of blood?

Blood Plasma

More than half of the total volume of blood is plasma. The plasma itself is 90% water. Many different substances, dissolved or suspended in the water, make up the other 10%. The plasma content may vary somewhat because substances are removed and added as the blood circulates to and from the tissues. However, the body tends to maintain a fairly constant level of most substances. For example, the level of glucose, a simple sugar, is maintained at a remarkably constant level of about one tenth of one percent (0.1%) in solution.

After water, the next largest percentage of material in the plasma is *protein.* Proteins are the principal constituents of cytoplasm and are essential to the growth and the rebuilding of body tissues. The plasma proteins include the following:

- *Albumin* (al-BU-min), the most abundant protein in plasma, is important for maintaining the osmotic pressure of the blood. This protein is manufactured in the liver.
- *Clotting factors,* necessary for blood coagulation, are also manufactured in the liver.
- *Antibodies* combat infection.
- A system of enzymes made of several proteins, collectively known as *complement,* helps antibodies in their fight against pathogens (see Chap. 15).

Nutrients are also found in the plasma. The principal carbohydrate found in the plasma is *glucose,* which is absorbed by the capillaries of the intestine after digestion. Glucose is stored mainly in the liver as glycogen and is released as needed to supply energy.

Amino acids, the products of protein digestion, are also found in the plasma. These are also absorbed into the blood through the intestinal capillaries.

Lipids constitute a small percentage of blood plasma. Lipid components include fats, cholesterol, and lipoproteins, which are proteins bound to cholesterol.

The *electrolytes* in the plasma appear primarily as chloride, carbonate, or phosphate salts of sodium, potassium, calcium, and magnesium. These salts have a variety of functions, including the formation of bone (calcium and phosphorus), the production of certain hormones (such as iodine for the production of thyroid hormones), and the maintenance of the acid–base balance (sodium and potassium carbonates and phosphates).

Other materials, such as vitamins, hormones, waste products, and drugs, also are transported in the plasma.

✔ CHECKPOINT **3**:

Next to water, what is the most abundant type of substance in plasma?

The Formed Elements

Erythrocytes

Erythrocytes, the red blood cells (RBCs, or red cells), are tiny, disk-shaped bodies with a central area that is thinner than the edges (Fig. 12-1). They are different from other cells in that the mature form found in the circulating blood is lacking a nucleus and most of the other organelles commonly found in cells. As red cells mature, these components are lost to provide more space for the cells to carry oxygen. This vital gas is bound in the red cells to **hemoglobin** (he-mo-GLO-bin), a protein that contains iron (see Hemoglobin). Hemoglobin, combined with oxygen, gives the blood its characteristic red color. The more oxygen carried by the hemoglobin, the brighter is the red color of the blood. Therefore, the blood that goes from the lungs to the tissues is a bright red because it carries a great supply of oxygen; in contrast, the blood that returns to the lungs is a much darker red because it has given up much of its oxygen to the tissues.

Hemoglobin has two lesser functions in addition to the transport of oxygen. Hemoglobin that has given up its oxygen is able to carry hydrogen ions. In this way, hemoglobin acts as a buffer and plays an important role in acid–base balance (see Chap. 19). Hemoglobin also carries some carbon dioxide from the tissues to the

Hemoglobin

The hemoglobin molecule is a protein made of four chains of amino acids (the "globin" part of the molecule), each of which holds an iron-containing "heme" unit. It is the heme portion that binds oxygen.

Hemoglobin allows the blood to carry much more oxygen than it could carry simply dissolved in the plasma. Hemoglobin picks up oxygen in the lungs and releases it in the body tissues. When cells are active, they need more oxygen. At the same time, they generate heat and acidity. These changing conditions promote the release of oxygen from hemoglobin.

Hemoglobin is produced by red cells in the red bone marrow. It is constantly broken down as the red cells die and disintegrate. Some of its components are recycled, but dietary protein and iron are still essential to maintain supplies.

12

lungs for elimination. The carbon dioxide is bound to a different part of the molecule than the part that holds oxygen, so that it does not interfere with oxygen transport.

The ability of hemoglobin to carry oxygen can be blocked by carbon monoxide. This harmful gas combines with hemoglobin to form a stable compound that can severely restrict the ability of the erythrocytes to carry oxygen. Carbon monoxide is a byproduct of the incomplete burning of fuels, such as gasoline and other petroleum products and coal, wood, and other carbon-containing materials. It also occurs in cigarette smoke and automobile exhaust.

The erythrocytes are by far the most numerous of the blood cells, averaging from 4.5 to 5 million per cubic millimeter (mm^3) of blood. (A cubic millimeter is the same as a microliter [uL], one millionth of a liter, another way of expressing the concentration of blood cells.) Because mature red cells have no nucleus and cannot divide, they must be replaced constantly. The production of red cells is stimulated by the hormone **erythropoietin** (eh-rith-ro-POY-eh-tin). This hormone is released from

neutrophil

eosinophil

basophil

blood smear

red blood cells and platelets

lymphocyte

A

monocyte

B

FIGURE 12•1   **(A)** Normal blood smear and close-up view of individual blood cells. **(B)** Red blood cells as seen by scanning electron microscopy.

the kidney in response to a decrease in oxygen supply.

✔ CHECKPOINT **4**:

Red cells are modified to carry a maximum amount of hemoglobin. What is the function of hemoglobin?

Leukocytes

The **leukocytes,** or white blood cells (WBCs, or white cells), are different from the erythrocytes in appearance, quantity, and function (see Fig. 12-1). The cells themselves are round, but they contain prominent nuclei of varying shapes and sizes. Occurring at a concentration of 5,000 to 10,000 per cubic millimeter of blood, leukocytes are outnumbered by red cells by about 700 to 1.

Although the red cells have a definite color, the leukocytes tend to be colorless.

The different types of white cells are identified by their size, the shape of the nucleus, and the appearance of granules in the cytoplasm when the cells are stained (Table 12-1). The stain commonly used for blood is Wright's stain. This is a mixture of dyes that differentiates the various cells in blood. The relative percentage of the different types of leukocytes is a valuable clue in arriving at a medical diagnosis.

The granular leukocytes, or **granulocytes** (GRAN-u-lo-sites), are so named because they show visible granules in the cytoplasm when stained. They include the following:

- **Neutrophils** (NU-tro-fils), which show lavender granules
- **Eosinophils** (e-o-SIN-o-fils), which have beadlike, bright pink granules
- **Basophils** (BA-so-fils), which have large, dark blue granules that often obscure the nucleus

The neutrophils, which are active in fighting infections, are the most numerous of the white cells, constituting up to 60% of all leukocytes. The eosinophils and basophils make up a small percentage of the white cells but increase in number during allergic reactions.

Because the nuclei of the neutrophils are of various shapes, they are also called **poly-morphs** (meaning "many forms") or simply *polys*. Other nicknames are *segs*, referring to the segmented nucleus, and *PMNs*, an abbreviation of *polymorphonuclear neutrophils*. Before reaching full maturity and becoming segmented, the nucleus of the neutrophil looks like a thick, curved band. An increase in the number of these **band cells** (also called *stab* or *staff cells*) is a sign of infection and active production of neutrophils.

The agranular leukocytes, or **agranulocytes,** are so named because they lack easily visible granules. There are two types:

- **Lymphocytes** (LIM-fo-sites) are the second most numerous of the white cells and are active in immunity.
- **Monocytes** (MON-o-sites) are the largest in size. They function as phagocytes.

Function of Leukocytes

The most important function of leukocytes is to destroy pathogens. Whenever pathogens enter the tissues, as through a wound, certain white cells (neutrophils and monocytes) are attracted to that area. They leave the blood vessels and proceed by ameboid (ah-ME-boyd), or ameba-like, motion to the area of infection. There, they engulf the invaders by the process of **phagocytosis** (fag-o-si-TO-sis) (Fig. 12-2). In battling pathogens, leukocytes may be destroyed. A mixture of dead and living bacteria, together with dead and living leukocytes, forms **pus**. A collection of pus localized in one area is known as an **abscess**.

Some monocytes enter the tissues, enlarge, and mature into **macrophages** (MAK-ro-faj-ez), which are highly active in disposing of invaders or foreign material. Some lymphocytes become **plasma cells,** active in the production of circulating antibodies needed for immunity. The activities of the various white cells are further discussed in Chapter 15.

Table 12•1	Leukocytes (White Blood Cells)	
TYPE OF CELL	RELATIVE PERCENTAGE (ADULT)	FUNCTION
Granulocytes		
Neutrophils (NU-tro-fils)	54%–62%	Phagocytosis
Eosinophils (e-o-SIN-o-fils)	1%–3%	Allergic reactions: defense against parasites
Basophils (BA-so-fils)	< 1%	Allergic reactions; inflammatory reactions
Agranulocytes		
Lymphocytes (LIM-fo-sites)	25%–38%	Immunity (T cells and B cells)
Monocytes (MON-o-sites)	3%–7%	Phagocytosis

✔ CHECKPOINT **5**:

What is the most important function of leukocytes?

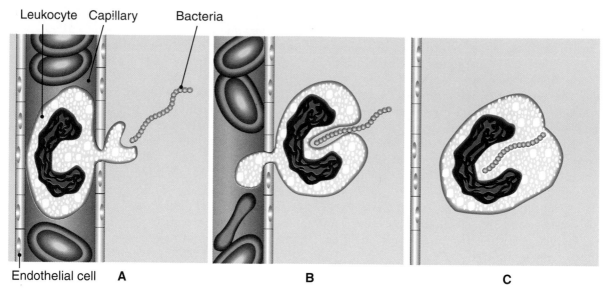

Leukocyte   Capillary   Bacteria

Endothelial cell   **A**   **B**   **C**

FIGURE **12•2**   Phagocytosis. **(A)** White blood cell squeezes through a capillary wall in the region of an infection. **(B, C)** White cells engulfs the bacteria.

Platelets

Of all the formed elements, the blood ***platelets*** (thrombocytes) are the smallest (see Fig. 12-1). These tiny structures are not cells in themselves but rather fragments of cells. The number of platelets in the circulating blood has been estimated to range from 150,000 to 450,000 per cubic millimeter.

Platelets are essential to blood ***coagulation*** (clotting). When, as a result of injury, blood comes in contact with any tissue other than the innermost lining of the blood vessels, the platelets stick together and form a plug that seals the wound. The platelets then release chemicals that participate in the formation of a clot to stop blood loss. More details on these reactions are given later.

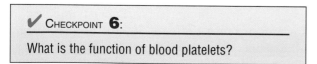

✔ CHECKPOINT **6**:

What is the function of blood platelets?

Origin of the Formed Elements

All of the formed elements of the blood are produced in red marrow, which is located in the ends of long bones and in the inner mass of all other bones. The ancestors of the blood cells are called ***stem cells.*** Each kind of stem cell develops into one of the blood cell types found within the red marrow.

One group of white cells, the lymphocytes, develops to maturity in lymphoid tissue and can multiply in this tissue as well (see Chap. 15). When an invader enters the tissues, the bone marrow and lymphoid tissue go into emergency production of white cells, and their number increases enormously as a result. Detection in a blood examination of an abnormally large number of white cells is an indication of infection.

The platelets are believed to originate in the red marrow as fragments of certain giant cells called ***megakaryocytes*** (meg-ah-KAR-e-o-sites), which are formed in the red marrow. Platelets do not have nuclei or DNA, but they do contain active enzymes and mitochondria.

Life-Span of the Blood Cells

The life-span of the different types of blood cells varies considerably. For example, after leaving the bone marrow, erythrocytes circulate in the bloodstream for about 120 days. Leukocytes may appear in the circulating blood for only 6 to 8 hours. They may then enter the tissues, where they survive for longer periods—days, months, or even years. Blood platelets have a life-span of about 10 days.

In comparison with other tissue cells, most of those in the blood are short lived. The need for constant replacement of blood cells means that normal activity of the red bone marrow is absolutely essential to life.

✔ CHECKPOINT **7**:

Where do blood cells form?

HEMOSTASIS

Hemostasis (he-mo-STA-sis) is the process that prevents the loss of blood from the circulation when a blood vessel is ruptured by an injury. Events in hemostasis include the following:

- *Contraction* of the smooth muscles in the wall of the blood vessel. This reduces the flow of blood and loss from the defect in the vessel wall. The term for this reduction in the diameter of a vessel is *vasoconstriction*.
- Formation of a *platelet plug*. Activated platelets become sticky and adhere to the defect to form a temporary plug.
- Formation of a *blood clot*.

Blood Clotting

The many substances necessary for blood clotting, or coagulation, are normally inactive in the bloodstream. A balance is maintained between compounds that promote clotting, known as *procoagulants,* and those that prevent clotting, known as *anticoagulants.* In addition, there are chemicals in the circulation that act to dissolve any clots that may form. Under normal conditions, the substances that prevent clotting prevail. When an injury occurs, however, the procoagulants are activated, and a clot is formed.

The clotting process is a well-controlled series of separate events involving 12 different factors. The final step in these reactions is the conversion of a plasma protein called *fibrinogen* (fi-

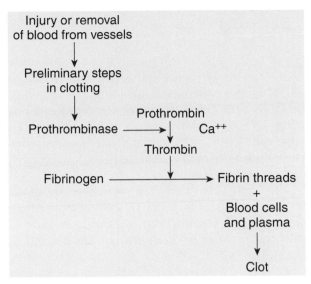

FIGURE **12•3**   Final steps in the formatin of a blood clot.

BRIN-o-jen) into solid threads of *fibrin,* which form the clot.

A few of the final steps involved in the formation of a blood clot are described below and diagrammed in Figure 12-3:

- Substances released from damaged tissues result in the formation of *prothrombinase* (pro-THROM-bih-nase), a substance that triggers the final clotting mechanism.
- Prothrombinase converts prothrombin in the blood to *thrombin.* Calcium is needed for this step.
- Thrombin, in turn, converts soluble fibrinogen into insoluble fibrin. *Fibrin* forms a network of threads that entraps plasma and blood cells to form a clot.

Blood clotting occurs in response to injury. Blood also clots when it comes into contact with some surface other than the innermost lining of a blood vessel, such as a glass or plastic tube used for a blood specimen. In this case, the preliminary steps of clotting are somewhat different and require more time. The fluid that remains after clotting has occurred is called *serum* (plural, *sera*). Serum contains all the components of blood plasma *except* the clotting factors.

Several methods used to measure the body's ability to coagulate blood are described later in this chapter.

BLOOD TYPES

If for some reason the amount of blood in the body is severely reduced, through **hemorrhage** (HEM-eh-rij) (excessive bleeding) or disease, the body cells suffer from lack of oxygen and nutrients. One possible measure to take in such an emergency is to administer blood from another person into the veins of the patient, a procedure called **transfusion.**

Care must be taken in transferring blood from one person to another, however, because the patient's plasma may contain substances, called *antibodies* or *agglutinins*, that can cause the red cells of the donor's blood to rupture and release their hemoglobin. Such cells are said to be **hemolyzed** (HE-mo-lized), and the resulting condition can be dangerous.

Certain proteins, called *antigens* (AN-ti-jens) or *agglutinogens,* on the surface of the red cells cause these incompatibility reactions. There are many types of these proteins on blood cells, but only two groups are particularly likely to cause a transfusion reaction, the so-called A and B antigens and the Rh factor.

The ABO Blood Type Group

Four blood types involving the A and B antigens have been recognized: A, B, AB, and O (Table 12-2). These letters indicate the type of antigen present on the red cells. If only the A antigen is present on the red cells, the person has type A blood; if only the B antigen is present, he or she has type B blood. Type AB red cells have both antigens, and type O have neither. Of course no one has antibodies to his or her own blood type antigens, or their plasma would destroy their own cells. Each person does, however, develop antibodies that react with the AB antigens he or she is lacking. It is these antibodies in the patient's plasma that can react the antigens on the donor's red cells to cause a transfusion reaction.

Testing for Blood Type

Blood sera containing antibodies to the A or B antigens are used to test for blood type. These antisera are prepared in animals using either the A or the B antigens to induce a response. Blood serum containing antibodies that can agglutinate and destroy red cells with A antigen on the surface is called **anti-A serum;** blood serum containing antibodies that can destroy red cells with B antigen on the surface is called **anti-B serum.** When combined with a blood sample in the laboratory, each antiserum causes the corresponding red cells to clump together in a process known as **agglutination** (ah-glu-tih-NA-shun). The blood's pattern of agglutination, when mixed *separately* with these two sera, reveals its blood type (Fig. 12-4). Type A reacts with anti-A serum only; type B reacts with anti-B serum only. Type AB agglutinates with both, and type O agglutinates with neither A nor B.

A blood specimen from any person who has had a prior blood transfusion or a pregnancy is tested further for the presence of any less common antibodies. Both the red cells and the serum are tested separately for any possible cross-reactions with donor blood.

Blood Compatibility

A person's blood type is determined by heredity, and the percentage of people with each of the different blood types varies in different populations. About 45% of the white population of the United States has type O blood.

In an emergency, type O blood can be given to any ABO type because the cells lack both A and

	RED BLOOD CELL	REACTS WITH	PLASMA	CAN TAKE	CAN
BLOOD TYPE	ANTIGEN	ANTISERUM	ANTIBODIES	FROM	DONATE TO
A	A	Anti-A	Anti-B	A, O	A, AB
B	B	Anti-B	Anti-A	B, O	B, AB
AB	A, B	Anti-A, Anti-B	None	AB, A, B, O	AB
O	None	None	Anti-A, anti-B	O	O, A, B, AB

Table 12•2 **The ABO Blood Group System**

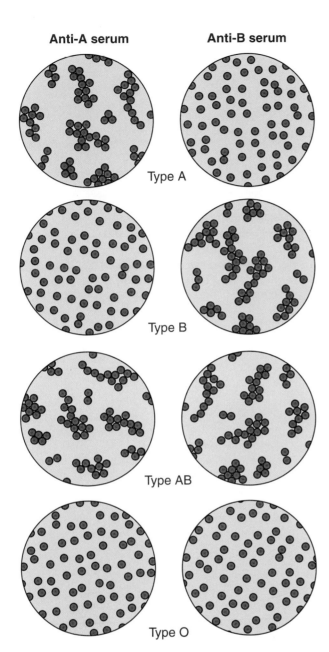

Anti-A serum   **Anti-B serum**

Type A

Type B

Type AB

Type O

FIGURE **12•4** Blood typing. Red cells in type A blood are agglutinated (clumped) by anti-A serum; those in type B blood are agglutinated by anti-B serum. Type AB blood cells are agglutinated by both sera, and type O blood is not agglutinated by either serum.

B antigens and will not react with either A or B antibodies. Conversely, type AB blood contains no antibodies to agglutinate red cells, and people with this blood type can therefore receive blood from any ABO type donor (see Table 12-2). Under normal circumstances, it is safest to give blood of the same type.

The Rh Factor

More than 85% of the population of the United States has another red cell antigen group called the **Rh factor,** named for *Rh*esus monkeys, in which it was first found. Rh is also known as the *D antigen*. People with this antigen are said to be **Rh positive;** those who lack this protein are said to be **Rh negative.** If Rh-positive blood is given to an Rh-negative person, he or she may produce antibodies to the "foreign" Rh antigens. The blood of this "Rh-sensitized" person will then destroy any Rh-positive cells received in a later transfusion.

Rh incompatibility is a potential problem in certain pregnancies. A mother who is Rh negative may develop antibodies to the Rh protein of an Rh-positive fetus (the fetus having inherited this factor from the father). Red cells from the fetus that enter the mother's circulation during pregnancy and childbirth evoke the response. In a subsequent pregnancy with an Rh-positive fetus, some of the anti-Rh antibodies may pass from the mother's blood into the blood of her fetus and destroy the fetus's red cells. This condition is called **hemolytic disease of the newborn** (HDN). HDN is now prevented by administration of immune globulin $Rh_o(D)$, trade name Rho-GAM, to the mother during pregnancy and shortly after delivery. These preformed antibodies clear the mother's circulation of Rh antigens and prevent stimulation of an immune system response. In many cases, a baby born with HDN could be saved by a transfusion during which much of the baby's blood is replaced with Rh-negative blood.

✔ CHECKPOINT **8**:

What are the blood antigens most often involved in incompatibility reactions?

BLOOD STUDIES

Many kinds of studies can be done on blood, and some of these have become a standard part of a routine physical examination. Machines that are able to perform several tests at the same time have largely replaced manual procedures, particularly in large institutions.

The Hematocrit

The **hematocrit** (he-MAT-o-krit), the volume percentage of red cells in whole blood, is determined by spinning of a blood sample in a high-speed centrifuge for 3 to 5 minutes. In this way, the cellular elements are separated out from the plasma.

The hematocrit is expressed as the volume of packed red cells per unit volume (100 mL) of whole blood. For example, if a laboratory report states "hematocrit, 38%," that means that there are 38 mL red cells per 100 mL whole blood. In other words, 38% of the whole blood is red cells. For adult men, the normal range is 42 to 54 mL per 100 mL blood, whereas for adult women the range is slightly lower, 36 to 46 mL per 100 mL blood. These normal ranges, like all normal ranges for humans, may vary depending on the method used and the interpretation of the results by an individual laboratory. Hematocrit values much below or much above these figures point to an abnormality requiring further study.

Hemoglobin Tests

A sufficient amount of hemoglobin in red cells is required for adequate delivery of oxygen to the tissues. To measure its level, the hemoglobin is released from the red cells, and the color of the blood is compared with a known color scale. Hemoglobin is expressed in grams per 100 mL (dL) whole blood. Normal hemoglobin concentrations for adult males range from 14 to 17 g per 100 mL blood. Values for adult women are in a somewhat lower range, at 12 to 15 g per 100 mL blood. A decrease in hemoglobin to below normal levels signifies anemia.

Normal and abnormal types of hemoglobin can be separated and measured by the process of **electrophoresis** (e-lek-tro-fo-RE-sis). In this procedure, an electric current is passed through the liquid that contains the hemoglobin. This test is useful in the diagnosis of sickle cell anemia and other disorders caused by abnormal types of hemoglobin.

See Preventing Nutritional Anemia.

Preventing Nutritional Anemia

The term "anemia" has long been misused as a primary diagnosis. In its correct usage, the term refers to a set of complex signs and symptoms that are generally related to a decrease in numbers of red blood cells (RBC) and/or hemoglobin (Hb) in the blood. Nutritional anemias may be caused by deficiencies of iron, vitamin C, vitamin B_{12}, and folate. They are usually easily controlled through changes in dietary intake. Not recognizing and therefore not treating even mild anemias could be a serious mistake, since the presence of any type of anemia indiciates an underlying disorder. To avoid nutritional anemias:

- Make sure your diet contains ample iron. Because iron is poorly absorbed from the intestines, most individuals barely meet the recommended dietary allowance (RDA). This can be especially important in women who lose iron through menstruation, lactation, or any other blood loss. The best sources of dietary iron are red meats; although vegetables and bran also contain iron, it is not as readily absorbed as the iron in meat.

- Increase vitamin C intake if needed. Vitamin C (ascorbic acid) is known to directly effect absorption of iron from the intestinal tract. Vitamin C deficiency inevitably leads to anemia. Eating citrus fruits and green leafy vegetables will ensure enough vitamin C to have adequate iron absorption.

- Build up stores of vitamin B_{12} in your body. Vitamin B_{12} deficiency also leads to anemia. This vitamin is found in red meats (especially liver), eggs, milk, and red vegetables, such as red cabbage and beets. B_{12} can only be absorbed from a full stomach as digestive proteins and enzymes are necessary for its absorption.

- Take in plenty of folate. Both vitamin B_{12} and folate are needed for the maturation of red cells. Folate is found in many plant and animal tissues and is absorbed from the large intestine. Foods high in folate are green leafy vegetables, yeasts, liver, and mushrooms. Inadequate intake of folate is common and many medications interfere with its absorption, as does alcohol.

Blood Cell Counts

Most laboratories use automated methods for obtaining the data for blood counts. Visual counts are sometimes done using a **hemocytometer** (he-mo-si-TOM-eh-ter), a ruled slide used to count the cells in a given volume of blood under the microscope.

The normal count for red cells varies from 4.5 to 5.5 million cells per cubic millimeter (µL) of blood. The leukocyte count varies from 5000 to 10,000 cells per cubic millimeter of blood.

It is difficult to count platelets directly because they are so small. More accurate counts can be obtained with automated methods. These counts are necessary for the evaluation of platelet loss (thrombocytopenia) such as occurs after radiation therapy or cancer chemotherapy. The normal platelet count ranges from 150,000 to 450,000 per cubic millimeter of blood, but counts may fall to 100,000 or less without causing serious bleeding problems. If a count is very low, a platelet transfusion may be given.

The Blood Slide (Smear)

In addition to the above tests, the **complete blood count** (CBC) includes the examination of a stained blood slide. In this procedure, a drop of blood is spread thinly and evenly over a glass slide, and a special stain (Wright's) is applied to differentiate the otherwise colorless white cells. The slide is then studied under the microscope. The red cells are examined for abnormalities in size, color, or shape and for variations in the percentage of immature forms. The number of platelets is estimated. Parasites, such as the malarial organism and others, may be found. In addition, a **differential white count** is done. This is an estimation of the percentage of each type of white cell in the smear. Because each type of white cell has a specific function, changes in their proportions can be a valuable diagnostic aid.

✔ CHECKPOINT **9**:

The hematocrit is a common blood test. What is a hematocrit?

Blood Chemistry Tests

Batteries of tests on blood serum are often done by machine. One machine, the Sequential Multiple Analyzer (SMA), provides for the running of some 20 tests per minute. Tests for electrolytes, such as sodium, potassium, chloride, and bicarbonate, as well as for blood glucose, blood urea nitrogen (BUN), and **creatinine** (kre-AT-in-in), another nitrogen waste product, may be performed at the same time.

Other tests check for enzymes. Increased levels of **CPK** (creatine phosphokinase), **LDH** (lactic dehydrogenase), and other enzymes indicate tissue damage, such as that which may occur in heart disease. An excess of **alkaline phosphatase** (FOS-fah-tase) could indicate a liver disorder or cancer involving bone.

Blood can be tested for amounts of lipids, such as cholesterol, triglycerides (fats), and lipoproteins, or for amounts of plasma proteins. Many of these tests help in evaluating disorders that may involve various vital organs. For example, the presence of more than the normal amount of glucose (sugar) dissolved in the blood, a condition called **hyperglycemia** (hi-per-gli-SE-me-ah), is found most frequently in patients with unregulated diabetes. Sometimes, several evaluations of sugar content are done after the administration of a known amount of glucose. This procedure is called the **glucose tolerance test** and is usually given along with another test that determines the amount of sugar in the urine. This combination of tests can indicate faulty cell metabolism. The list of blood chemistry tests is extensive and is constantly increasing. We may now obtain values for various hormones, vitamins, antibodies, and toxic or therapeutic drug levels.

Coagulation Studies

Nature prevents the excessive loss of blood from small vessels by the formation of a clot. Before surgery and under some other circumstances, it is important to know that the time required for coagulation to take place is within normal limits. Because clotting is a rather complex process involving many reactants, a delay may be due to a number of different causes, including lack of certain hormonelike substances, calcium salts, or vitamin K.

Each of the various clotting factors has been designated by a Roman numeral, ranging from I to XIII. Factor I is fibrinogen, factor II is prothrombin, factor III is tissue factor, and factor IV is assigned to calcium ions. The amounts of all these factors may be determined and evaluated on a percentage basis, aiding in the diagnosis and treatment of some bleeding disorders.

Additional tests for coagulation include tests for bleeding time, clotting time, capillary strength, and platelet function.

Summary

I. Functions of the blood
  A. Transportation—of oxygen, carbon dioxide, nutrients, minerals, vitamins, hormones, waste
  B. Regulation—of pH, fluid balance, body temperature
  C. Protection—against foreign organisms, blood loss

II. Blood constituents
  A. Plasma—liquid component
    1. Water—main ingredient
    2. Proteins—albumin, clotting factors, antibodies, complement
    3. Nutrients—carbohydrates, lipids, amino acids
    4. Electrolytes (minerals)
    5. Waste products
    6. Hormones and other materials
  B. The formed elements
    1. Erythrocytes (red cells)—carry oxygen bound to hemoglobin
    2. Leukocytes (white cells)
      a. Granulocytes—neutrophils (polymorphs, segs, PMNs), eosinophils, basophils
      b. Agranulocytes—lymphocytes, monocytes
    3. Platelets (thrombocytes)—necessary for blood clotting
  C. Origin of formed elements—produced in red bone marrow from stem cells

III. Hemostasis—prevention of blood loss
    1. Contraction of blood vessels
    2. Formation of platelet plug
    3. Formation of blood clot
  A. Blood clotting
    1. Regulators
      a. Procoagulants—promote clotting
      b. Anticoagulants—prevent clotting
    2. 12 clotting factors (I–XII)
    3. Final steps in blood clotting
      a. Prothrombinase converts prothrombin to thrombin
      b. Thrombin converts fibrinogen to solid threads of fibrin
      c. Threads form clot
    4. Serum—fluid that remains after blood has clotted

IV. Blood types
  A. ABO blood type group—types A, B, AB, and O
    1. Tested by mixing blood sample with antisera to different antigens
    2. Incompatible transfusions cause destruction of donor red cells
  B. Rh factor—positive or negative

V. Blood studies
  A. Hematocrit—measures percentage of packed red cells in whole blood
  B. Hemoglobin tests—color test, electrophoresis
  C. Blood cell counts
  D. Blood slide (smear)
  E. Blood chemistry tests—electrolytes, waste products, enzymes, glucose, hormones
  F. Coagulation studies—clotting factor assays, bleeding time, clotting time, capillary strength, platelet function

Questions for Study and Review

1. How does the color of blood vary with the amount of oxygenation?
2. What is the average total quantity of circulating blood?
3. Name the three main purposes of blood.
4. Name the two main fractions of blood.
5. Name four main types of proteins in blood plasma. What are their purposes?
6. Name some substances carried in blood plasma other than proteins.
7. Name and describe the three main types of formed elements in blood.
8. Describe the structure and function of erythrocytes.
9. Name and give the functions of the five types of leukocytes.
10. What are platelets and what is their function?
11. Where are blood cells formed?
12. Define *hemostasis*. Describe the three main steps in hemostasis.
13. Describe the three final steps in blood clotting.
14. Name the four blood types in the ABO system. What determines the different types?
15. What is the Rh factor? What proportion of the population of the United States possesses this factor? In what situations is this factor of medical importance? Why?
16. What does the hematocrit measure? Cite normal hematocrit ranges for males and females.
17. What can be learned by studying the blood smear? What is determined by a differential white count?
18. What are some evaluations made by blood chemistry tests?

✔ ANSWERS TO CHECKPOINTS

1. Some substances transported in blood are oxygen, carbon dioxide, nutrients, electrolytes, vitamins, hormones, urea, and toxins.
2. The two main divisions of the blood are the liquid portion or plasma, and the formed elements, which include the cells and cell fragments.
3. Protein is the most abundant type of substance in plasma aside from water.
4. The function of hemoglobin is to carry oxygen in the blood.
5. The main function of leukocytes is to destroy pathogens.
6. The blood platelets are essential to blood coagulation (clotting).
7. Blood cells form in the red bone marrow.
8. The blood antigens most often involved in incompatibility reactions are the A antigen, the B antigen, and the Rh antigen.
9. The hematocrit is the volume percentage of red cells in whole blood.

The Heart

SELECTED KEY TERMS

The following terms are defined in the Glossary:

atrium

coronary

diastole

echocardiograph

electrocardiograph

endocardium

epicardium

murmur

myocardium

pericardium

septum

systole

valve

ventricle

BEHAVIORAL OBJECTIVES

After careful study of this chapter, you should be able to:

1. Describe the three layers of the heart wall

2. Compare the functions of the right heart and left heart

3. Name the four chambers of the heart

4. Name the valves at the entrance and exit of each ventricle

5. Briefly describe blood circulation through the myocardium

6. Briefly describe the cardiac cycle

7. Name the components of the heart's conduction system

8. Explain the effects of the autonomic nervous system on the heart rate

9. List and define several terms that describe variations in heart rates

10. Explain what produces the two main heart sounds

11. Briefly describe four methods for studying the heart

CIRCULATION AND THE HEART

The next two chapters investigate the manner in which the blood delivers oxygen and nutrients to the cells and carries away the waste products of cell metabolism. This continuous one-way movement of the blood is known as its *circulation.* The prime mover that propels blood throughout the body is the *heart.* We shall have a look at the heart before going into the subject of the blood vessels in detail.

The heart is a muscular pump that drives the blood through the blood vessels. Slightly bigger than a fist, this organ is located between the lungs in the center and a bit to the left of the midline of the body. The strokes (contractions) of this pump average about 72 per minute and are carried on unceasingly for the whole of a lifetime.

The importance of the heart has been recognized for centuries. The fact that its rate of beating is affected by the emotions may be responsible for the frequent references to the heart in song and poetry. However, the vital functions of the heart and its disorders are of more practical importance to us.

STRUCTURE OF THE HEART

Layers of the Heart Wall

The heart is a hollow organ, the walls of which are formed of three different layers. Just as a warm coat might have a smooth lining, a thick and bulky interlining, and an outer layer of a third fabric, so the heart wall has three tissue layers (Fig. 13-1). Starting with the innermost layer, these are as follows:

- The *endocardium* (en-do-KAR-de-um) is a thin, smooth layer of cells that resembles squamous epithelium. This membrane lines the interior of the heart. Reinforced folds of this material form the valves of the heart.
- The *myocardium* (mi-o-KAR-de-um), the muscle of the heart, is the thickest layer and is responsible for pumping blood through the vessels. The unique structure of cardiac muscle is described in more detail later.
- The *epicardium* (ep-ih-KAR-de-um) forms the thin, outermost layer of the heart wall and is continuous with the serous lining of the fibrous sac that encloses the heart. These membranes together make up the *pericardium* (per-ih-KAR-de-um). The serous lining of the pericardial sac is separated from the epicardium on the heart surface by a thin film of fluid.

Special Features of the Myocardium

Cardiac muscle cells are lightly striated (striped) and have specialized partitions between the cells that appear faintly under the light microscope. These *intercalated*

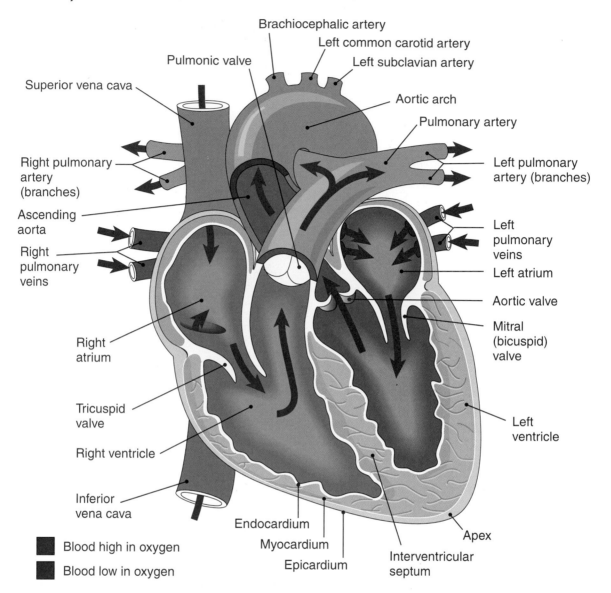

Brachiocephalic artery
Left common carotid artery
Left subclavian artery
Pulmonic valve
Aortic arch
Pulmonary artery
Superior vena cava
Right pulmonary artery (branches)
Left pulmonary artery (branches)
Ascending aorta
Right pulmonary veins
Left pulmonary veins
Left atrium
Aortic valve
Mitral (bicuspid) valve
Right atrium
Tricuspid valve
Right ventricle
Left ventricle
Inferior vena cava

Blood high in oxygen
Blood low in oxygen

Endocardium
Myocardium
Epicardium
Interventricular septum
Apex

FIGURE **13•1**   Heart and great vessels.

(in-TER-cah-la-ted) *disks* are actually modified cell membranes that allow for rapid transfer of electrical impulses between the cells. The adjective *intercalated* means "inserted between."

Another feature of cardiac muscle tissue is the branching of the muscle fibers (cells). These fibers are interwoven so that the stimulation that causes the contraction of one fiber results in the contraction of a whole group. These structural features play an important role in the working of the heart muscle.

 CHECKPOINT **1**:

What are the names of the innermost, middle, and outermost layers of the heart?

Two Hearts and a Partition

Health care professionals often refer to the *right heart* and the *left heart*. This is because the human heart is really a double pump (Fig. 13-2).

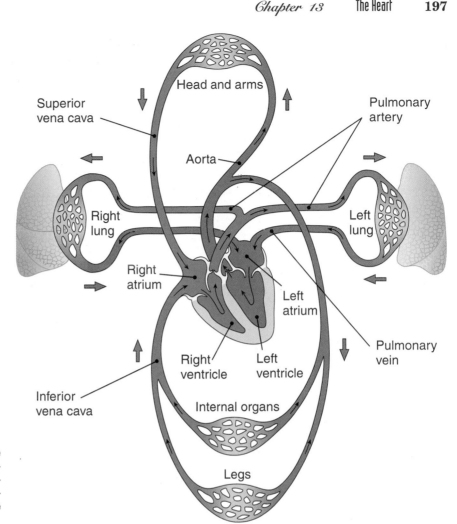

FIGURE **13•2** The heart is a double pump. The pulmonary circuit carries blood to the lungs to be oxygenated; the systemic circuit carries blood to all other parts of the body.

The right side pumps blood low in oxygen to the lungs through the ***pulmonary circuit.*** The left side pumps oxygenated blood to the remainder of the body through the ***systemic circuit.*** The two sides are completely separated from each other by a partition called the ***septum.*** The upper part of this partition is called the ***interatrial*** (in-ter-A-tre-al) ***septum,*** and the larger, lower portion is called the ***interventricular*** (in-ter-ven-TRIK-u-lar) ***septum.*** The septum, like the heart wall, consists largely of myocardium.

Four Chambers

On either side of the heart are two chambers. The upper chamber is a receiving chamber, the ***atrium*** (A-tre-um); the lower one is a pumping chamber, the ***ventricle*** (VEN-trih-kl) (see Fig. 13-1). The chambers, listed in the order in which blood flows through them, are as follows:

1. The ***right atrium*** is a thin-walled chamber that receives the blood returning from the body tissues. This blood, which is low in oxygen, is carried in veins, the blood vessels leading back to the heart from the body tissues. The superior vena cava brings blood from the head, chest, and arms; the inferior vena cava delivers blood from the trunk and legs.
2. The ***right ventricle*** pumps the venous blood received from the right atrium into the lungs. It pumps into a large pulmonary trunk, which then divides into right and left pulmonary arteries, which branch to

Coronary arteries

Aortic
(semilunar) valve

Tricuspid valve

Mitral valve

FIGURE **13•3** Valves of the heart, seen from above, in the closed position.

the lungs. An artery is a vessel that takes blood from the heart to the tissues.

3. The *left atrium* receives blood high in oxygen content as it returns from the lungs in pulmonary veins.

4. The *left ventricle,* which is the chamber with the thickest wall, pumps oxygenated blood to all parts of the body. This blood goes first into the aorta (a-OR-tah), the largest artery, and then into the branching systemic arteries that take blood to the tissues. The lower pointed region of the heart, the *apex,* is formed by the left ventricle (see Fig. 13-1).

The chambers of the heart can be seen in anterior and posterior views in Figure 13-4, shown later.

✔ CHECKPOINT **2**:

The heart is divided into four chambers. What is the upper receiving chamber on each side called? What is the lower pumping chamber called?

Four Valves

One-way valves that direct the flow of blood through the heart are located at the entrance and the exit of each ventricle. The entrance valves are the *atrioventricular* (a-tre-o-ven-TRIK-u-lar) *valves;* the exit valves are the *semilunar* (sem-e-LU-nar) *valves.* (So named because each flap of these valves resembles a half-moon.) Each valve has a specific name, as follows:

- The *right atrioventricular (AV) valve* is also known as the *tricuspid* (tri-KUS-pid) *valve* because it has three cusps, or flaps, that open and close. When this valve is open, blood flows freely from the right atrium into the right ventricle. When the right ventricle begins to contract, however, the valve closes so that blood cannot return to the right atrium; this ensures forward flow into the pulmonary artery.

- The *left atrioventricular (AV) valve* is the bicuspid valve, but it is usually referred to as the *mitral* (MI-tral) *valve* (named for a miter, the pointed, two-sided hat worn by bishops). It has two heavy cusps that permit blood to flow freely from the left atrium into the left ventricle. The cusps close when the left ventricle begins to contract; this closure prevents blood from returning to the left atrium and ensures the forward flow of blood into the aorta. Both the tricuspid and mitral valves are attached by means of thin fibrous threads to muscles in the walls of the ventricles (shown in Fig. 13-6). The function of these threads, called the *chordae tendineae* (KOR-de ten-DIN-e-e), is to stabilize the valve flaps when the ventricles contract so that the force of the blood will not push them up into the atria. In this manner, they help to prevent a backflow of blood when the heart beats.

- The *pulmonic* (pul-MON-ik) *valve,* also called the *pulmonary valve,* is a semilunar valve located between the right ventricle and the pulmonary artery that leads to the lungs. As soon as the right ventricle has finished emptying itself, the valve closes to prevent blood on its way to the lungs from returning to the ventricle.

- The **aortic** (a-OR-tik) **valve** is a semilunar valve located between the left ventricle and the aorta. After contraction of the left ventricle, the aortic valve closes to prevent the flow of blood back from the aorta to the ventricle.

The appearance of the heart valves in the closed position is illustrated in Figure 13-3.

> ✔ CHECKPOINT **3**:
>
> What is the purpose of valves in the heart?

Blood Supply to the Myocardium

Only the endocardium comes into contact with the blood that flows through the heart chambers. Therefore, the myocardium must have its own blood vessels to provide oxygen and nourishment and to remove waste products. Together, these blood vessels provide the **coronary circulation.**

The main arteries that supply blood to the muscle of the heart are the **right** and **left coronary arteries** (Fig. 13-4). These arteries, which are the first to branch off the aorta, arise just above the aortic semilunar valve (see Fig. 13-3). They receive blood when the heart relaxes and branch to all regions of the heart muscle. After passing through capillaries in the myocardium, blood drains into the cardiac veins and finally into the **coronary sinus** for return to the right atrium.

> ✔ CHECKPOINT **4**:
>
> The heart must have its own system of vessels to supply it with blood. What name is given to this blood supply to the heart?

FUNCTION OF THE HEART

The Work of the Heart

Although the right and left sides of the heart are separated from each other, they work together. Blood is squeezed through the chambers

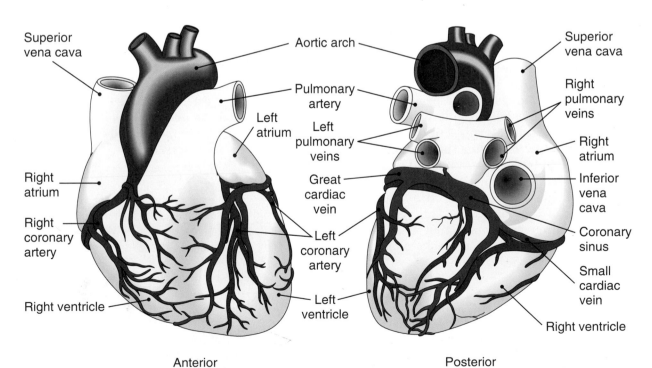

FIGURE **13•4** Coronary arteries and cardiac veins. (*left*) Anterior view, (*right*) Posterior view.

Diastole
Atria fill with blood which begins to flow into ventricles as soon as their walls relax.

Atrial systole
Contraction of atria pumps blood into the ventricles.

Ventricular systole
Contraction of ventricles pumps blood into aorta and pulmonary arteries.

FIGURE **13•5** Pumping cycle of the heart.

by a contraction of heart muscle beginning in the thin-walled upper chambers, the atria, followed by a contraction of the thick muscle of the lower chambers, the ventricles. This active phase is called *systole* (SIS-to-le), and in each case, it is followed by a resting period known as *diastole* (di-AS-to-le). The contraction of the walls of the atria is completed at the time the contraction of the ventricles begins. Thus, a resting phase (diastole) begins in the atria at the same time that a contraction (systole) begins in the ventricles. After the ventricles have emptied, both chambers are relaxed for a short period as they fill with blood. Then another beat begins with contraction of the atria followed by contraction of the ventricles. This sequence of heart relaxation and contraction is called the *cardiac cycle.* At rest, each cycle takes an average of 0.8 seconds (Fig. 13-5).

Cardiac Output

A unique property of heart muscle is its ability to adjust the strength of contraction to the amount of blood received. When the heart chamber is filled and the wall stretched (within limits), the contraction is strong. As less blood enters the heart, the contraction becomes less forceful. Thus, as more blood enters the heart, as occurs during exercise, the muscle contracts with greater strength to push the larger volume of blood out into the blood vessels.

The volume of blood pumped by each ventricle in 1 minute is termed the *cardiac output.* It is the product of the *stroke volume*—the volume of blood ejected from the ventricle with each beat—and the *heart rate*—the number of times the heart beats per minute (See Cardiac Reserve).

✔ CHECKPOINT **5**:

The cardiac cycle consists of an alternating pattern of contraction and relaxation. What name is given to the contraction phase? to the relaxation phase?

✔ CHECKPOINT **6**:

Cardiac output is the amount of blood pumped by each ventricle in 1 minute. What two factors determine cardiac output?

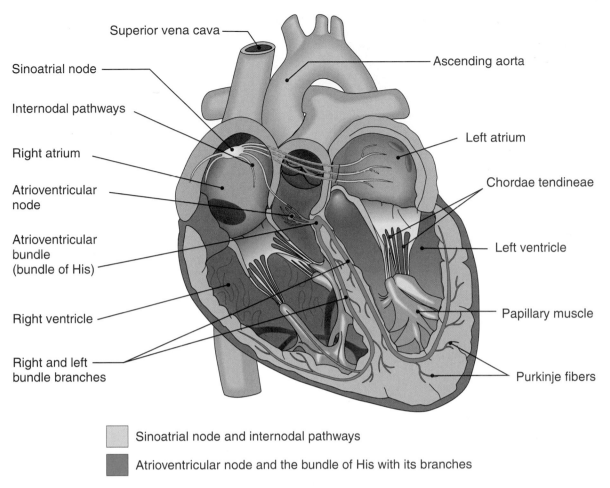

Superior vena cava

Sinoatrial node

Internodal pathways

Right atrium

Atrioventricular node

Atrioventricular bundle (bundle of His)

Right ventricle

Right and left bundle branches

Ascending aorta

Left atrium

Chordae tendineae

Left ventricle

Papillary muscle

Purkinje fibers

☐ Sinoatrial node and internodal pathways

■ Atrioventricular node and the bundle of His with its branches

FIGURE **13•6** Conduction system of the heart.

The Conduction System of the Heart

Like other muscles, the heart muscle is stimulated to contract by a wave of electrical energy that passes along the cells. This action potential is generated by specialized tissue within the heart and spreads over structures that form the heart's conduction system (Fig. 13-6). Two of these structures are tissue masses called *nodes.* In addition to the two nodes, there is a group of fibers called the *atrioventricular bundle,* which subdivides to branch through the myocardium.

The *sinoatrial (SA) node* is located in the upper wall of the right atrium. This node initiates the heartbeats by generating an action potential at regular intervals. Because the SA node sets the rate of heart contractions, it is called the *pacemaker.* The second node, located in the interatrial septum at the bottom of the right atrium, is called the *atrioventricular (AV) node.*

The *atrioventricular bundle,* also known as the *bundle of His,* is located at the top of the interventricular septum; it has branches that extend to all parts of the ventricular walls. Fibers travel first down both sides of the interventricular septum in groups called the *right* and *left bundle branches.* Smaller *Purkinje* (pur-KIN-je) *fibers* then travel in a branching network throughout the myocardium of the ventricles.

The special membranes between the cells (intercalated disks) allow the rapid flow of impulses throughout the heart muscle.

Cardiac Reserve

Like many other organs, the heart has great reserves of strength. The **cardiac reserve** is a measure of how many times more than average the heart can produce when needed. Based on a heart rate of 75 beats/minute and a stroke volume of 70 mL/beat, the average cardiac output for an adult at rest is about 5L/minute. This means that *at rest,* the heart pumps the equivalent of the total blood volume each minute.

During mild exercise, this volume might double and even double again during strenuous exercise. For most people the cardiac reserve is 4 to 5 times the resting output. In athletes exercising vigorously, the ratio may reach 6 to 7 times. In contrast, those with heart disease may have little or no cardiac reserve. They may be fine at rest but quickly become short of breath or fatigued when exercising.

The Conduction Pathway

The order in which impulses travel through the heart is as follows:

1. The sinoatrial node generates the electrical impulse that begins the heartbeat.

2. The excitation wave travels throughout the muscle of each atrium, causing the atria to contract.

3. The atrioventricular node is stimulated. The relatively slower conduction through this node allows time for the atria to contract and complete the filling of the ventricles.

4. The excitation wave travels rapidly through the bundle of His and then throughout the ventricular walls by means of the bundle branches and Purkinje fibers. The entire musculature of the ventricles contracts practically at once.

As a safety measure, a region of the conduction system other than the sinoatrial node can generate a heartbeat if the sinoatrial node fails, but it does so at a slower rate. A normal heart rhythm originating at the SA node is termed a *sinus rhythm.*

✔ CHECKPOINT **7**:

The heartbeat is started by a small mass of tissue in the upper right atrium. This is commonly called the pacemaker, but what is its scientific name?

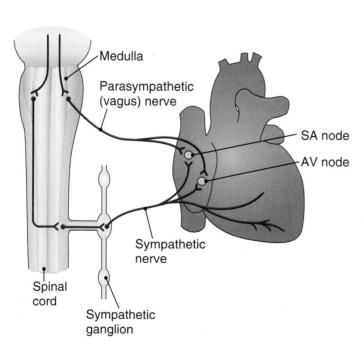

FIGURE **13•7**   Nervous stimulation of the heart.

Control of the Heart Rate

Although the fundamental beat of the heart originates within the heart itself, the heart rate can be influenced by the nervous system and by other factors in the internal environment.

The autonomic nervous system (ANS) plays a major role in modifying the heart rate according to need (Fig. 13-7). Stimulation from the sympathetic nervous system increases the heart rate. During a fight-or-flight response, the sympathetic nerves can boost the cardiac output two to three times the resting value. Sympathetic fibers increase the rate of contraction by stimulating the SA and AV nodes. They also increase the force of contraction by acting directly on the fibers of the myocardium. These actions translate into increased cardiac output. Stimulation from the parasympathetic nervous system decreases the heart rate to restore homeostasis. The parasympathetic nerve that supplies the heart is the vagus nerve (cranial nerve X). It slows the heart rate by acting on the SA and AV nodes.

These ANS influences allow the heart to meet changing needs rapidly. The heart rate is also affected by substances circulating in the blood, including hormones, ions, and drugs. Regular exercise strengthens the heart and increases the amount of blood ejected with each beat. At rest, the needs of the body then can be met with a lower heart rate. Trained athletes usually have a low resting heart rate.

Variations in Heart Rates

- ***Bradycardia*** (brad-e-KAR-de-ah) is a relatively slow heart rate of less than 60 beats/minute. During rest and sleep, the heart may beat less than 60 beats/minute but usually does not fall below 50 beats/minute.
- ***Tachycardia*** (tak-e-KAR-de-ah) refers to a heart rate of more than 100 beats/minute. Tachycardia is normal during exercise or stress but may also occur under abnormal conditions.
- ***Sinus arrhythmia*** (ah-RITH-me-ah) is a regular variation in heart rate due to changes in the rate and depth of breathing. It is a normal phenomenon.
- ***Premature beat,*** also called *extrasystole,* is a beat that comes before the expected normal beat. These may occur in normal people initiated by caffeine, nicotine, or psychological stresses. They are also common in people with heart disease.

Heart Sounds

The normal heart sounds are usually described by the syllables "lubb" and "dupp." The first is a longer, lower-pitched sound that occurs at the start of ventricular systole. It is probably caused by a combination of things, mainly closure of the atrioventricular valves. The second, or "dupp," sound is shorter and sharper. It occurs at the beginning of ventricular relaxation and is due in large part to sudden closure of the semilunar valves.

Murmurs

An abnormal sound is called a ***murmur*** and is usually due to faulty action of a valve. For example, if a valve fails to close tightly and blood leaks back, a murmur is heard. Another condition giving rise to an abnormal sound is the narrowing (stenosis) of a valve opening.

The many conditions that can cause abnormal heart sounds include congenital defects, disease, and physiologic variations. An abnormal sound caused by any structural change in the heart or the vessels connected with the heart is called an ***organic murmur.*** Certain normal sounds heard while the heart is working may also be described as murmurs, such as the sound heard during rapid filling of the ventricles. To differentiate these from abnormal sounds, they are more properly called ***functional murmurs.***

✔ CHECKPOINT **8**:

What is a heart murmur?

THE HEART IN THE ELDERLY

As a person ages, the heart becomes smaller, and there is a decrease in the strength of heart muscle contraction. The valves become less flexible, and incomplete closure may produce an audible murmur. By 70 years of age, the cardiac output may decrease by as much as 35%. Damage within the conduction system can produce abnormal rhythms, including extra beats, rapid atrial beats, and slowing of ventricular rate. Temporary failure of the conduction system (heart block) can cause periodic loss of consciousness. Due to the decrease in the reserve strength of the heart, elderly people are often limited in their ability to respond to physical or emotional stress

See Managing Cardiac Risk Factors.

HEART STUDIES

Experienced listeners can gain much information about the heart using a *stethoscope* (STETH-o-skope). This is a relatively simple instrument used to convey sounds from within the patient's body to the ear of an examiner.

The *electrocardiograph* (*ECG* or *EKG*) is used for making records of the changes in electrical currents produced by the contracting heart muscle. It may thus reveal certain myocardial injuries. Electrical activity is picked up by electrodes placed on the surface of the skin and appears as *waves* on the ECG tracing. The P wave represents the activity of the atria; the QRS and T waves represent the activity of the ventricles (Fig. 13-8). Changes in the waves and the intervals between them are used to diagnose heart damage and arrhythmias.

Many people with heart disease undergo *catheterization* (kath-eh-ter-i-ZA-shun). In right heart catheterization, an extremely thin tube (catheter) is passed through the veins of the right arm or right groin and then into the right side of heart. A *fluoroscope* (flu-OR-o-scope), an instrument for examining deep structures with x-rays, is used to show the route taken by the catheter. The tube is passed all the way through the pulmonic valve into the large lung arteries. Blood samples are obtained along the way for testing, and pressure readings are taken.

In left heart catheterization, a catheter is passed through an artery in the left groin or arm to the heart. Dye can then be injected into the coronary arteries to map damage to the vessels. The tube may also be passed through the

Managing Cardiac Risk Factors

Management of those risk factors for cardiac disease that we have some control over is essential to good health. Modification of these risk factors can significantly delay the onset of disease by 12 to 20 years. Each of the following modifications can have some effect by itself; however, used together the effects can be dramatic:

- Stop smoking; nicotine has been shown to increase sclerosis of the coronary arteries as well as to increase irritability of the arterial wall, leading to coronary artery spasm.
- Gain control over your weight; even marginal obesity, less than 20 pounds over your ideal weight, increases the workload on your heart by 3 times and significant obesity (more than 20 pounds) eventually leads to heart failure. If you need to lose weight, do so gradually, most physicians recommend no more than 2 to 3 pounds per week.
- Watch your diet: reduce overall intake of fats and cholesterol, paying special attention to saturated fats. Increase items that are high in monounsaturated fat (fish oils and olive oil), and vitamins A, E, and C. Increase the number of servings of grains in your diet and include plenty of vegetables while avoiding red meats.
- Exercise! A good aerobic/cardiovascular work-out, such as walking or bicycling, 3 times a week allows the heart muscle to become stronger and pump more efficiently. Remember to begin slowly and work yourself up to a regular regimen and don't forget the warm-up and cool-down parts of the routine.

The key to making any significant, lasting modifications is to do so in moderation. Drastic changes will undoubtedly be short-term and have little benefit.

aortic valve into the left ventricle for further studies.

Ultrasound consists of sound waves generated at a frequency above the range of sensitivity of the human ear. In *echocardiography* (ek-o-kar-de-OG-rah-fe), also known as *ultrasound cardiography,* high-frequency sound waves are sent to the heart from a small instrument on the surface of the chest. The ultra-

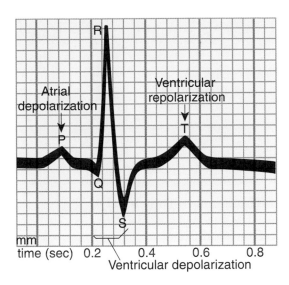

FIGURE **13•8** Normal EKG showing one cardiac cycle.

sound waves bounce off the heart and are recorded as they return, showing the heart in action. Movement of the echoes is traced on an electronic instrument called an *oscilloscope* and recorded on film. (The same principle is employed by submarines to detect ships.) The method is safe and painless, and it does not use x-rays. It provides information on the size and shape of heart structures, on cardiac function, and on possible heart defects.

✔ CHECKPOINT **9**:

What does ECG stand for?

Summary

I. Circulation and the heart—heart contractions drive blood through the blood vessels

II. Structure of the heart
  A. Layers of the heart wall
    1. Endocardium—thin inner layer
    2. Myocardium—thick muscle layer
      a. Lightly striated, intercalated disks, branching of fibers
    3. Epicardium—thin outer layer
      a. Pericardium—membrane-lined sac that encloses the heart
  B. Two hearts and a partition—left and right sides divided by a septum
  C. Four chambers
    1. Atria—left and right receiving chambers
    2. Ventricles—left and right pumping chambers
  D. Four valves—prevent backflow of blood
    1. Tricuspid—right atrioventricular valve
    2. Mitral (bicuspid)—left atrioventricular valve
    3. Pulmonic (semilunar) valve—at entrance to pulmonary artery
    4. Aortic (semilunar) valve—at entrance to aorta
  E. Blood supply to the myocardium
    1. Coronary arteries—first branches of aorta; fill when heart relaxes
    2. Coronary sinus—collects venous blood from heart and empties into right atrium

III. Function of the heart
  A. The work of the heart—cardiac cycle
    1. Phases
      a. Diastole—relaxation phase
      b. Systole—contraction phase
    2. Cardiac output—volume pumped by each ventricle per minute
      a. Stroke volume—amount pumped with each beat
      b. Heart rate—number of beats per minute
  B. Conduction system of the heart

1. Sinoatrial node (pacemaker)—at top of right atrium
2. Atrioventricular node—between atria and ventricles
3. Atrioventricular bundle (bundle of His)—at top of interventricular septum
   a. Bundle branches—right and left, on either side of septum
   b. Purkinje fibers—branch through myocardium of ventricles

C. Control of the heart rate
   1. Autonomic nervous system
      a. Sympathetic system—speeds heart rate
      b. Parasympathetic system—slows heart rate through vagus nerve
   2. Others—hormones, ions, drugs
   3. Variations in heart rates
      a. Bradycardia—slower rate than normal; less than 60 beats/minute
      b. Tachycardia—faster rate than normal; more than 100 beats/minute

   c. Sinus arrhythmia—related to breathing changes
   d. Premature beat—extrasystole

D. Heart sounds
   1. Normal
      a. "Lubb"—occurs at closing of atrioventricular valves
      b. "Dupp"—occurs at closing of semilunar valves
   2. Abnormal—murmur

IV. The heart in the elderly

V. Heart studies
   1. Stethoscope—used to listen to heart sounds
   2. Electrocardiograph (ECG, EKG)—records electrical activity as waves
   3. Catheterization—thin tube inserted into heart for blood samples, pressure readings, and other tests
   4. Fluoroscope—examines deep tissue with x-rays; used to guide catheter
   5. Echocardiography—uses ultrasound to record pictures of heart in action

Questions for Study and Review

1. What are the three layers of the heart wall?
2. Describe the characteristics of heart muscle tissue.
3. Name the sac around the heart.
4. What is a partition in the heart called? Name two such partitions.
5. Name the chambers of the heart and tell what each does.
6. Explain the purpose of valves in the heart and name the four valves in the heart.
7. Why does the myocardium need its own blood supply? Name the arteries that supply blood to the heart.
8. Explain the contraction pattern of the cardiac cycle.
9. Define *cardiac output*. What determines cardiac output?
10. What are the parts of the heart's conduction system called and where are these structures located? Outline the order in which the excitation waves travel.
11. Compare the effects of the sympathetic and parasympathetic nervous systems on the working of the heart.
12. What two syllables are used to indicate normal heart sounds and at what times in the heart cycle can they be heard?
13. What changes occur in the heart with age?
14. What is a stethoscope?
15. What is an electrocardiograph and what is its purpose?

16. Of what value is heart catheterization and how is it carried out?
17. How is echocardiography used to study the heart?
18. Differentiate between the terms in each of the following pairs:
    a. *pulmonary* and *systemic circuit*
    b. *interatrial* and *interventricular*
    c. *systole* and *diastole*
    d. *stroke volume* and *heart rate*
    e. *tachycardia* and *bradycardia*
    f. *functional murmur* and *organic murmur*

✔ Answers to Checkpoints
_____

1. The innermost layer of the heart is the endocardium, the middle is the myocardium, and the outermost is the epicardium.
2. The upper chamber on each side of the heart is the atrium; each lower chamber is the ventricle.
3. Valves direct the flow of blood through the heart.
4. The coronary circulation is the blood supply to the heart.
5. The contraction phase of the cardiac cycle is systole; the relaxation phase is diastole.
6. Cardiac output is determined by the stroke volume, the volume of blood ejected from the ventricle with each beat, and by the heart rate, the number of times the heart beats per minute.
7. The small mass of tissue that starts the heartbeat is the sinoatrial (SA) node.
8. A heart murmur is an abnormal heart sound.
9. ECG stands for electrocardiography.

13

Blood Vessels and Blood Circulation

SELECTED KEY TERMS

The following terms are defined in the Glossary:

anastomosis

aorta

arteriole

artery

capillary

endothelium

pulse

sinusoid

sphygmomanometer

vasoconstriction

vasodilation

vein

venule

BEHAVIORAL OBJECTIVES

After careful study of this chapter, you should be able to:

1. Differentiate among the three main types of vessels in the body with regard to structure and function

2. Compare the locations and functions of the pulmonary and systemic circuits

3. Name the four sections of the aorta and list the main branches of each section

4. Define *anastomosis*. Cite the function of anastomoses and give several examples

5. Compare superficial and deep veins and give examples of each type

6. Name the main vessels that drain into the superior and inferior venae cavae

7. Define *venous sinus* and give four examples

8. Describe the structure and function of the hepatic portal system

9. Explain how materials are exchanged across the capillary wall

10. Describe the factors that regulate blood flow

11. Define *pulse* and list factors that affect the pulse rate

12. List several factors that affect blood pressure

13. Explain how blood pressure is commonly measured

The blood vessels, together with the four chambers of the heart, form a closed system in which blood is carried to and from the tissues. Although whole blood does not leave the vessels, components of the plasma and tissue fluids can be exchanged through the walls of the tiniest vessels, the capillaries.

The vascular system is easier to understand if you refer to the appropriate illustrations in this chapter as the vessels are described. When this information is added to what you already know about the blood and the heart, a picture of the cardiovascular system as a whole will emerge.

BLOOD VESSELS

Types of Blood Vessels

On the basis of function, blood vessels may be divided into three groups:

- *Arteries* carry blood away from the heart and toward the capillaries in the tissues. Blood is pumped out of the ventricles into the arteries. The smallest arteries are called *arterioles* (ar-TE-re-olz).
- *Veins* drain capillaries in the tissues and return the blood to the heart. The smallest veins are the *venules* (VEN-ulz).
- *Capillaries* allow for exchanges between

the blood and body cells, or between the blood and air in the lung tissues. The capillaries connect the arterioles and venules.

> ✔ CHECKPOINT **1**:
>
> What are the three main groups of blood vessels?

Blood Circuits

The vessels together may be subdivided into two groups or circuits: pulmonary and systemic. The vessels in these two circuits are shown in Figure 14-1; the anatomic relation of the circuits to the heart is shown in Figure 13-2 in Chapter 13.

The Pulmonary Circuit

The *pulmonary circuit* eliminates carbon dioxide from the blood and replenishes its supply of oxygen. The pulmonary vessels that carry blood to and from the lungs include the following:

- The pulmonary artery and its branches, which carry blood from the right ventricle to the lungs
- The capillaries in the lungs, through which gases are exchanged
- The pulmonary veins, which carry blood back to the left atrium

FIGURE **14•1** Blood vessels form a closed system for the flow of blood. Blood high in oxygen (oxygenated) is shown in red; blood low in oxygen (deoxygenated) is shown in blue. Changes in oxygen content occur as blood flows through capillaries.

The pulmonary vessels differ from those in the systemic circuit in that the pulmonary arteries carry blood that is *low* in oxygen, and the pulmonary veins carry blood that is *high* in oxygen. All the remaining arteries carry highly oxygenated blood, and all remaining veins carry blood that is low in oxygen.

The Systemic Circuit

The *systemic* (sis-TEM-ik) *circuit* serves the rest of the body. These vessels supply nutrients and oxygen to all the tissues and carry waste materials away from the tissues for disposal. The systemic vessels include the following:

- The aorta, which receives blood from the left ventricle and then branches into the systemic arteries carrying blood to the tissues

- The systemic capillaries, through which materials are exchanged
- The systemic veins, which carry blood back toward the heart. The venous blood flows into the right atrium of the heart through the superior vena cava and inferior vena cava.

✔ CHECKPOINT **2**:

What are the two blood circuits and what do they do?

Vessel Structure

Artery Walls

The arteries have thick walls because they must be strong enough to receive blood pumped under pressure from the ventricles of the heart (Fig. 14-2). The three coats (tunics) of the arteries resemble the three tissue layers of the heart:

- The innermost membrane of simple, flat epithelial cells makes up the ***endothelium*** (en-do-THE-le-um), forming a smooth surface over which the blood flows easily.
- The middle and thickest layer is made of smooth (involuntary) muscle, which is under the control of the autonomic nervous system. Elastic tissue between the layers of the arterial wall allows these vessels to stretch when receiving blood and then return to their original size. The amount of elastic tissue diminishes as the arteries branch and become smaller.
- An outer tunic is made of a supporting connective tissue.

The largest artery, the ***aorta*** (a-OR-tah), is about 2.5 cm (1 inch) in diameter and has the thickest wall because it receives blood under the highest pressure from the left ventricle. The smallest subdivisions of arteries, the arterioles, have thinner walls in which there is little elastic connective tissue but relatively more smooth muscle.

See Keeping Your Arteries Clean.

Artery
Vein
Elastic tissue
Tunica interna (endothelium)
Tunica media (smooth muscle)
Tunica externa (connective tissue)
Blood flow
Arteriole
Venule
Capillary

FIGURE **14•2** Sections of small blood vessels showing the thick arterial wall, the thin wall of a vein, and the single-layered wall of a capillary. A venous valve also is shown. The arrow indicates the direction of blood flow.

Capillary Walls

The microscopic branches of these tiny connecting vessels have the thinnest walls of any vessels: one cell layer. The capillary walls are transparent and are made of smooth, platelike cells that continue from the lining of the arteries. Because of the thinness of these walls, exchanges between the blood and the body cells are possible. The capillary boundaries are the most important center of activity for the entire circulatory system. Their function is explained later in this chapter.

Vein Walls

The smallest veins, the **venules,** are formed by the union of capillaries, and their walls are only slightly thicker than those of the capillaries. As veins become larger, their walls become thicker. The wall of a vein, however, is much thinner than the wall of an artery of comparable size and has less elastic tissue. As a result, the blood within the veins is carried under much lower pressure.

Although there are the same three layers of tissue in the walls of the larger veins, as in the artery walls, the middle tunic is relatively thin in the veins. Therefore, veins are easily collapsed, and only slight pressure on a vein by a tumor or other mass may interfere with return blood flow. Most veins are equipped with one-way valves that permit blood to flow in only one direction: toward the heart (see Fig. 14-2). Such valves are most numerous in the veins of the extremities.

Figure 14-3 is a cross-section of an artery and a vein as seen through a microscope.

✔ CHECKPOINT **3**:

What type of tissue makes up the middle layer of arteries and veins, and how is this tissue controlled?

14

Keeping Your Arteries Clean

With age, arteries accumulate fatty deposits referred to as *plaque*. The first step in the buildup of plaque is thought to be microscopic damage to the inner wall of the arteries, the endothellium. This damage is thought to be caused by direct contact with LDL (the "bad" cholesterol), oxidizing chemicals, such as free-radicals, and some proteins. LDL invades the endothelium, causing an accumulation of lipids in the wall of the artery. This is followed by aggregation of platelets and macrophages. The endothelium starts to divide in an attempt to seal itself off. This leads to the incorporation of all of the above substances within the arterial wall. The wall soon bulges into the lumen and obstructs blood flow. This obstruction then leads to the formation of clots that may further close off the flow of blood through the vessel. Arteries in the heart, brain, kidneys, and the extremities seem to be especially vulnerable to this process. To help slow this degenerative process, one should:

- Reduce fat intake; cut intake of foods high in LDL—the saturated fats
- Increase intake of soluble fibers, such as oat, bran, and fruit fibers, which have been shown to decrease cholesterol levels in the blood
- Take in adequate amounts of vitamin E, vitamin C, folic acid, and calcium; each has been shown to have beneficial effects on the heart
- Add vitamins B_6 and B_{12} to your diet; both are thought to help the heart by lowering levels of an enzyme considered to be harmful to the heart
- Take one low-dose aspirin a day (check with your doctor first!); aspirin helps to block platelet aggregation in the arterial wall, preventing clot formation.

SYSTEMIC ARTERIES

The Aorta and Its Parts

The aorta extends upward and to the right from the left ventricle. Then it curves backward and to the left. It continues down behind the heart just in front of the vertebral column, through the diaphragm, and into the abdomen (Figs. 14-4 and 14-5). The aorta is one continuous artery, but it may be divided into sections:

- The *ascending aorta* is near the heart and inside the pericardial sac.
- The *aortic arch* curves from the right to the left and also extends backward.
- The *thoracic aorta* lies just in front of the vertebral column behind the heart and in the space behind the pleura.
- The *abdominal aorta* is the longest section of the aorta, spanning the abdominal cavity.

The thoracic and abdominal aorta together make up the descending aorta.

Branches of the Ascending Aorta and Aortic Arch

The first, or ascending, part of the aorta has two branches near the heart, called the *left* and *right coronary arteries,* which supply the heart muscle. These form a crown around the base of the heart and give off branches to all parts of the myocardium.

The arch of the aorta, located immediately beyond the ascending aorta, gives off three large branches.

- The *brachiocephalic* (brak-e-o-seh-FAL-ik) *trunk* is a short artery formerly called the *innominate.* Its newer name means that it supplies the head and the arm. After extending upward somewhat less than 5 cm (2 inches), it divides into the *right subclavian* (sub-KLA-ve-an) *artery,* which supplies the right upper extremity (arm), and the *right common carotid* (kah-ROT-id) *artery,* which supplies the right side of the head and the neck. Note that the brachiocephalic artery is unpaired.
- The *left common carotid artery* extends upward from the highest part of the aortic arch. It supplies the left side of the neck and the head.
- The *left subclavian artery* extends under the left clavicle (collar bone) and supplies the left upper extremity. This is the last branch of the aortic arch.

smooth muscle

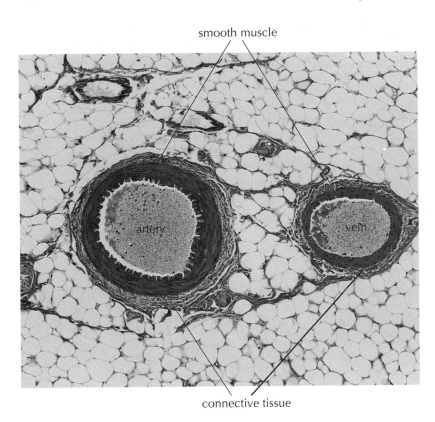

connective tissue

FIGURE **14•3** Cross section of an artery and a vein as seen through a microscope. (Cormack DH: Essential Histology, Plate 11–1. Philadelphia, JB Lippincott, 1993)

14

Branches of the Thoracic Aorta

The thoracic aorta supplies branches to the chest wall, to the *esophagus* (e-SOF-ah-gus), and to the bronchi (the subdivisions of the trachea) and their treelike subdivisions in the lungs. There are usually 9 to 10 pairs of *intercostal* (in-ter-KOS-tal) *arteries* that extend between the ribs, sending branches to the muscles and other structures of the chest wall.

Branches of the Abdominal Aorta

As in the case of the thoracic aorta, there are unpaired branches extending forward and paired arteries extending toward the side. The unpaired vessels are large arteries that supply the abdominal viscera. The most important of these visceral branches are as follows:

- The *celiac* (SE-le-ak) *trunk* is a short artery about 1.25 cm (½ inch) long that subdivides into three branches: the *left gastric artery* goes to the stomach, the *splenic* (SPLEN-ik) *artery* goes to the spleen, and the *hepatic* (heh-PAT-ik)

artery carries oxygenated blood to the liver.

- The *superior mesenteric* (mes-en-TER-ik) *artery,* the largest of these branches, carries blood to most of the small intestine and to the first half of the large intestine.
- The much smaller *inferior mesenteric artery,* located below the superior mesenteric and near the end of the abdominal aorta, supplies the second half of the large intestine.

The paired lateral branches of the abdominal aorta include the following right and left vessels:

- The *phrenic* (FREN-ik) *arteries* supply the diaphragm.
- The *suprarenal* (su-prah-RE-nal) *arteries* supply the adrenal (suprarenal) glands.
- The *renal* (RE-nal) *arteries,* the largest in this group, carry blood to the kidneys.
- The *ovarian arteries* in the female and *testicular* (tes-TIK-u-lar) *arteries* in the

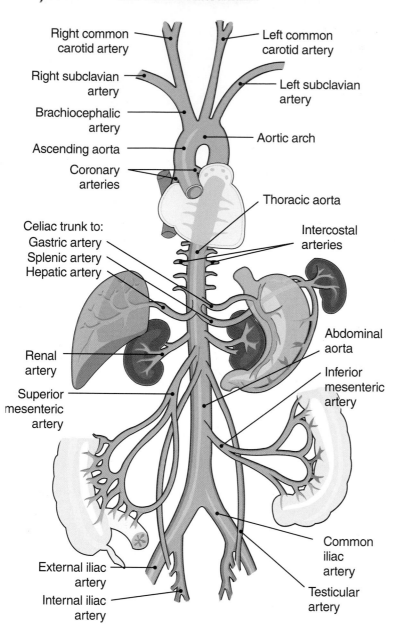

FIGURE **14•4** Aorta and its branches.

male (formerly called the *spermatic arteries*), supply the sex glands.

• Four pairs of **lumbar** (LUM-bar) **arteries** extend into the musculature of the abdominal wall.

✔ CHECKPOINT **4**:

What are the subdivisions of the aorta, the largest artery?

The Iliac Arteries and Their Subdivisions

The abdominal aorta finally divides into two **common iliac** (IL-e-ak) **arteries.** Both of these vessels, about 5 cm (2 inches) long, extend into the pelvis, where each one subdivides into an **internal** and an **external iliac artery.**

The internal iliac vessels then send branches to the pelvic organs, including the urinary blad-

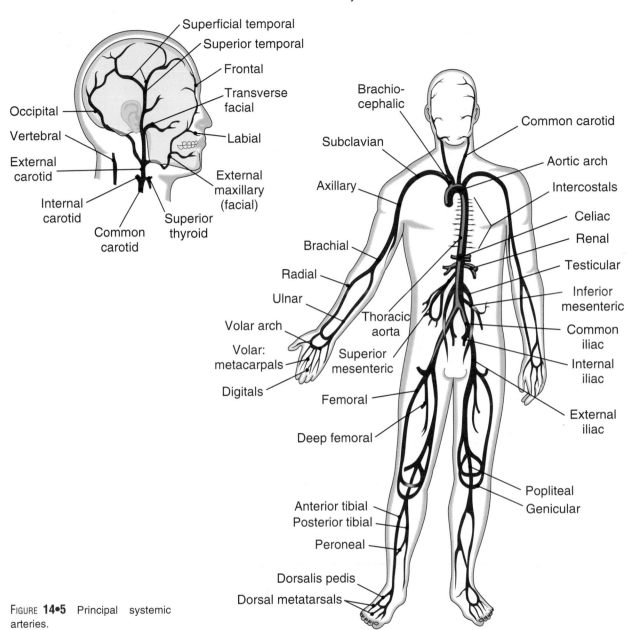

FIGURE **14•5** Principal systemic arteries.

der, the rectum, and some of the reproductive organs.

Each external iliac artery continues into the thigh as the ***femoral*** (FEM-or-al) ***artery.*** This vessel gives off branches in the thigh and then becomes the ***popliteal*** (pop-LIT-e-al) ***artery,*** which subdivides below the knee. The subdivisions include the ***tibial artery*** and the ***dorsalis pedis*** (dor-SA-lis PE-dis), which supply the leg and the foot.

Arteries That Branch to the Head and Arm

Each common carotid artery gives off branches to the thyroid gland and other structures in the neck before dividing into the ***external*** and ***internal carotid arteries,*** which supply parts of the head.

The arm and hand receive blood from the ***subclavian*** (sub-KLA-ve-an) ***artery***, which becomes the ***axillary*** (AK-sil-ar-e) ***artery*** in the axilla (armpit). The longest part of this vessel, the ***brachial*** (BRA-ke-al) ***artery,*** is in the arm proper. It subdivides into two branches near the elbow: the ***radial artery,*** which continues down the thumb side of the forearm and wrist, and the ***ulnar artery,*** which extends along the medial or little finger side into the hand.

Just as the larger branches of a tree give off limbs of varying sizes, so the arterial tree has a multitude of subdivisions. Hundreds of names might be included. We have mentioned only some of them.

Anastomoses

A communication between two vessels is called an ***anastomosis*** (ah-nas-to-MO-sis). By means of arterial anastomoses, blood reaches vital or-gans by more than one route. Some examples of such unions of end arteries are as follows:

- The ***circle of Willis*** (Fig. 14-6) receives blood from the two internal carotid arteries and from the ***basilar*** (BAS-il-ar) ***artery,*** which is formed by the union of two verte-bral arteries. This arterial circle lies just under the center of the brain and sends branches to the cerebrum and other parts of the brain.
- The ***volar*** (VO-lar) ***arch*** is formed by the union of the radial and ulnar arteries in the hand. It sends branches to the hand and the fingers.
- The ***mesenteric arches*** are made of com-munications between branches of the ves-sels that supply blood to the intestinal tract.
- ***Arterial arches*** are formed by the union

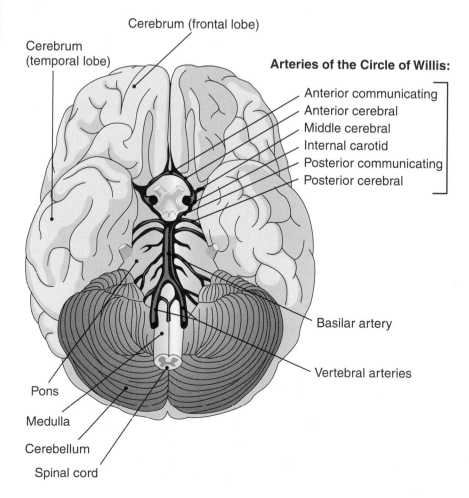

Cerebrum (frontal lobe)

Cerebrum (temporal lobe)

Arteries of the Circle of Willis:

Anterior communicating
Anterior cerebral
Middle cerebral
Internal carotid
Posterior communicating
Posterior cerebral

Basilar artery

Vertebral arteries

Pons

Medulla

Cerebellum

Spinal cord

FIGURE **14•6** Arteries that supply the brain, showing the arteries that make up the circle of Willis.

of branches of the tibial arteries in the foot. Similar anastomoses are found in other parts of the body.

Arteriovenous anastomoses are blood shunts found in a few areas, including the external ears, the hands, and the feet. Vessels with muscular walls connect arteries directly with veins and thus bypass the capillaries (Fig. 14-7). This provides a more rapid flow and a greater volume of blood to these areas than elsewhere, thus protecting these exposed parts from freezing in cold weather.

✔ CHECKPOINT **5**:

What is an anastomosis?

SYSTEMIC VEINS

Whereas most arteries are located in protected and rather deep areas of the body, many veins are found near the surface (Fig. 14-8). The most important of these **superficial veins** are in the extremities. These include the following:

- The veins on the back of the hand and at the front of the elbow. Those at the elbow are often used for removing blood samples for test purposes as well as for intravenous injections. The largest of this group of veins

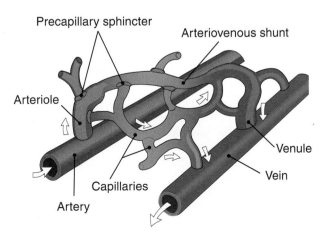

FIGURE **14•7** Capillary network showing an arteriovenous shunt (anastomosis).

are the **cephalic** (seh-FAL-ik), the **basilic** (bah-SIL-ik), and the **median cubital** (KU-bih-tal) **veins.**

- The **saphenous** (sah-FE-nus) **veins** of the lower extremities, which are the longest veins of the body. The great saphenous vein begins in the foot and extends up the medial side of the leg, the knee, and the thigh. It finally empties into the femoral vein near the groin.

The **deep veins** tend to parallel arteries and usually have the same names as the corresponding arteries. Examples of these include the **femoral** and the **iliac** vessels of the lower part of the body and the **brachial, axillary,** and **subclavian** vessels of the upper extremities. Exceptions are found in the veins of the head and the neck. The **jugular** (JUG-u-lar) **veins** drain the areas supplied by the carotid arteries. Two **brachiocephalic** (innominate) **veins** are formed, one on each side, by the union of the subclavian and the jugular veins. (Remember, there is only *one* brachiocephalic artery.)

The Venae Cavae and Their Tributaries

The veins of the head, neck, upper extremities, and chest all drain into the **superior vena cava** (VE-nah KA-vah), which goes to the heart. It is formed by the union of the right and left brachiocephalic veins, which drain the head, neck, and upper extremities. The **azygos** (AZ-ih-gos) **vein** drains the veins of the chest wall and empties into the superior vena cava just before the latter empties into the heart (see Fig. 14-8).

The **inferior vena cava,** which is much longer than the superior vena cava, returns the blood from the parts of the body below the diaphragm. It begins in the lower abdomen with the union of the two common iliac veins. It then ascends along the back wall of the abdomen, through a groove in the posterior part of the liver, through the diaphragm, and finally through the lower thorax to empty into the right atrium of the heart.

Drainage into the inferior vena cava is more complicated than drainage into the superior

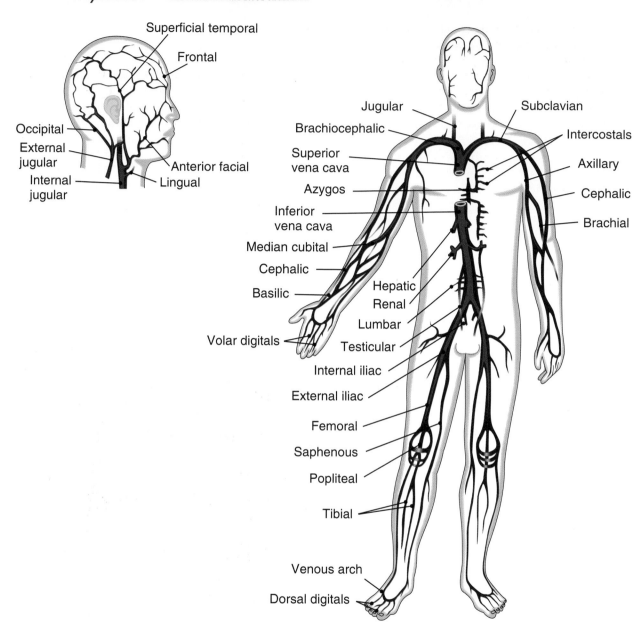

FIGURE **14•8** Principal systemic veins.

vena cava. The large veins below the diaphragm may be divided into two groups:

- The right and left veins that drain paired parts and organs. They include the *iliac veins* from near the groin, four pairs of *lumbar veins* from the dorsal part of the trunk and from the spinal cord, the *testicular veins* from the testes of the male and the *ovarian veins* from the ovaries of the

female, the *renal* and *suprarenal veins* from the kidneys and adrenal glands near the kidneys, and finally the large *hepatic veins* from the liver. For the most part, these vessels empty directly into the inferior vena cava. The left testicular in the male and the left ovarian in the female empty into the left renal vein, which then takes this blood to the inferior vena cava; these veins thus constitute exceptions to the rule that the paired veins empty directly into the vena cava.

- Unpaired veins that come from the spleen and from parts of the digestive tract (stomach and intestine) empty into a vein called the **hepatic portal vein.** Unlike other lower veins, which empty into the inferior vena cava, the hepatic portal vein is part of a special system that enables blood to circulate through the liver before returning to the heart.

✔ CHECKPOINT **6**:

Veins are described as superficial or deep. What does superficial mean?

Venous Sinuses

The word *sinus* means "space" or "hollow." A **venous sinus** is a large channel that drains deoxygenated blood but does not have the usual tubular structure of the veins.

One example of a venous sinus is the **coronary sinus,** which receives most of the blood from the veins of the heart wall (see Fig. 13-4 in Chap. 13). It lies between the left atrium and left ventricle on the posterior surface of the heart, and it empties directly into the right atrium along with the two venae cavae.

Other important venous sinuses are the **cranial venous sinuses,** which are located inside the skull and drain the veins that come from all over the brain (Fig. 14-9). The largest of the cranial venous sinuses are the following:

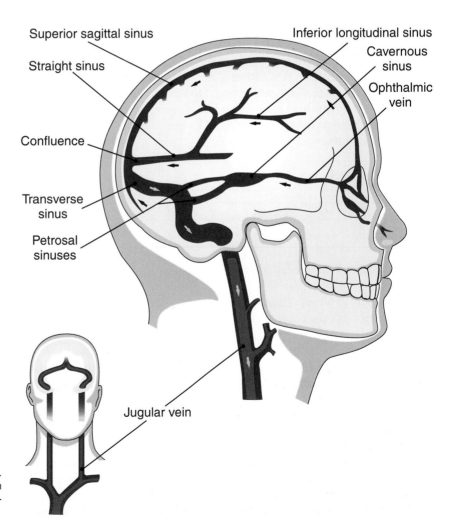

Superior sagittal sinus
Straight sinus
Confluence
Transverse sinus
Petrosal sinuses
Inferior longitudinal sinus
Cavernous sinus
Ophthalmic vein
Jugular vein

FIGURE **14•9** Cranial venous sinuses. The paired transverse sinuses, which carry blood from the brain to the jugular veins, are shown in the inset.

- The two **cavernous sinuses,** situated behind the eyeballs, serve to drain the **ophthalmic** (of-THAL-mik) **veins** of the eyes.
- The **superior sagittal** (SAJ-ih-tal) **sinus** is a single long space located in the midline above the brain and in the fissure between the two hemispheres of the cerebrum. It ends in an enlargement called the **confluence** (KON-flu-ens) **of sinuses.**
- The two **transverse sinuses,** also called the **lateral sinuses,** are large spaces between the layers of the dura mater (the outermost membrane around the brain). They begin posteriorly, in the region of the confluence of sinuses, and then extend toward either side. As each sinus extends around the inside of the skull, it receives blood draining those parts not already drained by the superior sagittal and other sinuses that join the back portions of the transverse sinuses. This means that nearly all the blood that comes from the veins of the brain eventually empties into one or the other of the transverse sinuses. On either side, the sinus extends far enough forward to empty into an internal jugular vein, which then passes through a hole in the skull to continue downward in the neck.

✔ CHECKPOINT **7**:

What is a venous sinus?

The Hepatic Portal System

Almost always, when blood leaves a capillary bed, it flows directly back to the heart. In a portal system, however, blood circulates through a second capillary bed, usually in a second organ, before it returns to the heart. A portal system is a kind of detour in the pathway of venous return that transports materials directly from one organ to another.

The largest portal system in the body is the **hepatic portal system,** which carries blood from the abdominal organs to the liver (Fig. 14-10). In a similar fashion, a small, local portal system is located in the brain to carry substances from the hypothalamus to the pituitary

(see Chap. 11). The hepatic portal system includes the veins that drain blood from capillaries in the spleen, stomach, pancreas, and intestine. Instead of emptying their blood directly into the inferior vena cava, they deliver it by way of the hepatic portal vein to the liver. The largest tributary of the portal vein is the **superior mesenteric vein,** which drains blood from the proximal portion of the intestine. It is joined by the **splenic vein** just under the liver. Other tributaries of the portal circulation are the **gastric, pancreatic,** and **inferior mesenteric veins.**

On entering the liver, the portal vein divides and subdivides into ever smaller branches. Eventually, the portal blood flows into a vast network of sinuslike vessels called **sinusoids** (SI-nus-oyds). These enlarged capillary channels allow liver cells close contact with the blood coming from the abdominal organs. (Similar blood channels are found in the spleen and endocrine glands, including the thyroid and adrenals.) After leaving the sinusoids, blood is finally collected by the hepatic veins, which empty into the inferior vena cava.

The purpose of the hepatic portal system of veins is to transport blood from the digestive organs and the spleen to the liver sinusoids, so that the liver cells can carry out their functions. For example, when food is digested, most of the end products are absorbed from the small intestine into the bloodstream and transported to the liver by the portal system. In the liver, these nutrients are processed, stored, and released as needed into the general circulation.

✔ CHECKPOINT **8**:

The hepatic portal system takes blood from the abdominal organs to what organ?

THE PHYSIOLOGY OF CIRCULATION

In a general way, the circulating blood might be compared to a train that travels around the country, loading and unloading freight in each of the cities it serves. For example, as blood

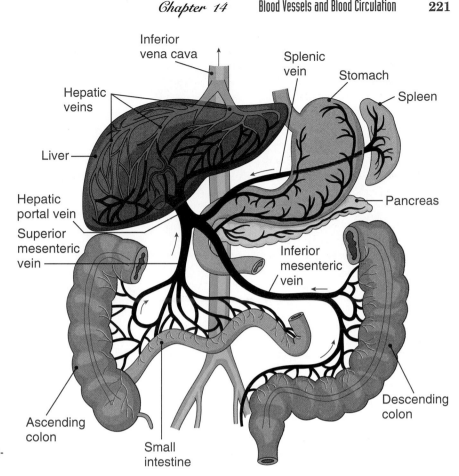

Figure **14•10** Hepatic portal circulation.

flows through capillaries surrounding the air sacs in the lungs, it picks up oxygen and unloads carbon dioxide. Later, when this oxygenated blood is pumped to capillaries in other parts of the body, it unloads the oxygen and picks up carbon dioxide and other substances resulting from cellular activities (Fig. 14-11). The microscopic capillaries are of fundamental importance in these activities. It is only through and between the cells of these thin-walled vessels that the necessary exchanges can occur. See The Blood–Brain Barrier.

All living cells are immersed in a slightly salty liquid called *tissue fluid* or *interstitial fluid*. Looking again at Figure 14-11, one can see how this fluid serves as "middleman" between the capillary membrane and the neighboring cells. As water, oxygen, and other materials necessary for cellular activity pass through the capillary walls, they enter the tissue fluid. Then, these substances make their

way by diffusion to the cells. At the same time, carbon dioxide and other end products of cell metabolism come from the cells and move in the opposite direction. These substances enter the capillary and are carried away in the bloodstream, to reach other organs or to be eliminated from the body.

Capillary Exchange

Diffusion is the main process by which substances move between the cells and the capillary blood. A secondary force is the pressure of the blood as it flows through the capillaries. Blood pressure acts to filter, or "push," water and dissolved materials out of the capillary into the tissue fluid. Fluid is drawn back into the capillary by osmotic pressure, the "pulling force" of substances dissolved and suspended in the blood. Osmotic pressure is maintained by

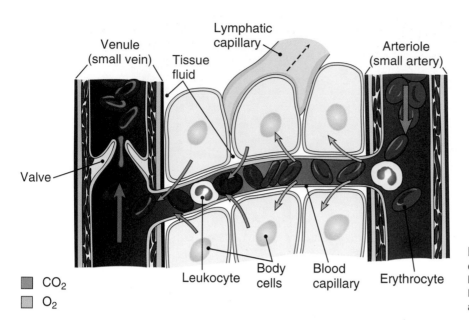

FIGURE **14•11** Diagram showing the connection between the small blood vessels through capillaries. Note the lymphatic capillary, which aids in tissue drainage.

14

plasma proteins (mainly albumin), which are too large to go through the capillary wall. These processes result in the constant exchange of fluids across the capillary wall.

The movement of blood through the capillaries is relatively slow, owing to the much larger size of the cross-sectional area of the capillaries compared with that of the larger vessels from which capillaries branch. This slow progress through the capillaries allows time for exchanges to occur.

> ✔ CHECKPOINT **9**:
>
> As materials diffuse back and forth between the blood and tissue fluid across the capillary wall, what force helps to push materials out of the capillary? What force helps to draw materials into the capillary?

The Dynamics of Blood Flow

The flow of blood is carefully regulated to supply the needs of the tissues without unnecessary burden on the heart. Some organs, such as the brain, liver, and kidneys, require large quantities of blood even at rest. The require-

ments of some tissues, such as those of skeletal muscles and digestive organs, increase greatly during periods of activity. (The blood flow in muscle can increase 25 times during exercise.) The volume of blood flowing to a particular organ can be regulated by changing the size of the blood vessels supplying that organ.

An increase in the diameter of a blood vessel is called **vasodilation.** This change allows for the delivery of more blood to an area. **Vasoconstriction** is a decrease in the diameter of a blood vessel, causing a decrease in blood flow. These *vasomotor activities* result from the contraction or relaxation of smooth muscle in the walls of the blood vessels, mainly the arterioles. A **vasomotor center** in the medulla of the brain stem regulates these activities, sending its messages through the autonomic nervous system.

The flow of blood into an individual capillary is regulated by a **precapillary sphincter** of smooth muscle that encircles the entrance to the capillary (see Fig. 14-7). This widens to allow more blood to enter when tissues need oxygen.

> ✔ CHECKPOINT **10**:
>
> Where are vasomotor activities regulated?

The Blood–Brain Barrier

The blood–brain barrier (BBB) is an adaptation of the circulation that protects the central nervous system from harmful substances traveling in the blood. It acts as a barrier to hormones, drugs, neurotransmitters, and other substances that might harm the brain or adversely affect its function. The barrier is formed by special cells in the brain capillaries. These cells are joined by tight junctions that limit the passage of materials between them. Also contributing to this barrier are astrocytes, specialized glial (connective tissue) cells that wrap around the capillaries to limit their permeability.

Pathogens are excluded by the blood–brain barrier, although some viruses, including poliovirus and herpesvirus, can get around it by traveling along peripheral nerves into the central nervous system. Also, some streptococci have the ability to get through the tight capillary junctions.

The blood–brain barrier can be an obstacle to getting drugs into the brain. Some antibiotics can cross the barrier, whereas others cannot. In Parkinson's disease, there is a deficiency of the neurotransmitter dopamine in the brain. The neurotransmitter itself will not pass through the barrier, but a related compound, L-dopa, is administered instead. L-dopa can cross the blood–brain barrier and is then converted to dopamine in the brain.

Return of Blood to the Heart

By the time blood arrives in the veins, little force remains from the pumping action of the heart. Also, because the veins tend to expand under pressure, considerable amounts of blood are stored in the venous system. Blood is moved back toward the heart by several mechanisms:

- **Contraction of skeletal muscles.** As skeletal muscles contract, they compress the veins and squeeze blood forward.
- **Valves** in the veins prevent backflow and keep blood flowing toward the heart.
- **Breathing.** Changes in pressures in the abdominal and thoracic cavities during breathing also promote return of blood in the venous system. During inhalation, the diaphragm flattens and puts pressure on the large abdominal veins. At the same time, expansion of the chest causes pressure to drop in the thorax. Together, these actions serve to both push and pull blood through these cavities and return it to the heart.

As evidence of these effects, if a person stands completely motionless, especially on a hot day when the superficial vessels dilate, enough blood can accumulate in the lower extremities to cause fainting from insufficient oxygen to the brain.

The Pulse

The ventricles pump blood into the arteries regularly about 70 to 80 times a minute. The force of ventricular contraction starts a wave of increased pressure that begins at the heart and travels along the arteries. This wave, called the *pulse,* can be felt in any artery that is relatively close to the surface, particularly if the vessel can be pressed down against a bone. At the wrist, the radial artery passes over the bone on the thumb side of the forearm, and the pulse is most commonly obtained here. Other vessels sometimes used for obtaining the pulse are the carotid artery in the neck and the dorsalis pedis on the top of the foot.

Normally, the pulse rate is the same as the heart rate. Only if a heartbeat is abnormally weak, or if the artery is obstructed, may the beat not be detected as a pulse. In checking the pulse of another person, it is important to use your second or third finger. If you use your thumb, you may find that you are getting your own pulse. When taking a pulse, it is important to gauge the strength as well as the regularity and the rate.

Pulse Rate

Various factors may influence the pulse rate. We describe just a few here:

- The pulse is somewhat faster in small people than in large people and usually is slightly faster in women than in men.
- In a newborn infant, the rate may be from 120 to 140 beats/minute. As the

child grows, the rate tends to become slower.

- Muscular activity influences the pulse rate. During sleep, the pulse may slow down to 60 beats/minute, whereas during strenuous exercise, the rate may go up to well over 100 beats/minute. For a person in good condition, the pulse does not go up as rapidly as it does in an inactive person, and it returns to a resting rate more quickly after exercise.
- Emotional disturbances may increase the pulse rate.
- In many infections, the pulse rate increases with the increase in temperature.
- An excessive amount of secretion from the thyroid gland may cause a rapid pulse.

✔ CHECKPOINT **11**:

What is the definition of *pulse?*

Blood Pressure

Blood pressure is the force exerted by the blood against the walls of the vessels. Blood pressure is the product of the output of the heart and the resistance in the vessels. The output of the heart is influenced by the following factors:

- Strength of the contraction of the heart
- Total blood volume, which controls the volume each beat pushes out

The resistance in the vessels is affected by the following factors:

- Vasomotor changes. Vasoconstriction increases resistance to flow; vasodilation lowers resistance.
- Elasticity of blood vessels. Blood vessels lose elasticity and often become hard as a part of aging, thus increasing resistance.
- Thickness of the blood, called *viscosity*. In-

creased numbers of red blood cells increase viscosity.

Measurement of Blood Pressure

The measurement and careful interpretation of blood pressure may prove a valuable guide in the care and evaluation of a person's health. Because blood pressure decreases as the blood flows from arteries into capillaries and finally into veins, measurements ordinarily are made of arterial pressure only. The instrument used is called a *sphygmomanometer* (sfig-mo-mah-NOM-eh-ter), and two variables are measured:

- *Systolic pressure,* which occurs during heart muscle contraction, averages about 120 and is expressed in millimeters of mercury (mmHg).
- *Diastolic pressure,* which occurs during relaxation of the heart muscle, averages about 80 mmHg.

The sphygmomanometer is essentially a graduated column of mercury connected to an inflatable cuff. The cuff is wrapped around the patient's upper arm and inflated with air until the brachial artery is compressed and the blood flow is cut off. Then, listening with a stethoscope, the doctor or nurse slowly lets air out of the cuff until the first pulsations are heard. At this point, the pressure in the cuff is equal to the systolic pressure, and this pressure is read off the mercury column. Then, more air is let out until a characteristic muffled sound indicates the point at which the diastolic pressure is to be read. Considerable experience is required to ensure an accurate reading. The blood pressure is reported as a fraction, with the systolic pressure above and the diastolic pressure below, such as 120/80 mmHg. Note that blood pressure varies throughout the day, so a single reading does not give a complete picture.

✔ CHECKPOINT **12**:

What is the definition of blood pressure?

Summary

I. Blood vessels

A. Types of blood vessels
1. Arteries—carry blood away from heart
   a. Arterioles—small arteries
2. Veins—carry blood toward heart
   a. Venules—small veins
3. Capillaries—allow for exchanges between blood and tissues, or blood and air in lungs; connect arterioles and venules

B. Blood circuits
1. Pulmonary circuit—carries blood to and from lungs
2. Systemic circuit—carries blood to and from rest of body

C. Vessel structure
1. Artery walls—layers
   a. Innermost—single layer of flat epithelial cells (endothelium)
   b. Middle—thicker layer of smooth muscle and elastic connective tissue
   c. Outer—connective tissue
2. Arterioles—thinner walls, less elastic tissue, more smooth muscle
3. Capillaries—only endothelium; single layer of cells
4. Venules—wall slightly thicker than capillary wall
5. Veins—all three layers; thinner walls than arteries, less elastic tissue

II. Systemic arteries

A. The aorta and its parts
1. Largest artery
2. Divisions
   a. Ascending aorta
      (1) Left and right coronary arteries
   b. Aortic arch
      (1) Brachiocephalic trunk—branches to head and arm
      (2) Left common carotid artery—supplies left side of neck and the head
      (3) Left subclavian artery—supplies left arm
   c. Descending aorta
      (1) Thoracic aorta—branches to chest wall, esophagus, bronchi
      (2) Abdominal aorta—supplies abdominal viscera

B. Iliac arteries and their subdivisions
1. Final divisions of aorta
2. Branch to pelvis and legs

C. Arteries that branch to the head and arm—carotid, subclavian, brachial

D. Anastomoses—communications between vessels

III. Systemic veins

1. Superficial—near surface
2. Deep—usually parallel to arteries with same names as corresponding arteries

A. The venae cavae and their tributaries
1. Superior vena cava—drains upper part of body
2. Inferior vena cava—drains lower part of body

B. Venous sinuses—enlarged venous channels

C. Hepatic portal system—carries blood from abdominal organs to liver, where it is processed before returning to heart

IV. The physiology of circulation

A. Capillary exchange
1. Primary method—diffusion
2. Medium—tissue fluid
3. Blood pressure—drives fluid into tissues
4. Osmotic pressure—pulls fluid into capillary

B. Dynamics of blood flow
1. Vasomotor activities
   a. Vasodilation—increase in diameter of blood vessel
   b. Vasoconstriction—decrease in diameter of blood vessel
   c. Vasomotor center—in medulla; controls contraction and relax-

ation of smooth muscle in vessel wall
2. Precapillary sphincter—regulates blood flow into capillary
3. Return of blood to heart
   a. Pumping action of heart
   b. Pressure of skeletal muscles on veins
   c. Valves in veins
   d. Breathing—changes in pressure move blood toward heart

C. **The pulse**
   1. Wave of pressure that travels along arteries as ventricles contract
   2. Rate affected by size, age, sex, activity, and other factors

D. Blood pressure
   1. Force exerted by blood against vessel walls
   2. Product of cardiac output, vascular resistance
   3. Measured in arm with sphygmomanometer
      a. Systolic pressure
         (1) Occurs during heart contraction
         (2) Averages 120 mmHg
      b. Diastolic pressure
         (1) Occurs during heart relaxation
         (2) Averages 80 mmHg

Questions for Study and Review

1. Name the three main groups of blood vessels and describe their functions.
2. Compare the oxygen content of blood in the pulmonary and systemic vessels.
3. How does the structure of the vessels correlate with their function?
4. Name the main branches of the aorta.
5. Describe an arterial anastomosis and give several examples.
6. Trace a drop of blood through the shortest possible route from the capillaries of the foot to the capillaries of the head.
7. What are the names and functions of some cranial venous sinuses? Where is the coronary venous sinus and what does it do?
8. What large vessels drain the blood low in oxygen from most of the body into the right atrium? What vessels carry blood high in oxygen into the left atrium?
9. Trace a drop of blood from capillaries in the wall of the small intestine to the right atrium. What is the purpose of going through the liver on this trip?
10. Define *portal system*. Name the largest portal system in the body.
11. What is the purpose of interstitial fluid?
12. What substances diffuse into the tissues from the capillaries? into the capillaries from the tissues?
13. What force pushes fluid out of the capillaries? What force pulls fluid back into the capillaries?
14. What actions help force blood back to the heart?
15. What is meant by *pulse?* Where is the pulse usually determined? If a large part of the body were burned, leaving only the lower extremities accessible for obtaining the pulse, what vessel would you try to use?
16. What are some factors that cause an increase in the pulse rate?
17. List five factors that can change blood pressure.
18. What instrument is used for measuring blood pressure? What are the two values usually obtained called and what does each represent?

19. Explain the difference between the terms in the following pairs:
    a. *pulmonary circuit* and *systemic circuit*
    b. *arteriole* and *venule*
    c. *vasodilation* and *vasoconstriction*

✔ ANSWERS TO CHECKPOINTS

1. The three main groups of blood vessels are arteries, veins, and capillaries.
2. The pulmonary circuit carries blood from the heart to the lungs and back to the heart; the systemic circuit carries blood to and from all remaining tissues in the body.
3. Smooth muscle makes up the middle layer of arteries and veins. Smooth muscle is involuntary muscle controlled by the autonomic nervous system.
4. The aorta is divided into the ascending aorta, aortic arch, thoracic aorta, and abdominal aorta.
5. An anastomosis is a communication between two vessels.
6. Superficial means near the surface.
7. A venous sinus is a large channel that drains deoxygenated blood.
8. The hepatic portal system takes blood from the abdominal organs to the liver.
9. As materials diffuse across the capillary wall, blood pressure helps to push materials out of the capillaries, and osmotic pressure of the blood helps to draw materials into the capillaries.
10. Vasomotor activities are regulated in the medulla of the brain stem.
11. The pulse is the wave of pressure that begins at the heart and travels along the arteries.
12. Blood pressure is the force exerted by blood against the walls of the vessels.

14

The Lymphatic System and Immunity

SELECTED KEY TERMS

The following terms are defined in the Glossary:

antibody

antigen

antiserum

B cell

chyle

complement

gamma globulin

immunity

immunization

lacteal

lymph

lymphatic duct

lymph node

macrophage

plasma cell

spleen

thymus

tonsil

vaccine

BEHAVIORAL OBJECTIVES

After careful study of this chapter, you should be able to:

1. List the functions of the lymphatic system

2. Explain how lymphatic capillaries differ from blood capillaries

3. Name the two main lymphatic ducts and describe the area drained by each

4. List the major structures of the lymphatic system and give the locations and functions of each

5. Describe the composition and function of the reticuloendothelial system

6. Differentiate between nonspecific and specific body defenses and give examples of each.

7. List several types of inborn immunity

8. Define *antigen* and *antibody*

9. Compare T cells and B cells with respect to development and type of activity

10. Describe the reaction between an antigen and an antibody

11. Differentiate between natural and artificial acquired immunity

12. Differentiate between active and passive immunity

13. Differentiate between a vaccine and an immune serum

As noted in the preceding chapter, body cells live in tissue fluid, a liquid derived from the bloodstream. Water and dissolved substances, such as oxygen and nutrients, are constantly filtering through capillary walls into the spaces between cells and constantly adding to the volume of tissue fluid. Under normal conditions, fluid is also constantly removed, so that it does not accumulate in the tissues. Part of this fluid simply diffuses back into the capillary bloodstream, taking with it some of the end products of cellular metabolism, including carbon dioxide and other substances.

THE LYMPHATIC SYSTEM

A second pathway for the drainage of tissue fluid involves the *lymphatic system* (Fig. 15-1). In the tissues, in addition to the blood-carrying capillaries, there are microscopic vessels called *lymphatic capillaries*, which drain excess fluid that does not return to the blood. The lymphatic capillaries also absorb any proteins suspended in this interstitial (tissue) fluid and return them to the bloodstream. Figure 15-2 shows the lymphatic capillaries and the pathway of lymphatic drainage within the tissues.

Lymph

As soon as tissue fluid enters the lymphatic capillary, it is called *lymph.* The lymphatic cap-

illaries join to form the larger lymphatic vessels, or ducts, and these vessels (which we shall have a closer look at in a moment) eventually empty into veins near the heart. Before the lymph reaches these veins, it flows through a series of filters called *lymph nodes,* where bacteria and other foreign particles are trapped and destroyed. The lymph nodes may be compared in a simple way to the oil filter in an automobile.

✔ CHECKPOINT **1**:

What are some functions of the lymphatic system?

Lymphatic Capillaries

The lymphatic capillaries resemble the blood capillaries in that they are made of one layer of flattened (squamous) epithelial cells, also called *endothelium,* which allows for easy passage of soluble materials and water (Fig. 15-3). The gaps between these endothelial cells in the lymphatic capillaries are larger than those of the blood capillaries to allow easier entrance of proteins and other relatively large suspended particles (see How Lymphatic Capillaries Work). They are more permeable than the blood capillaries; that is, materials can pass through them more easily.

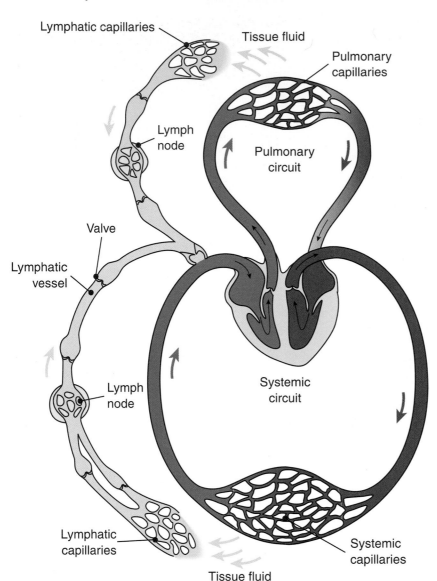

Lymphatic capillaries

Tissue fluid

Pulmonary capillaries

Lymph node

Pulmonary circuit

Valve

Lymphatic vessel

Systemic circuit

Lymph node

Lymphatic capillaries

Systemic capillaries

Tissue fluid

FIGURE **15•1** The lymphatic system in relation to the cardiovascular system.

Unlike the capillaries of the bloodstream, the lymphatic capillaries begin blindly; that is, they are closed at one end and do not serve to bridge two larger vessels. Instead, one end simply lies within a lake of tissue fluid, and the other communicates with a larger lymphatic vessel that transports the lymph toward the heart (see Fig. 15-1).

In the small intestine are some specialized lymphatic capillaries, called ***lacteals*** (LAK-te-als), which act as a pathway for the transfer of digested fats into the bloodstream. This process is covered in the chapter on digestion (see Chap. 17).

✔ CHECKPOINT **2**:

What are two differences between blood capillaries and lymphatic capillaries?

See How Lymphatic Capillaries Work.

Lymphatic Vessels

The lymphatic vessels are thin walled and delicate and have a beaded appearance because of indentations where valves are located (see Fig.

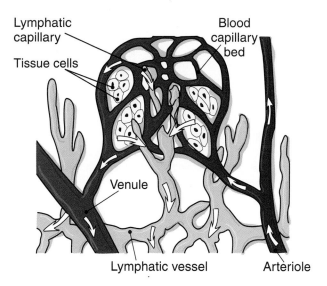

FIGURE **15•2**   Pathway of lymphatic drainage in the tissues.

How Lymphatic Capillaries Work

Lymphatic capillaries are more permeable than blood capillaries because the junctions between the cells are wider and because there is less basement membrane underlying the cells. Proteins and other large molecules that escape from the bloodstream can enter the lymphatic capillaries more easily than they can return to the blood capillaries.

Why don't substances that get into the lymphatic capillaries flow right out again? The cells that form the capillary wall overlap slightly to function as one-way valves. Pressure outside the vessel forces materials in. Once fluid enters the capillary, pressure against the cells in the capillary wall blocks its return.

15-1). These valves prevent backflow in the same way as do those found in some veins.

Lymphatic vessels (Fig. 15-4) include *superficial* and *deep* sets. The surface lymphatics are immediately below the skin, often lying near the superficial veins. The deep vessels are usually larger and accompany the deep veins.

Lymphatic vessels are named according to location. For example, those in the breast are called *mammary* lymphatic vessels, those in the thigh *femoral* lymphatic vessels, and those

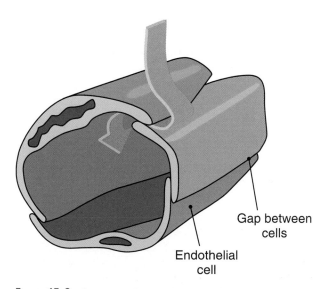

FIGURE **15•3**   Structure of a lymphatic capillary.

in the leg *tibial* lymphatic vessels. All the lymphatic vessels form networks, and at certain points, they carry lymph into the regional nodes (the nodes that "service" a particular area). For example, nearly all the lymph from the upper extremity and the breast passes through the *axillary lymph nodes,* whereas that from the lower extremity passes through the *inguinal nodes.* Lymphatic vessels carrying lymph away from the regional nodes eventually drain into one of the two terminal vessels, the right lymphatic duct or the thoracic duct, both of which empty into the bloodstream.

The *right lymphatic duct* is a short vessel about 1.25 cm (½ inch) long that receives only the lymph that comes from the upper right quadrant of the body: the right side of the head, neck, and thorax, as well as the right upper extremity. It empties into the right subclavian vein. Its opening into this vein is guarded by two pocketlike semilunar valves to prevent blood from entering the duct. The rest of the body is drained by the thoracic duct.

The Thoracic Duct

The *thoracic duct* is the larger of the two terminal vessels; it is about 40 cm (16 inches) in length. As shown in Figure 15-4, the thoracic duct receives lymph from all parts of the body except those above the diaphragm on the right side. This duct begins in the posterior part of

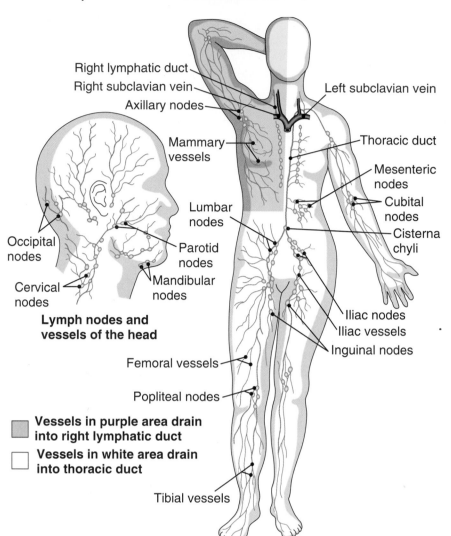

Lymph nodes and vessels of the head

Right lymphatic duct

Right subclavian vein

Axillary nodes

Mammary vessels

Lumbar nodes

Occipital nodes

Parotid nodes

Cervical nodes

Mandibular nodes

Left subclavian vein

Thoracic duct

Mesenteric nodes

Cubital nodes

Cisterna chyli

Iliac nodes

Iliac vessels

Inguinal nodes

Femoral vessels

Popliteal nodes

Tibial vessels

▨ **Vessels in purple area drain into right lymphatic duct**

☐ **Vessels in white area drain into thoracic duct**

Figure **15•4** Lymphatic system.

the abdominal cavity, below the attachment of the diaphragm. The first part of this duct is enlarged to form a cistern, or temporary storage pouch, called the *cisterna chyli* (sis-TER-nah KI-li). *Chyle* (kile) is the milky fluid, formed by the combination of fat globules and lymph, that comes from the intestinal lacteals. Chyle passes through the intestinal lymphatic vessels and the lymph nodes of the mesentery, finally entering the cisterna chyli. In addition to chyle, all the lymph from below the diaphragm empties into the cisterna chyli by way of the various clusters of lymph nodes and then is carried by the thoracic duct into the bloodstream.

The thoracic duct extends upward through the diaphragm and along the back wall of the thorax up into the root of the neck on the left side. Here, it receives the left jugular lymphatic vessels from the head and neck, the left subclavian vessels from the left upper extremity, and other lymphatic vessels from the thorax and its parts. In addition to the valves along the duct, there are two valves at its opening into the left subclavian vein to prevent the passage of blood into the duct.

✔ CHECKPOINT **3**:

What are the two main lymphatic vessels?

Movement of Lymph

The segments of lymphatic vessels located between the valves contract rhythmically, propelling the lymph along. The rate of these contractions is related to the volume of fluid in the vessel—the more fluid, the more rapid the contractions of the vessel.

Lymph is also moved by the same mechanisms that promote venous return of blood to the heart. As skeletal muscles contract during movement, they compress the lymphatic vessels and drive lymph forward. Changes in pressures within the abdominal and thoracic cavities due to breathing aid the movement of lymph during passage through these body cavities.

LYMPHOID TISSUE

The previous section was a brief survey of the system of lymph vessels and lymph transport. Although the lymph nodes were mentioned, they are described in greater detail in this section, along with discussion of other organs made of similar tissue.

Lymphoid (LIM-foyd) *tissue* is distributed throughout the body and makes up the specialized organs of the lymphatic system. We will look at some of these organs, but first let us consider some properties of lymphoid tissue to see what characteristics these organs have in common.

Some of the general functions of lymphoid tissue include the following:

- Removal of impurities, such as carbon particles, cancer cells, pathogenic organisms, and dead blood cells. These materials are filtered out of body fluids and then destroyed by phagocytes that ingest and destroy foreign matter.
- Processing of lymphocytes, cells of the immune system. Some of these lymphocytes produce antibodies, substances in the blood that aid in combating infection; others attack foreign invaders directly. Lymphocytes and the immune system are discussed later in this chapter.

Lymph Nodes

The lymph nodes, as we have seen, are designed to filter the lymph once it is drained from the tissues (Fig. 15-5). The lymph nodes are small, rounded masses varying from pinhead size to as long as 2.5 cm (1 inch). Each has a fibrous connective tissue capsule from which partitions (trabeculae) extend into the substance of the node. Inside the node are masses of lymphatic tissue, which include lymphocytes and

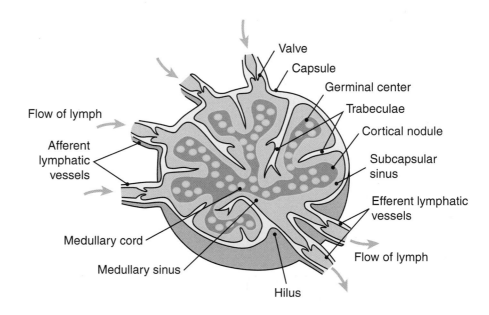

FIGURE **15•5**   Structure of a lymph node.

Valve
Capsule
Germinal center
Trabeculae
Cortical nodule
Subcapsular sinus
Efferent lymphatic vessels
Flow of lymph
Hilus
Medullary sinus
Medullary cord
Afferent lymphatic vessels
Flow of lymph

macrophages, white blood cells active in immunity.

At various points in the surface of the node, afferent lymphatic vessels pierce the capsule to carry lymph into the spaces inside the pulplike nodal tissue. An indented area called the **hilus** (HI-lus) serves as the exit for efferent lymphatic vessels carrying lymph out of the node. At this region, other structures, including blood vessels and nerves, connect with the node.

Lymph nodes are seldom isolated. As a rule, they are massed together in groups, the number in each group varying from 2 or 3 to well over 100. Some of these groups are placed deeply, whereas some are superficial. The main groups include the following:

*   **Cervical nodes,** located in the neck in deep and superficial groups, drain various parts of the head and neck. They often become enlarged during upper respiratory infections.
*   **Axillary nodes,** located in the axillae (armpits), may become enlarged after infections of the upper extremities and the breasts. Cancer cells from the breasts often metastasize (spread) to the axillary nodes.
*   **Tracheobronchial** (tra-ke-o-BRONG-ke-al) **nodes** are found near the trachea and around the larger bronchial tubes. In people living in highly polluted areas, these nodes become so filled with carbon particles that they are solid black masses resembling pieces of coal.
*   **Mesenteric** (mes-en-TER-ik) **nodes** are found between the two layers of peritoneum that form the mesentery (membrane around the intestines). There are some 100 to 150 of these nodes.
*   **Inguinal nodes,** located in the groin region, receive lymph drainage from the lower extremities and from the external genital organs. When they become enlarged, they are often referred to as **buboes** (BU-bose), from which bubonic plague got its name.

✔ CHECKPOINT **4**:
_____
What is the function of the lymph nodes?

The Tonsils

There are masses of lymphoid tissue that are designed to filter not lymph, but tissue fluid. Found beneath certain areas of moist epithelium that are exposed to the outside, and hence to contamination, these masses include parts of the digestive, urinary, and respiratory tracts. Associated with the latter system are those well-known masses of lymphoid tissue called the **tonsils,** which include the following:

*   The **palatine** (PAL-ah-tine) **tonsils,** oval bodies located at each side of the soft palate. These are generally meant when one refers to "the tonsils."
*   The **pharyngeal** (fah-RIN-je-al) **tonsil,** commonly referred to as the **adenoids** (from a general term that means "gland-like"). It is located behind the nose on the back wall of the upper pharynx.
*   The **lingual** (LING-gwal) **tonsils,** little mounds of lymphoid tissue at the back of the tongue.

Any or all of these tonsils may become so loaded with bacteria that the pathogens gain the upper hand; removal then is advisable. A slight enlargement of any of them is not an indication for surgery. All lymphoid tissue masses tend to be larger in childhood, so that a physician must consider the patient's age in determining whether these masses are enlarged abnormally. Because the tonsils function in immunity during early childhood, efforts are made *not* to remove them unless absolutely necessary.

✔ CHECKPOINT **5**:
_____
Tonsils filter tissue fluid. What is the general location of the tonsils?

The Thymus

Because of its appearance under the microscope, the **thymus** (THI-mus), located in the upper thorax beneath the sternum, has been considered part of the lymphoid system. Recent studies, however, suggest that this structure has a much wider function than other lymphoid tissue. It appears that the thymus plays a key role in the development of the immune system before birth and during the first few months of infancy. Certain lymphocytes must mature in the thymus gland before they can perform their functions in the immune system. These T cells (T lymphocytes) develop under the effects of the hormone from the thymus gland called ***thymosin*** (THI-mo-sin), which also promotes the growth and activity of lymphocytes in lymphoid tissue throughout the body. Removal of the thymus causes a decrease in the production of T cells as well as a decrease in the size of the spleen and of lymph nodes throughout the body.

The thymus is most active during early life. After puberty, the tissue undergoes changes; it shrinks in size and is replaced by connective tissue and fat.

✔ CHECKPOINT **6**:

What kind of immune system cells develop in the thymus?

The Spleen

The spleen is an organ that contains lymphoid tissue designed to filter blood. It is located in the upper left hypochondriac region of the abdomen, high up under the dome of the diaphragm, and normally is protected by the lower part of the rib cage. The spleen is a soft, purplish, and somewhat flattened organ about 12.5 to 16 cm (5 to 6 inches) long and 5 to 7.5 cm (2 to 3 inches) wide. The capsule of the spleen, as well as its framework, is more elastic than that of the lymph nodes. It contains involuntary muscle, which enables the splenic capsule to contract and also to withstand some swelling.

The spleen has an unusually large blood supply, considering its size. The organ is filled with a soft pulp, one of the functions of which is to filter out worn-out red blood cells. The spleen also harbors phagocytes, which engulf bacteria and other foreign particles. The spleen is classi-

fied as part of the lymphatic system because it contains prominent masses of lymphoid tissue. However, it has wider functions than other lymphatic structures, including the following:

* Cleansing the blood by filtration and phagocytosis
* Destroying old, worn-out red blood cells. The iron and other breakdown products of hemoglobin are carried to the liver by the hepatic portal system to be reused or eliminated from the body.
* Producing red blood cells before birth
* Serving as a reservoir for blood, which can be returned to the bloodstream in case of hemorrhage or other emergency

---

✔ CHECKPOINT **7**:

What is filtered by the spleen?

THE RETICULOENDOTHELIAL SYSTEM

The ***reticuloendothelial*** (reh-tik-u-lo-en-do-THE-le-al) ***system*** consists of related cells concerned with the destruction of worn-out blood cells, bacteria, cancer cells, and other foreign substances that are potentially harmful to the body. Included among these cells are monocytes, relatively large white blood cells (see Fig. 12-1 in Chap. 12) that are formed in the bone marrow and then circulate in the bloodstream to various parts of the body. On entering the tissues, monocytes develop into ***macrophages*** (MAK-ro-faj-ez), a term that means "big eaters."

Some monocytes are given special names; ***Kupffer's*** (KOOP-ferz) ***cells,*** for example, are located in the lining of the liver sinusoids (blood channels). Other parts of the reticuloendothelial system are found in the spleen, bone marrow, lymph nodes, and brain. Some macrophages are located in the lungs, where they are called *dust cells* because they ingest solid particles that enter the lungs; others are found in soft connective tissues all over the body.

This widely distributed protective system has

been called by several other names, including tissue macrophage system, mononuclear phagocyte system, and monocyte-macrophage system. These names describe the type of cells found in this system.

IMMUNITY

The reticuloendothelial system is but one of the body's mechanisms for fighting disease and ridding itself of impurities. Because this system is active against any harmful agent entering the body, it is described as a ***nonspecific*** defense. Other nonspecific defenses include the skin and mucous membranes, body secretions such as tears and digestive juices, and the imflammatory response.

Our final line of defense against disease, however, is the immune system, which is referred to as ***specific*** because it acts against particular harmful agents. Immunity is a selective process; that is, immunity to one disease does not necessarily cause immunity to another.

There are two main categories of immunity:

- ***Inborn immunity*** is inherited along with other characteristics in a person's genes.
- ***Acquired immunity*** develops after birth. Acquired immunity may be obtained by ***natural*** or ***artificial*** means; in addition, acquired immunity may be either ***active*** or ***passive***.

Figure 15-6 is a summary of the different types of immunity. Refer to this diagram as we investigate each category in turn.

Inborn Immunity

Both humans and animals have what is called a ***species immunity*** to many of each other's diseases. Although certain diseases found in animals may be transmitted to humans, many infections, such as chicken cholera, hog cholera, distemper, and other animal diseases, do not affect human beings. However, the constitutional differences that make human beings immune to these disorders also make them susceptible to others that do not affect the lower animals.

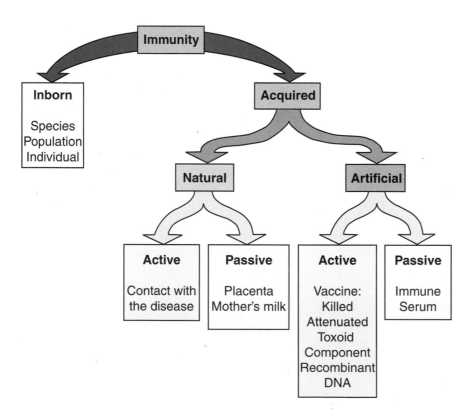

FIGURE **15•6** Types of immunity.

Such infections as measles, scarlet fever, diphtheria, and influenza do not appear to affect animals in contact with humans who have these illnesses.

Another form of inborn immunity is **population immunity.** Some groups appear to have a greater inborn immunity to certain diseases than others. Although measles, for example, is generally a mild disease in Europeans, it became a serious and often fatal disease among people of the Pacific Islands when foreigners brought it there. These populations had never been exposed to the measles virus and had not developed genetic resistance to the disease over time. When poliomyelitis was a public health threat in the United States, American blacks were apparently more resistant to the disease than whites. Some populations are more resistant to malaria and yellow fever than others.

Of course, it is often difficult to tell how much of this variation in resistance to infection is due to environment and how much is due to inborn traits of the various groups.

Some members of a given group have a more highly developed **individual immunity** to specific diseases. For example, some people are prone to cold sores (fever blisters) caused by herpes virus, whereas others have never experienced this type of infection. Newspapers and magazines sometimes feature the advice of an elderly person who is asked to give her secret for living to a ripe old age. One elderly person may say that he practiced temperance and lived a carefully regulated life with the right amount of rest, exercise, and work, whereas the next may boast of her use of alcoholic beverages, constant smoking, lack of exercise, and other kinds of reputedly unhealthy behavior. However, it is possible that the latter person had lived through the onslaughts of toxins and disease organisms, resisted infection, and maintained health despite her habits, rather than because of them, thanks to the resistance factors and immunity to disease she inherited.

✔ CHECKPOINT **8**:

What are some types of inborn immunity?

Acquired Immunity

Unlike inborn immunity, which is due to inherited factors, acquired immunity develops during a person's lifetime as that person encounters various specific harmful agents.

If the following description of the immune system seems complex, bear in mind that from infancy on, your immune system is able to protect you from millions of foreign substances, even synthetic compounds and substances not found in nature. All the while, the system is kept in check, so that it does not usually overreact to produce allergies or mistakenly attack and damage your own body tissues.

Antigens
An **antigen** (AN-te-jen) **(Ag)** is any foreign substance that enters the body and induces an immune response. Most antigens are large protein molecules, but carbohydrates and some lipids may act as antigens. Antigens may be found on the surface of pathogenic (harmful) organisms, on the surface of red blood cells and tissue cells, on pollens, in toxins (poisons), and in foods. The critical feature of any substance described as an antigen is that it stimulates the activity of certain lymphocytes classified as T or B cells.

T Cells
Both T and B cells come from stem cells in bone marrow, as do all blood cells. They differ, however, in their development and their method of action. Some of the immature stem cells migrate to the thymus gland and become T cells, which constitute about 80% of the lymphocytes in the circulating blood. While in the thymus, these T lymphocytes multiply and become capable of combining with specific foreign antigens, at which time they are described as **sensitized.** These thymus-derived cells produce an immunity that is said to be **cell-mediated immunity.**

There are several types of T cells, each with different functions. Some of these functions and the T cell type involved in each are as follows:

- To destroy foreign cells directly. These are the **cytotoxic T cells.**

- To release substances known as *interleukins* (in-ter-LU-kinz) that stimulate other lymphocytes and macrophages and thereby assist in the destruction of foreign cells. There are several subtypes of these *helper T cells,* one of which is infected and destroyed by the AIDS virus (HIV). These targeted cells have a special surface receptor (CD_4) to which the virus attaches.
- To suppress the immune response in order to regulate it. These *suppressor T cells* may inhibit or destroy active lymphocytes.
- To remember an antigen and start a rapid response if that antigen is met again. These are *memory T cells.*

The T cell portion of the immune system is generally responsible for defense against cancer cells, certain viruses, and other pathogens that grow within cells (intracellular parasites), as well as for the rejection of tissue transplanted from another person.

The Role of Macrophages

Macrophages are phagocytic white blood cells derived from monocytes (their name means "big eater"). They ingest foreign proteins, such as disease organisms, and break them down. For a T cell to react with an antigen, that antigen must be presented to the T cell on the surface of a macrophage in combination with proteins that the T cell can recognize as belonging to the "self" (Fig. 15-7). Self antigens are known as MHC (major histocompatibility complex) antigens because of their importance in cross-matching for tissue transplantation. They are also known as HLAs (human leukocyte antigens) because white blood cells are used in testing tissues for compatibility. Macrophages and other cells that present antigens to T cells are known as APCs (antigen-presenting cells).

After combining with T cells, the macrophages also release interleukins (the name means "between white blood cells"). These substances stimulate the growth of T cells and

FIGURE **15•7**   Activation of a helper T cell by a macrophage.

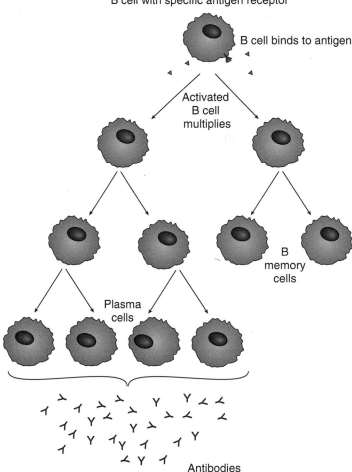

B cell with specific antigen receptor

B cell binds to antigen

Activated
B cell
multiplies

B
memory
cells

Plasma
cells

Antibodies

FIGURE **15•8** Activation of B cells. The B cell combines with a specific antigen. The cell divides to form plasma cells, which produce antibodies. Memory cells are also formed; these protect against reinfection.

have been used medically in efforts to boost the immune system.

✔ CHECKPOINT **9**:

What is the difference between inborn and acquired immunity?

✔ CHECKPOINT **10**:

What is an antigen?

B Cells and Antibodies

An *antibody (Ab)*, also known as an *immunoglobulin (Ig)*, is a substance produced in response to an antigen. Antibodies are manufactured by *B cells* (B lymphocytes), another type of lymphocyte active in the immune system. B cells must mature in the fetal liver or in lymphoid tissue before becoming active in the blood.

B cells have surface receptors that bind with a specific type of antigen (Fig. 15-8). Exposure to the antigen stimulates the cells to multiply rapidly and produce large numbers (clones) of *plasma cells*. Plasma cells produce antibodies against the original antigen and release these antibodies into the blood, providing the form of immunity described as ***humoral immunity*** (the term humoral refers to body fluids).

Humoral immunity generally protects against circulating antigens and bacteria that grow outside the cells (extracellular parasites). All antibodies are contained in a portion of the blood plasma called the ***gamma globulin*** fraction.

Some antibodies produced by B cells remain in the blood to give long-term immunity. In addition, some of the activated B cells do not become plasma cells but, like certain T cells, become memory cells. On repeated contact with an antigen, these cells are ready to produce antibodies immediately. Because of this "immunologic memory," one is usually immune to a childhood disease after having it.

> ✔ CHECKPOINT **11**:
>
> Immunity is based on the actions of two types of lymphocytes. What are these two types of cells called?

The Antigen–Antibody Reaction

The antibody that is produced in response to a specific antigen, such as a bacterial cell or a toxin, has a shape that matches some part of that antigen, much in the same way that the shape of a key matches the shape of its lock. The antibody can bind specifically to the antigen that caused its production and thereby destroy or inactivate it. In the laboratory, this can be seen as a settling (precipitation) or a clumping (agglutination) of the antigen–antibody combination, as is seen in the typing of red blood cells.

Complement

The destruction of foreign cells sometimes requires the enzymatic activity of a group of nonspecific proteins in the blood, together called ***complement.*** Complement proteins boost immunity by lysing (destroying) organisms that have been coated with antibody. They can also attract and activate phagocytes.

> ✔ CHECKPOINT **12**:
>
> What is complement?

Naturally Acquired Immunity

Active

Immunity may be acquired naturally through contact with a specific disease organism. In this case, antibodies manufactured by the infected person's cells act against the infecting agent or its toxins. The infection that calls forth the immunity may be a subclinical or inapparent infection that is so mild as to cause no symptoms. Nevertheless, it stimulates the host's cells to produce an active immunity.

Each time a person is invaded by disease organisms, his or her cells manufacture antibodies that provide immunity against the infection. Such immunity may last for years and in some cases lasts for life. Because the host is actively involved in the production of antibodies, this type of immunity is called ***active immunity.*** See Stress and the Immune System.

Passive

Immunity also may be acquired naturally by the passage of antibodies from a mother to her fetus through the placenta. Because these antibodies come from an outside source, this type of immunity is called ***passive immunity.*** The antibodies obtained in this way do not last as long as actively produced antibodies, but they do help protect the infant for about 6 months, at which time the child's own immune system begins to function. Nursing an infant can lengthen this period of protection owing to the presence of specific antibodies in breast milk and colostrum (the first breast secretion). These are the only known examples of naturally acquired passive immunity.

> ✔ CHECKPOINT **13**:
>
> What is the difference between the active and passive forms of naturally acquired immunity?

Stress and the Immune System

The effects of stress on the immune system may be the most wide ranging and significant of its many effects on the body. Stressors such as trauma, infection, debilitating disease, surgery, pain, extreme environmental conditions, and emotional distress all have significant effects on the immune system's ability to function fully and correctly.

The predominant effects of stress on the immune system are caused by an increase in the hormone cortisol, which is secreted in response to ACTH from the anterior pituitary. This increase parallels the release of norepinephrine and epinephrine from the sympathetic nervous system. The combined effect of these secretions is to increase the total number of white blood cells in circulation. The increase, however, occurs primarily in neutrophils, while eosinophils and basophils are reduced. In addition, lymphocyte maturation in the lymph nodes is halted since epinephrine decreases blood flow to the nodes in favor of flow to the heart, lungs, brain and muscles. Cortisol also reduces production of interleukins and antibodies, affecting both cellular and humoral immunity. These changes leave the body less capable of fighting off the effects of injury and disease, and, indeed, stress itself.

The increase in cortisol levels, initiated by stress, is an integral part of one's immediate ability to fight off a life-or-death stressor. Continued stress, however, even at low levels, leads to accumulated decreases in immune function.

Artificially Acquired Immunity

Active Immunization

A person who has not been exposed to repeated small doses of a particular organism has no antibodies against that organism and is defenseless against a heavy infection. Therefore, artificial measures may be taken to cause a person's tissues to manufacture antibodies. The administration of virulent pathogens obviously would be dangerous. Instead, the harmful agent is treated to reduce its virulence and then administered. In this way, the immune system is made to produce antibodies without causing a serious illness. This protective process is known as *vaccination* (vak-sin-A-shun), or *immunization,* and the solution used is called a *vaccine* (vak-SENE). Ordinarily, the administration of a vaccine is a preventive measure designed to provide protection in anticipation of invasion by a certain disease organism.

Types of Vaccines

Vaccines can be made with live organisms or with organisms killed by heat or chemicals. If live organisms are used, they must be nonvirulent (harmless) for humans, such as the cowpox virus used for smallpox immunization, or they must be treated in the laboratory to weaken them as human pathogens. An organism weakened for use in vaccines is described as *attenuated.* In some cases, just an antigenic component of the pathogen is used as a vaccine. Another type of vaccine is made from a form of the toxin produced by a disease organism. The toxin is altered with heat or chemicals to reduce its harmfulness, but it can still function as an antigen to induce immunity. Such an altered toxin is called a *toxoid.*

The newest types of vaccines are produced from antigenic components of pathogens or by genetic engineering. By techniques of *recombinant DNA,* the genes for specific disease antigens are inserted into the genetic material of harmless organisms. The antigens produced by these organisms are extracted and purified and used for immunization. The hepatitis B vaccine is produced in this manner.

Boosters

A final word about the long-term efficacy of vaccines: in many cases, an active immunity acquired by artificial (or even natural) means does not last a lifetime. Circulating antibodies can decline with time. To help maintain a high titer (level) of antibodies in the blood, repeated inoculations, called *booster shots,* are administered at intervals. The number of booster injections recommended varies with the disease and with the environment or range of exposure of the individual.

The successful completion of childhood immunizations can be a public health concern. States have different requirements for preschool immunizations and for vaccinations and boosters

15

for older children. On occasion, epidemics in high schools or colleges may prompt recommendations for specific boosters.

Passive Immunization

It takes several weeks to produce a naturally acquired active immunity and even longer to produce an artificial active immunity through the administration of a vaccine. Therefore, a person who receives a large dose of virulent organisms and has no established immunity to them is in great danger. To prevent illness, the person must quickly receive a counteracting dose of borrowed antibodies. This is accomplished through the administration of an ***immune serum,*** or ***antiserum.*** The "ready-made" serum gives short-lived but effective protection against the invaders in the form of an artificially acquired passive immunity. Immune sera are used in emergencies, that is, in situations in which there is no time to wait until an active immunity has developed.

Summary

15

I. **Lymphatic system**
   1. Functions
     a. Drainage of excess fluid and protein from tissues
     b. Filtration of body fluids
     c. Absorption of fats from small intestine
  A. Lymph—fluid in lymphatic system
  B. Lymphatic capillaries—made of endothelium (simple squamous epithelium)
  C. Lymphatic vessels
     a. Superficial
     b. Deep
     c. Right lymphatic duct—drains upper right part of body and empties into right subclavian vein
     d. Thoracic duct—drains remainder of body and empties into left subclavian vein
  D. Movement of lymph
    1. Valves in vessels
    2. Contraction of vessels
    3. Muscle contraction
    4. Breathing

II. **Lymphoid tissue**—distributed throughout body
   1. General functions
     a. Removal of impurities by filtration and phagocytosis
     b. Processing of lymphocytes of immune system
  A. Lymph nodes—filtration of lymph
  B. Tonsils—filtration of tissue fluid
  C. Thymus
    1. Processing of T lymphocytes (T cells)
    2. Secretion of thymosin—stimulates T lymphocytes in lymphoid tissue
  D. Spleen
    1. Filtration of blood
    2. Destruction of old red cells
    3. Production of red cells before birth
    4. Storage of blood

III. **The reticuloendothelial system**—cells throughout body that remove impurities

IV. **Immunity**—specific defense against disease
  A. Inborn immunity—inherited
    1. Types: species, population, individual
  B. Acquired immunity—develops after birth
    1. Antigens—stimulate lymphocyte activity
    2. Antibodies—inactivate pathogens or neutralize toxins
    3. T cells (T lymphocytes)
     a. Processed in thymus
     b. Types: cytotoxic, helper, suppressor, memory

c. Helper T cells produce interleukins (immune stimulants)
d. Involved in cell-mediated immunity
4. Macrophages
a. Derived from monocytes
b. Present antigen to T cells in combination with MHC ("self") proteins
5. B cells (B lymphocytes)
a. Mature in lymphoid tissue
b. Develop into plasma cells that
produce circulating antibodies
c. Also develop into memory cells
d. Involved in humoral immunity
C. The antigen–antibody reaction
1. Shape of antibody matches shape of
antigen

2. Complement—group of proteins
a. Aids in destroying foreign cells
b. Boosts immune response
D. Naturally acquired immunity
1. Active—acquired through contact
with the disease
2. Passive—acquired from antibodies
obtained through placenta and
mother's milk
E. Artificially acquired immunity
1. Active—immunization with vaccines
a. Types: live (attenuated), killed,
toxoid, recombinant DNA
b. Boosters—keep antibody titers
high
2. Passive—administration of immune
serum (antiserum)

Questions for Study and Review

1. What is lymph? How is it formed?
2. Briefly describe the system of lymph circulation.
3. Describe the lymphatic vessels with respect to structure and location.
4. Name the two main lymphatic ducts. What part of the body does each drain, and into what blood vessel does each empty?
5. Describe two functions of lymphoid tissue.
6. What is the cisterna chyli and what are its purposes?
7. Describe the structure of a typical lymph node.
8. Describe the location of the main groups of lymph nodes.
9. Name some conditions that cause enlargement of lymph nodes in specific regions.
10. What are the different tonsils called and where are they located? What is the purpose of these structures?
11. What is the function of the thymus?
12. Give the location of the spleen and name several of its functions.
13. Describe the reticuloendothelial system.
14. What is meant by a *nonspecific defense* against disease? Give several examples of nonspecific defenses.
15. Define *immunity.*
16. Give three examples of inborn immunity.
17. What is the difference between inborn and acquired immunity?
18. Define *antigen* and *antibody.* Why is the reaction between and antigen and antibody described as specific?
19. How do T and B cells differ? In what ways are they the same?
20. Name four types of T cells.
21. What is the role of macrophages in immunity?
22. What is complement?
23. Compare active and passive immunity.

24. What is a vaccine? a toxoid?
25. Why are booster shots given?
26. What is an immune serum?

✔ ANSWERS TO CHECKPOINTS

1. The lymphatic system drains excess fluid and proteins from the tissues and filters impurities from body fluids.
2. The lymphatic capillaries are more permeable than blood capillaries and begin blindly. They are closed at one end and do not bridge two vessels.
3. The two main lymphatic vessels are the right lymphatic duct and the thoracic duct.
4. The lymph nodes filter lymph.
5. Tonsils are located in the vicinity of the throat (pharynx).
6. T cells of the immune system develop in the thymus.
7. Blood is filtered by the spleen.
8. Some types of inborn immunity are species, population, and individual immunity.
9. Inborn immunity is inherited in a person's genetic material; acquired immunity develops during an individual's lifetime.
10. An antigen is any foreign substance, usually a protein, that induces an immune response.
11. The cells active in immunity are T cells and B cells.
12. Complement is a group of proteins in the blood that sometimes is required for the destruction of foreign cells.
13. The active form of naturally acquired immunity comes from contact with a disease organism; the passive form comes from the passage of antibodies from a mother to her fetus through the placenta or breast milk.

15

It is the purpose of the four chapters of this unit to show how oxygen and nutrients are processed, taken up by the body fluids, and used by the cells to yield energy. This unit also describes how the stability of body functions (homeostasis) is maintained and how waste products are eliminated.

Unit V

ENERGY: SUPPLY AND USE

Respiration

SELECTED KEY TERMS

The following items are defined in the Glossary:

alveolus (pl., alveoli)

bronchiole

bronchus (pl., bronchi)

chemoreceptor

compliance

diaphragm

epiglottis

hemoglobin

hilus (hilum)

larynx

lung

mediastinum

pharynx

pleura

respiration

surfactant

trachea

ventilation

BEHAVIORAL OBJECTIVES

After careful study of this chapter, you should be able to:

1. Define *respiration* and describe the three phases of respiration

2. Name and describe all the structures of the respiratory system

3. Explain the mechanism for pulmonary ventilation

4. List the ways in which oxygen and carbon dioxide are transported in the blood

5. Describe the ways in which respiration is regulated

Most people think of respiration simply as the process by which air moves into and out of the lungs, that is, *breathing*. By scientific definition, respiration is the process by which oxygen is obtained from the environment and delivered to the cells. Carbon dioxide is transported to the outside in a reverse pathway.

Respiration includes three phases:

- *Pulmonary ventilation,* which is the exchange of air between the atmosphere and the air sacs of the lungs. This is normally accomplished by the inspiration and expiration of breathing.
- The *diffusion* of gases, which includes the passage of oxygen from the air sacs into the blood and the passage of carbon dioxide out of the blood
- The *transport* of gases in the circulating blood. Oxygen is carried to the cells and carbon dioxide is transported from the cells to the lungs.

In the process of *cellular respiration,* oxygen is taken into the cell and used in the breakdown of nutrients with the release of energy. Carbon dioxide is the waste product of cellular respiration.

✔ CHECKPOINT **1**:

What are the three phases of respiration?

THE RESPIRATORY SYSTEM

The respiratory system is an intricate arrangement of spaces and passageways that conduct air into the lungs (Fig. 16-1). These spaces include the *nasal cavities;* the *pharynx* (FAR-inks), which is common to the digestive and respiratory systems; the voice box, or *larynx* (LAR-inks); the windpipe, or *trachea* (TRA-ke-ah); and the *lungs* themselves, with their conducting tubes and air sacs. The entire system might be thought of as a pathway for air between the atmosphere and the blood.

The Nasal Cavities

Air makes its initial entrance into the body through the openings in the nose called the *nostrils.* Immediately inside the nostrils, located between the roof of the mouth and the cranium, are the two spaces known as the *nasal cavities.* These two spaces are separated from each other by a partition, the *nasal septum.* The su-

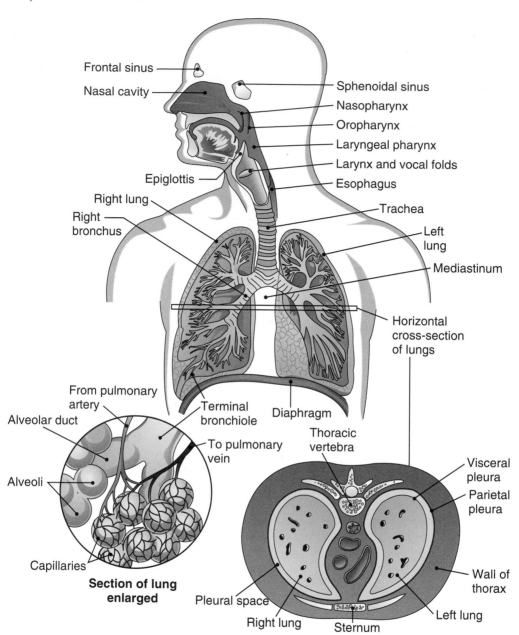

Frontal sinus
Nasal cavity
Sphenoidal sinus
Nasopharynx
Oropharynx
Laryngeal pharynx
Larynx and vocal folds
Epiglottis
Esophagus
Right lung
Trachea
Right bronchus
Left lung
Mediastinum
Horizontal cross-section of lungs
From pulmonary artery
Alveolar duct
Terminal bronchiole
Diaphragm
To pulmonary vein
Thoracic vertebra
Alveoli
Visceral pleura
Parietal pleura
Capillaries
Wall of thorax
Section of lung enlarged
Pleural space
Left lung
Right lung
Sternum

FIGURE **16•1** Respiratory system.

perior portion of the septum is formed by a thin plate of the ethmoid bone that extends downward, and the inferior portion is formed by the vomer (see Fig. 6-3A in Chap. 6). An anterior extension of the septum is made of hyaline cartilage. The septum and the walls of the nasal cavity are covered with mucous membrane. On the lateral (side) walls of each nasal cavity are three projections called the ***conchae*** (KONG-

ke) (see Figs. 6-3A and 6-6 in Chap. 6). The shell-like conchae greatly increase the surface over which air must travel on its way through the nasal cavities.

The mucous membrane lining the nasal cavities contains many blood vessels that deliver heat and moisture. The cells of this membrane secrete a large amount of fluid—up to 1 quart each day. The following changes are produced in the air as it comes in contact with the lining of the nose:

- Foreign bodies, such as dust particles and pathogens, are filtered out by the hairs of the nostrils or caught in the surface mucus.
- Air is warmed by the blood in the vascular membrane.
- Air is moistened by the liquid secretion.

To allow for these protective changes to occur, it is preferable to breathe through the nose rather than through the mouth.

The **sinuses** are small cavities lined with mucous membrane in the bones of the skull. The sinuses communicate with the nasal cavities, and they are highly susceptible to infection.

✔ CHECKPOINT **2**:

What happens to air as it passes over the nasal mucosa?

The Pharynx

The muscular **pharynx,** or throat, carries air into the respiratory tract and carries foods and liquids into the digestive system (see Fig. 16-1). The upper portion, located immediately behind the nasal cavity, is called the **nasopharynx** (na-zo-FAR-inks); the middle section, located behind the mouth, is called the **oropharynx** (o-ro-FAR-inks); and the lowest portion is called the **laryngeal** (lah-RIN-je-al) **pharynx.** This last section opens into the larynx toward the front and into the esophagus toward the back.

The Larynx

The **larynx,** commonly called the *voice box* (Fig. 16-2), is located between the pharynx and the trachea. It has a framework of cartilage, part of which is the thyroid cartilage that protrudes in the front of the neck. The projection formed by the thyroid cartilage is popularly called the *Adam's apple* because it is considerably larger in the male than in the female.

On both sides at the upper end of the larynx are folds of mucous membrane used in producing speech. These are the vocal folds, or **vocal cords** (Fig. 16-3). They are set into vibration by the flow of air from the lungs. A difference in the size of the larynx is what accounts for the difference between male and female voices; because a man's larynx is larger than a woman's, his voice is lower in pitch. The nasal cavities, the sinuses, and the pharynx all serve as resonating chambers for speech, just as the cabinet does for an audio speaker.

The space between the vocal cords is called

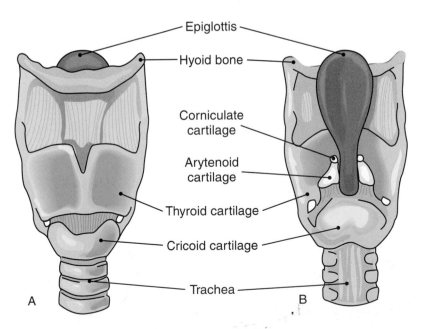

FIGURE **16•2** The larynx. **(A)** Anterior view. **(B)** Posterior view.

Epiglottis
Hyoid bone
Corniculate cartilage
Arytenoid cartilage
Thyroid cartilage
Cricoid cartilage
Trachea

A

B

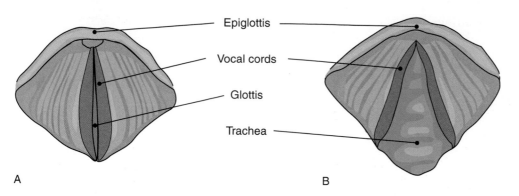

Epiglottis

Vocal cords

Glottis

Trachea

A

B

FIGURE **16•3** The vocal cords viewed from above. **(A)** The glottis in closed position. **(B)** The glottis in open position.

16

the **glottis** (GLOT-is), and the little leaf-shaped cartilage that covers the larynx during swallowing is called the **epiglottis** (ep-ih-GLOT-is). The glottis and epiglottis help keep food and liquids out of the remainder of the respiratory tract. As the larynx moves upward and forward during swallowing, the epiglottis moves downward, covering the opening into the larynx. The glottis assists by closing during swallowing. You can feel the larynx move upward toward the epiglottis during this process by placing the flat ends of your fingers on your larynx as you swallow.

The Trachea

The **trachea,** commonly called the *windpipe,* is a tube that extends from the lower edge of the larynx to the upper part of the chest above the heart. The purpose of the trachea is to conduct air between the larynx and the lungs.

The trachea has a framework of cartilages to keep it open. These cartilages, shaped somewhat like a tiny horseshoe or the letter C, are found along the entire length of the trachea. The open sections in the cartilages are lined up in the back so that the esophagus can bulge into this region during swallowing.

✔ CHECKPOINT **3**:

What are the scientific names for the throat, the voice box, and the windpipe?

The Bronchi

At its inferior end, the trachea divides into two primary, or main-stem, **bronchi** (BRONG-ki), which enter the lungs. The right bronchus is considerably larger in diameter than the left and extends downward in a more vertical direction. Therefore, if a foreign body is inhaled, it is likely to enter the right lung. Each bronchus enters the lung at a notch or depression called the **hilus** (HI-lus) or **hilum** (HI-lum). Blood vessels and nerves also connect with the lung in this region.

The Lining of the Air Passageways

The bronchi and other conducting passageways of the respiratory tract are lined with a special type of epithelium (Fig. 16-4). Basically, it is simple columnar epithelium, but the cells are arranged in such a way that they appear stratified. The tissue is thus described as *pseudostratified*, meaning "falsely stratified." These epithelial cells have cilia to filter out impurities and to create movement of fluids within the conducting tubes. The cilia beat to drive impurities toward the throat, where they can be eliminated by coughing, sneezing, or blowing the nose.

✔ CHECKPOINT **4**:

The cells that line the respiratory passageways help to keep impurities out of the lungs. What feature of these cells enables them to filter impurities and move fluids?

- cilia
- goblet cell (secretes mucus)
- columnar epithelium (pseudostratified)
- Trachea

FIGURE **16•4** Microscopic view of the ciliated epithelium that lines the respiratory passageways. (Cormack DH: Essential Histology, Plate 4-1D, Philadelphia, JB Lippincott, 1993)

The Lungs

The *lungs* are the organs in which the diffusion of gases takes place through the extremely thin and delicate lung tissues. The two lungs are set side by side in the thoracic (chest) cavity. On its medial side, the left lung has an indentation that accommodates the heart.

Each primary bronchus enters the lung at the hilus and immediately subdivides. The right bronchus divides into three secondary bronchi, each of which enters one of the three lobes of the right lung. The left bronchus gives rise to two secondary bronchi, which enter the two lobes of the left lung. Because the subdivisions of the bronchi resemble the branches of a tree, they have been given the common name *bronchial tree.* The bronchi subdivide again and again, becoming progressively smaller as they branch through lung tissue.

The smallest of these conducting tubes are called **bronchioles** (BRONG-ke-oles). The bronchi contain small bits of cartilage, which give firmness to the walls and serve to hold the passageways open so that air can pass in and out easily. As the bronchi become smaller, however, the cartilage decreases in amount. In the bronchioles, there is no cartilage at all; what remains is mostly smooth muscle, which is under the control of the autonomic (involuntary) nervous system.

The Alveoli

At the end of the **terminal bronchioles,** the smallest subdivisions of the bronchial tree, are the clusters of tiny air sacs in which most gas exchange takes place. These sacs are known as **alveoli** (al-VE-o-li). The wall of each alveolus is made of a single-cell layer of squamous (flat) epithelium. This thin wall provides easy passage for the gases entering and leaving the blood as the blood circulates through the millions of tiny capillaries covering the alveoli.

Certain cells in the alveolar wall produce **surfactant** (sur-FAK-tant), a substance that reduces the surface tension ("pull") of the fluids that line the alveoli. This surface action prevents collapse of the alveoli and eases expansion of the lungs.

There are millions of alveoli in the human lung. The resulting surface area in contact with gases approximates 60 square meters, about three times as much lung tissue as is necessary for life. Because of the many air spaces, the lung is light in weight; normally, a piece of lung tissue dropped into a glass of water will float. Figure 16-5 shows a microscopic view of lung tissue.

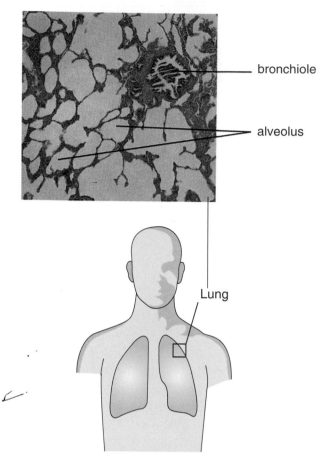

bronchiole

alveolus

Lung

FIGURE **16•5** Lung tissue as seen through a microscope, (Courtesy of Dana Morse Bittus and B.J. Cohen)

The pulmonary circuit brings blood to and from the lungs. In the lungs, the blood passes through the capillaries around the alveoli, where the gas exchange takes place (see Fig. 16-7, shown later).

The Lung Cavities and Pleura

The lungs occupy a considerable portion of the thoracic cavity, which is separated from the abdominal cavity by the muscular partition known as the **diaphragm.** A continuous doubled sac, known as the **pleura,** covers each lung. Each layer of the pleura is named according to its location. The portion of the pleura that is attached to the chest wall is the **parietal pleura,** and the portion that is attached to the surface of the lung is called the **visceral pleura.** Each closed sac completely surrounds the lung, except in the place where the

bronchus and blood vessels enter the lung, a region known as the *root* of the lung.

Between the two layers of the pleura is the **pleural space,** in which there is a thin film of fluid that lubricates the membranes. The effect is the same as between two flat pieces of glass joined by a film of water; that is, the surfaces slide easily on each other but strongly resist separation. Thus, the lungs are able to move and enlarge effortlessly in response to changes in the thoracic volume that occur during breathing.

The region between the lungs, the **mediastinum** (me-de-as-TI-num), contains the heart, great blood vessels, esophagus, trachea, and lymph nodes.

✔ CHECKPOINT **5**:

What is the name of the membrane that encloses the lung?

THE PROCESS OF RESPIRATION

Pulmonary Ventilation

Ventilation is the movement of air into and out of the lungs, as in breathing. There are two phases of ventilation (Fig. 16-6):

- **Inhalation** is the drawing of air into the lungs.
- **Exhalation** is the expulsion of air from the lungs.

In **inhalation,** the active phase of breathing, the respiratory muscles contract to enlarge the thoracic cavity. During quiet breathing, the movement of the diaphragm accounts for most of the increase in thoracic volume. The diaphragm is a strong, dome-shaped muscle attached to the body wall around the base of the rib cage. The contraction and flattening of the diaphragm cause a pistonlike downward motion that results in an increase in the vertical dimension of the chest. Other muscles that participate in enlarging the chest cavity during inhalation are the intercostal muscles. These muscles run at angles in two layers between the

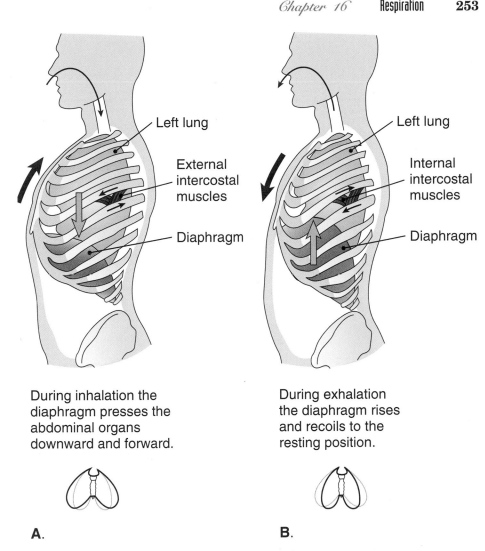

During inhalation the diaphragm presses the abdominal organs downward and forward.

A.

During exhalation the diaphragm rises and recoils to the resting position.

B.

FIGURE **16•6** Pulmonary ventilation. **(A)** Inhalation. **(B)** Exhalation.

16

ribs. As they contract, they lift the rib cage upward and outward. Put the palms of your hands on either side of the rib cage to feel this action as you inhale. During exertion, the rib cage is moved further up and out by contraction of muscles in the neck and chest wall.

As the thoracic cavity increases in size, gas pressure within the cavity decreases. When the pressure drops to slightly below atmospheric pressure, air is drawn into the lungs, as by suction.

The ease with which the lungs and thorax can be expanded is termed ***compliance.*** Normal elasticity of the lung tissue, aided by surfactant, allows the lungs to expand under pressure and fill adequately with air during inhalation. Compliance is decreased when the lungs resist ex-

pansion. Conditions that can decrease compliance include diseases that damage or scar lung tissue, accumulation of fluid in the lungs, deficiency of surfactant, and interference with the action of breathing muscles.

In ***exhalation,*** the passive phase of breathing, the muscles of respiration relax, allowing the ribs and diaphragm to return to their original positions. The tissues of the lung are elastic and recoil during exhalation. During forced exhalation, the internal intercostal muscles in the posterior of the rib cage and the muscles of the abdominal wall contract, pulling the bottom of the rib cage in and down, pushing the abdominal viscera upward against the relaxed diaphragm.

Air enters the respiratory passages and flows

through the ever-dividing tubes of the bronchial tree. As the air traverses this passage, it moves more and more slowly through the great number of bronchial tubes until there is virtually no forward flow as it reaches the alveoli. Here, the incoming air mixes with the existing air so that the gases soon are evenly distributed. Each breath causes relatively little change in the gas composition of the alveoli, but normal continuous breathing ensures the presence of adequate oxygen and the removal of carbon dioxide. See The Air We Breathe.

Table 16-1 gives the definitions and average values for some of the breathing volumes and capacities that are important in any evaluation of respiratory function. A lung *capacity* is a sum of volumes.

✔ CHECKPOINT **6**:

What are the two phases of breathing? Which is active and which is passive?

Gas Exchange in the Lungs

The barrier that separates alveolar air from the blood is composed of the wall of the alveolus and the wall of the capillary, both of which are extremely thin. This respiratory membrane is not only very thin, it is also moist. The moisture is important because the oxygen and carbon dioxide must go into solution before they can diffuse across the membrane. Recall that *diffusion* refers to the movement of molecules from an area in which they are in higher concentration to an area in which they are in lower con-

The Air We Breathe

The air we breathe comes under close inspection because of our increasing awareness of air pollution, both indoors and out. Automobile exhaust and industrial smoke pollute the air in many populated areas. The pronounced increase in asthma among children observed since 1980 is explained in part by increased exposure to allergens both within the home and in the general environment. Air in agricultural areas may include smoke from burning fields and drift of airborne pesticide applications far from the intended target. Lumber operations may burn scrap. Wind carries dust and pollen everywhere. Much work is being carried out to decrease these sources of airborne pollution.

Air inside homes or offices often carries a less visible burden of pollution. Many products give off invisible gases that tend to accumulate in modern buildings, which usually are tightly sealed. Unless adequate amounts of clean air are supplied, the occupants often complain of vague illnesses. Attention needs to be given to processing the air not only for temperature but also for humidity. Most important, the air must be filtered, so that undesirable pollutants are removed.

centration. Normally, inspired air contains about 21% oxygen and 0.04% carbon dioxide; expired air has only 16% oxygen and 3.5% carbon dioxide. These figures illustrate that a two-way diffusion takes place through the walls of the alveoli and capillaries.

In the tissues, also by the process of diffusion, oxygen leaves the blood, and carbon dioxide en-

VOLUME	DEFINITION	AVERAGE VALUE (mL)
Tidal volume	The amount of air moved into or out of the lungs in quiet, relaxed breathing	500
Residual volume	The volume of air that remains in the lungs after maximum exhalation	1200
Vital capacity	The volume of air that can be expelled from the lungs by maximum exhalation after maximum inhalation	4800
Total lung capacity	The total volume of air that can be contained in the lungs after maximum inhalation	6000
Functional residual capacity	The amount of air remaining in the lungs after normal exhalation	2400

Table 16•1   **Lung Volumes and Capacities**

ters. Therefore, blood returning from the tissues and entering the lung capillaries is relatively low in oxygen. Oxygen then diffuses from the alveolus, where its concentration is higher, into the blood. Again, based on relative concentration, carbon dioxide diffuses out of the blood into the air of the alveolus (Fig. 16-7).

✔ CHECKPOINT **7**:

Gases move between the alveoli and the blood by the process of diffusion. What is the definition of diffusion?

Gas Transport

Transport of Oxygen

Almost all the oxygen that diffuses into the capillary blood in the lungs is bound to the ***hemoglobin*** of the red blood cells. A small percentage is carried in solution in the plasma. The hemoglobin molecule is a large protein with four small iron-containing "heme" regions. The oxygen is bound to these heme portions.

Arterial blood (in systemic arteries and pulmonary veins) is 97% saturated with oxygen, whereas venous blood (in systemic veins and pulmonary arteries) is about 70% saturated with oxygen. This 27% difference represents the oxygen that has been taken up by the cells.

Note that in clinical practice, gas concentrations are expressed as pressure in millimeters of mercury (mmHg), just as blood pressure is reported. Because air is a mixture of gases, each gas exerts only a portion of the total pressure, or a ***partial pressure*** (P). The partial pressures of oxygen and carbon dioxide are symbolized as P_{O_2} and P_{CO_2} respectively.

To enter the cells, oxygen must separate from hemoglobin. Normally, the bond between oxygen and hemoglobin is easily broken, and oxygen is released as blood travels into areas where the oxygen concentration is relatively low. Cells are constantly using oxygen in metabolism and obtaining fresh supplies by diffusion from the blood.

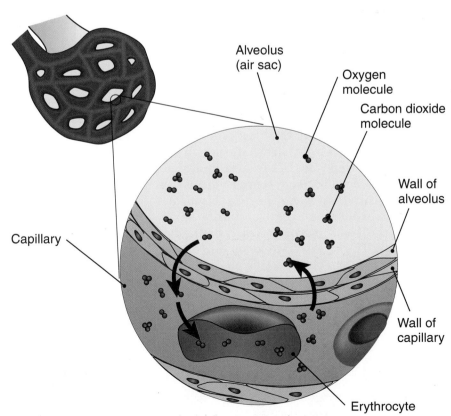

FIGURE **16•7** Diagram illustrating the diffusion of gas molecules in the lungs.

Alveolus (air sac)

Oxygen molecule

Carbon dioxide molecule

Wall of alveolus

Wall of capillary

Erythrocyte

Capillary

✔ CHECKPOINT **8**:

What substance in red blood cells carries almost all of the oxygen in the blood?

Transport of Carbon Dioxide

Carbon dioxide is produced continuously in the tissues as a byproduct of metabolism. It diffuses from the cells into the blood to be transported to the lungs in three ways:

- About 10% is dissolved in the plasma and the fluid in red blood cells.
- About 20% is combined with the protein portion of hemoglobin and plasma proteins.
- About 70% is transported as an ion, known as a *bicarbonate ion,* which is formed when carbon dioxide dissolves in blood fluids.

The bicarbonate ion is formed slowly in the plasma but much more rapidly inside the red blood cells, where an enzyme called *carbonic anhydrase* increases the speed of the reaction. The bicarbonate formed in the red blood cells moves to the plasma and then is carried to the lungs. Here, the process is reversed as bicarbonate reenters the red blood cells and releases carbon dioxide for diffusion into the alveoli and exhalation.

Carbon dioxide is important in regulating the pH (acid–base balance) of the blood. As a bicarbonate ion is formed from carbon dioxide in the plasma, a hydrogen ion (H^+) is also produced. Therefore, the blood becomes more acidic as the amount of carbon dioxide in the blood increases. The exhalation of carbon dioxide shifts the pH of the blood more toward the alkaline (basic) range. The bicarbonate ion is also an important buffer in the blood, acting chemically to help keep the pH of body fluids at a steady pH of 7.4.

✔ CHECKPOINT **9**:

What is the main form in which carbon dioxide is carried in the blood?

Regulation of Respiration

The respiratory pattern is controlled by centers in the central nervous system as modified in response to chemical stimuli detected by special receptors.

Nervous Control

Regulation of respiration is a complex process that must keep pace with moment-to-moment changes in cellular oxygen requirements and carbon dioxide production. Regulation depends primarily on a respiratory control center located partly in the medulla and partly in the pons of the brain stem. The main part of the control center, located in the medulla, sets the basic pattern of respiration. This pattern can be modified by centers in the pons. Breathing is regulated continuously, so that levels of oxygen, carbon dioxide, and acid are kept within normal limits.

✔ CHECKPOINT **10**:

What part of the brain stem sets the basic pattern of respiration?

From the respiratory center in the medulla, motor nerve fibers extend into the spinal cord. From the cervical (neck) part of the cord, these nerve fibers continue through the *phrenic* (FREN-ik) *nerve* to the diaphragm. The diaphragm and the other muscles of respiration are voluntary in the sense that they can be regulated consciously by messages from the higher brain centers, notably the cortex. It is possible for a person to deliberately breathe more rapidly or more slowly or to hold his or her breath and not breathe at all for a while. Most of the time, however, we breathe without thinking about it, and the respiratory center in the brain stem is in control.

✔ CHECKPOINT **11**:

What is the name of the motor nerve that controls the diaphragm?

Chemical Control

Of vital importance in the control of respiration are **chemoreceptors** (ke-mo-re-SEP-tors), which, like the receptors for taste and smell, are sensitive to chemicals dissolved in body fluids. The receptors that regulate respiration are found in structures called the *carotid* and *aortic bodies* as well as outside the medulla of the brain stem. The carotid bodies are located near the bifurcation (forking) of the common carotid arteries in the neck, whereas the aortic bodies are located in the aortic arch. These bodies contain many small blood vessels and sensory neurons, which respond to increases in carbon dioxide and acidity (H^+) and to decreases in oxygen supply.

Changes in the composition of the blood generate nerve impulses that are then sent to the brain. Because there is usually an ample reserve of oxygen in the blood, carbon dioxide has the most immediate effect in regulating respiration. When carbon dioxide levels increase, breathing must be increased to blow off the excess. It is only when oxygen levels fall considerably that this gas becomes a controlling factor. The receptor cells outside the medulla actually respond to the concentration of hydrogen ions in cerebrospinal fluid (CSF). The level of hydrogen ion increases as carbon dioxide dissolves in the blood.

✔ CHECKPOINT **12**:

What gas is the main chemical controller of respiration?

Breathing Rates

Normal rates of breathing vary from 12 to 20 times per minute for adults. In children, rates may vary from 20 to 40 times per minute, depending on age and size. In infants, the respiratory rate may be more than 40 times per minute. To determine the respiratory rate, one counts the subject's breathing for at least 30 seconds, usually by watching the rise and fall of the chest with each inhalation and exhalation. The count is then multiplied to obtain the rate in breaths per minute. It is best if the person does not realize that he or she is being observed because awareness of the measurement may cause a change in the breathing rate.

AGE AND THE RESPIRATORY TRACT

With age, the tissues of the respiratory tract lose elasticity and become more rigid. Similar rigidity in the chest wall, combined with arthritis and loss of strength in the breathing mus-

---

Recovering From Smoking: Yes You Can!

The damage to your respiratory system caused by smoking tobacco products is not necessarily permanent. Many studies have documented the following benefits of stopping smoking:

- Risk of having a heart attack returns to that of a nonsmoker within about 1 to 2 years.
- Risk of having a stroke returns to that of a nonsmoker within 1 to 3 years
- Rate of deterioration of lung function returns to that caused simply by age within about 3 years
- Risk of developing lung cancer returns to baseline in as little as 10 years
- Risk of developing rapidly advancing chronic obstructive pulmonary disease (COPD) returns to baseline after 5 years.

Of all patients who stop smoking each year, 90% do so with no medical assistance. However, in any given year, only 3.6% of all smokers succeed in their efforts to stop. To increase the chance of successful cessation, doctors advise the following:

- Select a specific quit date
- Use behavior modification to substitute for your normal cues to smoking
- Quit "cold turkey;" it works better than tapering off
- Manage tobacco withdrawal; nicotine gum or patches should be started on the quit date; the antidepressant medication buproprion may be started 1–2 weeks before the quit date

cles, results in an overall decrease in compliance and in lung capacity. Reduction in protective mechanisms, such as phagocytosis in the lungs, leads to increased susceptibility to infection. The incidence of emphysema increases with age, hastened by cigarette smoking and by exposure to other environmental irritants. Although there is much individual variation, especially related to how much activity one is accustomed to, these changes gradually lead to reduced capacity for exercise.

See Recovering From Smoking: Yes You Can!

Summary

I. The respiratory system
A. Nasal cavities—filter, warm, and moisten air
B. Pharynx (throat)—carries air into respiratory tract and food into digestive tract
C. Larynx (voice box)—contains vocal cords
  1. Epiglottis—covers larynx on swallowing to help prevent food from entering
D. Trachea (windpipe)
E. Bronchi—branches of trachea that enter lungs and then subdivide
  1. Bronchioles—smallest subdivisions
F. Lungs
  1. Organs of gas exchange
  2. Lobes: three on right; two on left
  3. Alveoli
    a. Tiny air sacs where gases are exchanged
    b. Surfactant—reduces surface tension in alveoli; eases expansion of lungs
  4. Pleura—membrane that encloses the lung
    a. Visceral pleura—attached to surface of lung
    b. Parietal pleura—attached to chest wall
    c. Pleural space—between layers
  5. Mediastinum—space and organs between lungs

II. The process of respiration
A. Pulmonary ventilation
  1. Inhalation—drawing of air into lungs
    a. Compliance—ease with which lungs and thorax can be expanded
  2. Exhalation—expulsion of air from lungs
  3. Lung volumes—used to evaluate respiratory function (*e.g.,* vital capacity, total lung capacity)
B. Gas exchange in the lungs
  1. Gases diffuse from area of higher concentration to area of lower concentration
  2. In lungs—oxygen enters blood and carbon dioxide leaves
  3. In tissues—oxygen leaves blood and carbon dioxide enters
C. Gas transport
  1. Oxygen—almost totally bound to heme portion of hemoglobin in red blood cells; separates from hemoglobin when oxygen concentration is low (in tissues)
  2. Carbon dioxide—most carried as bicarbonate ion; regulates pH of blood
D. Regulation of respiration
  1. Nervous control
    a. Controlled by center in medulla and pons

2. Chemical control
   a. Chemoreceptors detect changes in gas composition of blood
E. Breathing rates
   1. 12 to 20 times per minute in adult

2. 20 to 40 times per minute in children
3. Infants may be more than 40

III. Age and the respiratory tract

Questions for Study and Review

1. What is the definition of *respiration* and what are its three phases?
2. Trace the pathway of air from outside the body into the blood.
3. What is the purpose of the cilia on the cells that line the respiratory passageways?
4. What are the advantages of breathing through the nose?
5. What muscles are used for inhalation? forceful exhalation?
6. How is oxygen transported in the blood? What causes its release to the tissues?
7. How is carbon dioxide transported in the blood?
8. How does the pH of the blood change as the level of carbon dioxide increases? decreases?
9. What are chemoreceptors and how do they function to regulate breathing?
10. Define five volumes or capacities used to measure breathing.
11. Define:
   a. *epiglottis*
   b. *alveolus*
   c. *surfactant*
   d. *pleura*
   e. *mediastinum*
   f. *compliance*

✔ ANSWERS TO CHECKPOINTS

1. The three phases of respiration are pulmonary ventilation, diffusion of gases, and transport of gases in the blood.
2. As air passes over the nasal mucosa, it is filtered, warmed, and moistened.
3. The scientific name for the throat is pharynx, for the voice box is larynx, and for the windpipe is trachea.
4. The cells that line the respiratory passageways have cilia to filter impurities and to move fluids.
5. The pleura is the membrane that encloses the lung.
6. The two phases of breathing are inhalation, which is active, and exhalation, which is passive.
7. Diffusion is the movement of molecules from an area in which they are in higher concentration to an area where they are in lower concentration.
8. The substance in red blood cells that carries almost all of the oxygen in the blood is hemoglobin.
9. The main form in which carbon dioxide is carried in the blood is as bicarbonate ion.
10. The medulla of the brain stem sets the basic pattern of respiration.
11. The phrenic nerve is the motor nerve that controls the diaphragm.
12. Carbon dioxide is the main chemical controller of respiration.

Digestion

Chapter

17

SELECTED KEY TERMS

The following terms are defined in the Glossary:

absorption

bile

chyle

chyme

colon

defecation

deglutition

digestion

duodenum

emulsify

enzyme

esophagus

hydrolysis

lacteal

mastication

peristalsis

peritoneum

saliva

sphincter

ulcer

villi

BEHAVIORAL OBJECTIVES

After careful study of this chapter, you should be able to:

1. Name the two main functions of the digestive system
2. Describe the four layers of the digestive tract wall
3. Differentiate between the two layers of the peritoneum
4. Name and describe the functions of the organs of the digestive tract
5. Name and describe the functions of the accessory organs of digestion
6. Describe how bile functions in digestion
7. Name the ducts that carry bile from the liver into the digestive tract
8. Explain the role of enzymes in digestion and give examples of enzymes
9. Name the digestion products of fats, proteins, and carbohydrates
10. Define *absorption*
11. Define *villi* and state how villi function in absorption
12. Explain the use of feedback in regulating digestion and give several examples
13. List several hormones involved in regulating digestion

FUNCTION AND DESIGN OF THE DIGESTIVE SYSTEM

Every body cell needs a constant supply of nutrients to provide energy and to provide the building blocks for the manufacture of body substances. Food as we take it in, however, is too large to enter the cells. It must first be broken down into particles small enough to pass through the plasma membrane of the cell. This breakdown process is known as *digestion.*

After digestion, food must be carried to the cells in every part of the body by the circulation. The transfer of food into the circulation is called *absorption*. Digestion and absorption are the two chief functions of the digestive system.

For our purposes, the digestive system may be divided into two groups of organs:

- The *digestive tract,* a continuous passageway beginning at the mouth, where food is taken in, and terminating at the anus, where the solid waste products of digestion are expelled from the body
- The *accessory organs,* which are necessary for the digestive process but are not a direct part of the digestive tract. They release substances into the digestive tract through ducts. These organs are the salivary glands, liver, gallbladder, and pancreas.

✔ CHECKPOINT **1**:

Why does food have to be digested before it can be used by cells?

Before describing the individual organs of the digestive tract, we will pause to discuss the general pattern of the organs and also the large membrane (peritoneum) that lines the abdominopelvic cavity in which most of the digestive organs are contained.

The Wall of the Digestive Tract

Although modified for specific tasks in different organs, the wall of the digestive tract, from the esophagus to the anus, is similar in structure throughout. The general pattern consists of four layers:

- Mucous membrane
- Submucosa
- Smooth muscle
- Serous membrane

Refer to the diagram of the small intestine in Figure 17-1 as we describe the layers of this wall from the innermost to the outermost surface.

First is the *mucous membrane,* or *mucosa,* so called because its epithelial layer contains

261

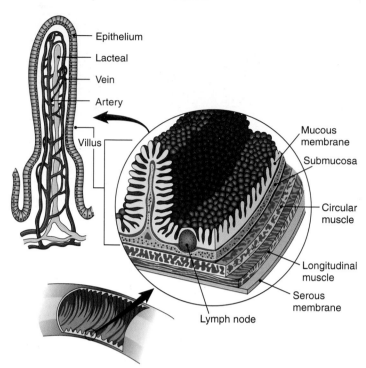

Epithelium

Lacteal

Vein

Artery

Villus

Mucous membrane

Submucosa

Circular muscle

Longitudinal muscle

Serous membrane

Lymph node

FIGURE **17•1** Diagram of the wall of the small intestine showing numerous villi. At the left is an enlarged drawing of a single villus.

many mucus-secreting cells. From the mouth through the esophagus, and also in the anus, the epithelium consists of multiple layers of squamous (flat) cells, which aid in protection of deeper tissues. Throughout the remainder of the digestive tract, the type of epithelium in the mucosa is simple columnar. Figure 17-2 is a microscopic view of the small intestine; the mucus-secreting cells appear as clear areas between epithelial cells.

The layer of connective tissue beneath the mucosa is the ***submucosa,*** which contains blood vessels and some of the nerves that help regulate digestive activity.

The next layer is composed of ***smooth muscle.*** Most of the digestive organs have two layers of smooth muscle: an inner layer of circular fibers, and an outer layer of longitudinal fibers. The alternate contractions of these muscles create the wavelike movement that propels food through the digestive tract and mixes it with digestive juices. This movement is called ***peristalsis*** (per-ih-STAL-sis).

The esophagus differs slightly from this pattern in having striated muscle in its upper portion, and the stomach has an additional third

layer of smooth muscle in its wall to add strength for churning food.

The digestive organs in the abdominopelvic cavity have an outermost layer of ***serous membrane,*** a thin, moist tissue composed of simple squamous epithelium and loose connective tissue. This membrane forms part of the peritoneum (per-i-to-NE-um). The esophagus above the diaphragm has instead an outer layer composed of fibrous connective tissue.

✔ CHECKPOINT **2**:

Most of the digestive tract has a wall that is similar throughout its length and is composed of four layers. What are the typical four layers of this wall?

The Peritoneum

The abdominopelvic cavity is lined with a thin, shiny serous membrane that also folds back to cover most of the organs contained within the cavity (Fig. 17-3). The outer portion of this

columnar epithelium

villa

goblet cells
(secrete mucus)

connective
tissue

digestive glands

smooth
muscle

mucous
glands

FIGURE **17•2** Microscopic view of the small intestine (duodenum). (Cormack DH: Essential HIstology, Plate 13-48. Philadelphia, JB Lippincott, 1993)

membrane, the layer that lines the cavity, is called the ***parietal peritoneum;*** that covering the organs is called the ***visceral peritoneum***. The peritoneum carries blood vessels, lymphatic vessels, and nerves. In some places, it serves to support the organs and to bind them to each other. Subdivisions of the peritoneum around the various organs have special names.

Subdivisions of the Peritoneum

The ***mesentery*** (MES-en-ter-e) is a double-layered portion of the peritoneum shaped somewhat like a fan. The handle portion is attached to the back wall, and the expanded long edge is attached to the small intestine. Between the two layers of membrane that form the mesentery are the vessels and nerves that supply the intestine. The section of the peritoneum that extends from the colon to the back wall is the ***mesocolon*** (mes-o-KO-lon).

A large double layer of the peritoneum containing much fat hangs like an apron over the front of the intestine. This ***greater omentum*** (o-MEN-tum) extends from the lower border of the stomach into the pelvic part of the abdomen

and then loops back up to the transverse colon. There is also a smaller membrane, called the ***lesser omentum,*** that extends between the stomach and the liver.

> ✔ CHECKPOINT **3**:
>
> What is the name of the large serous membrane that lines the abdominopelvic cavity and covers the organs it contains?

ORGANS OF THE DIGESTIVE TRACT

As we study the organs of the digestive system, locate each in Figure 17-4.

The digestive tract is a muscular tube extending through the body. It is composed of several parts: the ***mouth, pharynx, esophagus, stomach, small intestine,*** and ***large intestine.*** The digestive tract is sometimes called the ***alimentary tract,*** derived from a Latin word that means "food." It is more commonly referred to

Greater
peritoneal cavity

Lesser
peritoneal cavity

Liver

Stomach

Mesocolon

Greater omentum

Transverse colon

Small intestine

Uterus

Urinary
bladder

Lesser omentum

Pancreas

Duodenum

Retroperitoneal
space

Mesentery

Cul-de-sac

Rectum

FIGURE **17•3** Diagram of the abdominal cavity showing the peritoneum.

as the ***gastrointestinal (GI) tract*** because of the major importance of the stomach and intestine in the process of digestion.

The Mouth

The mouth, also called the ***oral cavity,*** is where a substance begins its travels through the digestive tract (Fig. 17-5). The mouth has three digestive functions:

- To receive food, a process called ***ingestion***
- To prepare food for digestion
- To begin the digestion of starch

Digestive activities in the mouth require saliva, a secretion that is produced by the sali-

vary glands and secreted into the mouth. The salivary glands are described with the other accessory organs.

The tongue, a muscular organ that projects into the mouth, is used as an aid in chewing and in swallowing and is one of the principal organs of speech. The tongue has on its surface a number of special organs, called *taste buds,* by means of which taste sensations (bitter, sweet, sour, or salty) can be differentiated.

The Teeth

The oral cavity also contains the teeth (see Fig. 17-5). A child between 2 and 6 years of age has 20 teeth, known as the baby teeth or ***deciduous*** (de-SID-u-us) teeth. (The word *deciduous* means "falling off at a certain time," such as the leaves that fall off the trees in autumn.) A com-

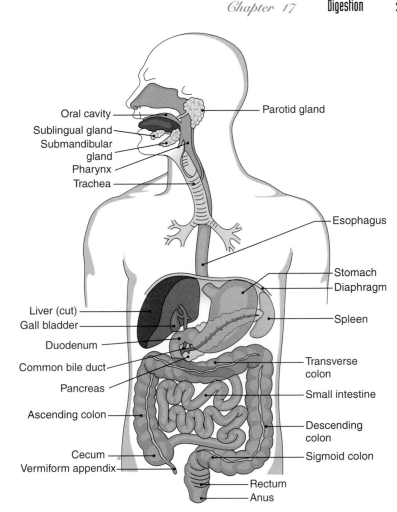

Oral cavity
Sublingual gland
Submandibular gland
Pharynx
Trachea
Parotid gland
Esophagus
Stomach
Diaphragm
Liver (cut)
Gall bladder
Duodenum
Common bile duct
Pancreas
Ascending colon
Cecum
Vermiform appendix
Spleen
Transverse colon
Small intestine
Descending colon
Sigmoid colon
Rectum
Anus

FIGURE **17•4** Digestive system.

plete set of adult permanent teeth numbers 32. Among these, the cutting teeth, or ***incisors,*** occupy the front part of the oral cavity, whereas the larger grinding teeth, the ***molars,*** are in the back.

The first eight deciduous (baby) teeth to appear through the gums are the incisors. Later, the ***cuspids*** (commonly called *canines* or *eyeteeth*) and molars appear. Usually, the 20 baby teeth have all appeared by the time a child has reached the age of 2 to 3 years. During the first 2 years, the permanent teeth develop within the upper jaw (maxilla) and lower jaw (mandible) from buds that are present at birth. The first permanent tooth to appear is the important 6-year molar. This permanent tooth comes in before the baby incisors are lost. Because decay and infection of adjacent deciduous molars may spread to and involve new, per-

manent teeth, deciduous teeth need proper care.

As a child grows, the jawbones grow, making space for additional teeth. After the 6-year molars have appeared, the baby incisors loosen and are replaced by permanent incisors. Next, the baby canines (cuspids) are replaced by permanent canines, and finally, the baby molars are replaced by the bicuspids (premolars) of the permanent teeth.

Now the larger jawbones are ready for the appearance of the 12-year, or second, permanent molar teeth. During or after the late teens, the third molars, or so-called *wisdom teeth,* may appear. In some cases, the jaw is not large enough for these teeth, or there are other abnormalities, so that the third molars may not erupt or may have to be removed. Figure 17-6 shows the parts of a molar.

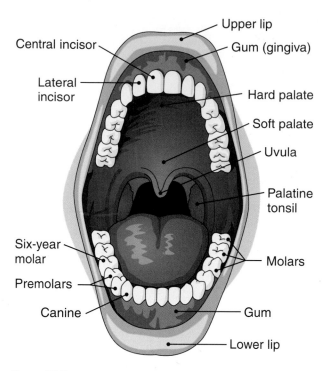

FIGURE **17•5** The mouth, showing the teeth and tonsils.

✔ CHECKPOINT **4**:

How many baby teeth are there and what is the scientific name for the baby teeth?

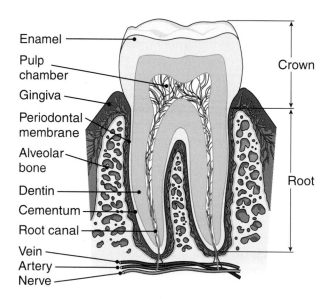

FIGURE **17•6** A molar tooth. (Cohen B: Medical Terminology: An Illustrated Guide, 3rd ed, p. 226. Philadelphia, Lippincott-Raven, 1998)

The Pharynx

The ***pharynx*** (FAR-inks) is commonly referred to as the *throat* (see Fig. 16-1 in Chap. 16). The oral part of the pharynx, the oropharynx, is visible when you look into an open mouth and depress the tongue. The palatine tonsils may be seen at either side of the oropharynx. The pharynx also extends upward to the nasal cavity as the nasopharynx and downward to the level of the larynx as the laryngeal pharynx. The ***soft palate*** is tissue that forms the back of the roof of the oral cavity. From it hangs a soft, fleshy, V-shaped mass called the ***uvula*** (U-vu-lah), which is used in speech production.

In swallowing, a ***bolus,*** a small portion of chewed food mixed with saliva, is pushed by the tongue into the pharynx. When the food reaches the pharynx, swallowing occurs rapidly by an involuntary reflex action. At the same time, the soft palate and uvula are raised to prevent food and liquid from entering the nasal cavity, and the tongue is raised to seal the back of the oral cavity. The entrance of the trachea is guarded during swallowing by a leaf-shaped cartilage, the ***epiglottis,*** which covers the opening of the larynx. The swallowed food is then moved into the esophagus.

The Esophagus

The ***esophagus*** (eh-SOF-ah-gus) is a muscular tube about 25 cm (10 inches) long. In the esophagus, food is lubricated with mucus and moved by peristalsis into the stomach. No additional digestion occurs in the esophagus.

Before joining the stomach, the esophagus must pass through the diaphragm. It travels through a space in the diaphragm called the ***esophageal hiatus*** (eh-sof-ah-JE-al hi-A-tus). If there is a weakness in the diaphragm at this point, a portion of the stomach or other abdominal organ may protrude through the space, a condition called ***hiatal hernia.***

The Stomach

The stomach is an expanded J-shaped organ in the upper left region of the abdominal cavity

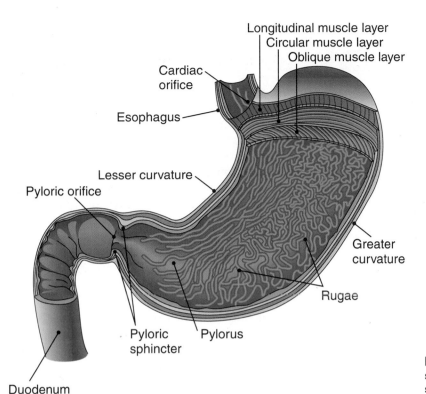

Longitudinal muscle layer
Circular muscle layer
Oblique muscle layer
Cardiac orifice
Esophagus
Lesser curvature
Pyloric orifice
Greater curvature
Rugae
Pyloric sphincter
Pylorus
Duodenum

FIGURE **17•7** Longitudinal section of the stomach and a portion of the duodenum showing the interior.

(Fig. 17-7). In addition to the two muscle layers already described, it has a third, inner oblique (angled) layer that aids in grinding food and mixing it with digestive juices. The left-facing arch of the stomach is the ***greater curvature,*** whereas the right surface forms the ***lesser curvature.***

Sphincters

A muscular ring, or ***sphincter*** (SFINK-ter), that permits the passage of substances in only one direction guards each end of the stomach.

Between the esophagus and the stomach is the ***lower esophageal sphincter (LES).*** This valve has also been called the ***cardiac sphincter*** because it separates the esophagus from the region of the stomach that is close to the heart. We are sometimes aware of the existence of this sphincter; sometimes, it does not relax as it should, producing a feeling of being unable to swallow past that point.

Between the distal, or far, end of the stomach and the small intestine is the ***pyloric*** (pi-LOR-ik) ***sphincter.*** The region of the stomach leading into this sphincter, the ***pylorus*** (pi-LOR-

us), is important in regulating how rapidly food moves into the small intestine.

Functions of the Stomach

The stomach serves as a storage pouch, digestive organ, and churn. When the stomach is empty, the lining forms many folds called ***rugae*** (RU-je). These folds disappear as the stomach expands. (It may be stretched to hold one half of a gallon of food and liquid.) Special cells in the lining of the stomach secrete substances that mix together to form ***gastric juice,*** the two main components of which are the following:

- Hydrochloric acid (HCl), a strong acid that softens the connective tissue in meat and destroys foreign organisms
- Pepsin, a protein-digesting enzyme produced in an inactive form and activated only when food enters the stomach and HCl is produced

The semiliquid mixture of gastric juice and food that leaves the stomach to enter the small intestine is called ***chyme*** (kime).

✔ CHECKPOINT **5**:

What type of food is digested in the stomach?

The Small Intestine

The small intestine is the longest part of the digestive tract. It is known as the small intestine because, although it is longer than the large intestine, it is smaller in diameter, with an average width of about 2.5 cm (1 inch). After death, when relaxed to its full length, the small intestine is about 6 m (20 feet) long. In life, the small intestine averages 3 m (10 feet) in length. The first 25 cm (10 inches) or so of the small intestine make up the **duodenum** (du-o-DE-num). Beyond the duodenum are two more divisions:

Surface Area and Transport

Whenever materials pass from one system to another, they must travel through a cellular membrane. A major factor in how much transport can occur per unit of time is the total surface area of the membrane.

The problem of packing a large amount of surface into a small space is solved in the body by folding the membranes. We do the same thing in everyday life. Imagine trying to store a bed sheet in the closet without folding it!

In the small intestine, where digested food must move into the bloodstream, there is folding of membranes down to the level of the single cells.

- The organ as a whole is coiled to fit its length into the abdominal cavity.
- The inner wall of the organ forms circular folds called *plicae circulares.*
- The projecting villi provide more surface area than a flat membrane would.
- The individual cells that line the small intestine have microvilli, tiny fingerlike folds of the cell membrane, that increase surface area tremendously.

Can you name other portions of the digestive tract or other systems that show this folding pattern and explain why it is there?

the **jejunum** (je-JU-num), which forms the next two fifths of the small intestine, and the **ileum** (IL-e-um), which constitutes the remaining portion.

Functions of the Small Intestine

The wall of the duodenum contains glands that secrete large amounts of mucus to protect the small intestine from the strongly acidic chyme entering from the stomach. Cells of the small intestine also secrete enzymes that digest proteins and carbohydrates. In addition, digestive juices from the liver and pancreas enter the small intestine through a small opening in the duodenum. Most of the digestive process takes place in the small intestine under the effects of these juices.

Most absorption of digested food also occurs through the walls of the small intestine. To increase the surface area of the organ for this purpose, the mucosa is formed into millions of tiny, fingerlike projections, called **villi** (VIL-li) (see Fig. 17-1), which give the inner surface a velvety appearance. In addition, each epithelial cell has small projecting folds of the cell membrane known as **microvilli.** These create a remarkable increase in the total surface area available in the small intestine for the absorption of nutrients (see Surface Area and Transport).

✔ CHECKPOINT **6**:

How does the small intestine function in the digestive process?

The Large Intestine

Any material that cannot be digested as it passes through the digestive tract must be eliminated from the body. In addition, most of the water secreted into the digestive tract for proper digestion must be reabsorbed into the bloodstream to prevent dehydration. The storage and elimination of undigested waste and the reabsorption of water are the functions of the large intestine.

The large intestine is about 6.5 cm (2.5 inches) in diameter and about 1.5 m (5 feet) long. The outer longitudinal muscle fibers in its wall form three separate bands on the surface. These bands draw up the wall of the organ to give it its distinctive puckered appearance.

Subdivisions of the Large Intestine

The large intestine begins in the lower right region of the abdomen. The first part is a small pouch called the *cecum* (SE-kum). Between the ileum of the small intestine and the cecum is a sphincter, the *ileocecal* (il-e-o-SE-kal) *valve,* that prevents food from traveling backward into the small intestine. Attached to the cecum is a small, blind tube containing lymphoid tissue; its full name is the *vermiform* (VER-mih-form) *appendix* (*vermiform* means "wormlike"). Inflammation of this tissue as a result of infection or obstruction is *appendicitis.*

The second portion, the *ascending colon,* extends upward along the right side of the abdomen toward the liver. The large intestine then bends and extends across the abdomen, forming the *transverse colon.* At this point, it bends sharply and extends downward on the left side of the abdomen into the pelvis, forming the *descending colon.* The lower part of the colon bends posteriorly in an S shape and continues downward as the *sigmoid colon.* The sigmoid colon empties into the *rectum,* which serves as a temporary storage area for indigestible or nonabsorbable food residue (see Fig. 17-4). Enlargement of the veins in this area constitutes *hemorrhoids.* A narrow portion of the distal large intestine is called the *anal canal.* This leads to the outside of the body through an opening called the *anus* (A-nus).

Functions of the Large Intestine

The large intestine secretes large quantities of mucus but no enzymes. Food is not digested in this organ, but water is reabsorbed, and undigested food is stored, formed into solid waste material called *feces* (FE-seze) or stool, and then eliminated.

At intervals, usually after meals, the involuntary muscles within the walls of the large intestine propel solid waste toward the rectum. Stretching of the rectum stimulates contraction of smooth muscle in the rectal wall. Aided by voluntary contractions of the diaphragm and the abdominal muscles, the feces are eliminated

from the body in a process called *defecation* (def-e-KA-shun). An anal sphincter provides voluntary control over defecation. See How to Increase Fiber in Your Diet

While the food residue is stored in the large intestine, bacteria that normally live in the colon act on it to produce vitamin K and some of the B-complex vitamins. As mentioned, systemic antibiotic therapy may destroy these symbiotic (helpful) bacteria and others living in the large intestine, causing undesirable side effects.

✔ CHECKPOINT **7**:

What are the functions of the large intestine?

How to Increase Fiber in Your Diet

Fiber in the diet has been deemed to be of benefit in decreasing colon cancer, improving bowel habits, and easing weight loss. Inadequate fiber is a predisposing cause in diverticulosis, bulging pouches in the large intestine.

Fiber is of plant origin and is a type of carbohydrate not digested by the gastrointestinal tract. The amount of fiber recommended for a 2000-calorie diet is 25 grams per day, but most people in the United States tend to get only half of this amount. Fiber-rich foods should be eaten throughout the day to meet the requirement. Note that it is best to increase fiber in the diet gradually to avoid unpleasant symptoms, such as intestinal bloating and flatulence. If your diet lacks fiber, try adding the following foods over a period of several weeks:

- Whole grain bread, cereals, pasta, and brown rice. These add 1 to 3 more grams of fiber per serving than the "white" product.
- Legumes, which include beans, peas, and lentils. These add 4 to 12 grams of fiber per serving.
- Fruits and vegetables. Whole, raw, unpeeled versions contain the most fiber, juices the least. Apple juice has no fiber, whereas a whole apple has 3 grams.
- Unprocessed bran. This can be sprinkled over almost any food: cereal, soups, casseroles. One tablespoon adds 2 grams of fiber. Be sure to take adequate fluids with bran.

THE ACCESSORY ORGANS

The Salivary Glands

While food is in the mouth, it is mixed with *saliva,* one purpose of which is to moisten the food and facilitate the processes of chewing, or *mastication* (mas-tih-KA-shun), and swallowing, or *deglutition* (deg-lu-TISH-un). Saliva also helps keep the teeth and mouth clean and helps reduce bacterial growth.

This watery mixture contains mucus and an enzyme called *salivary amylase* (AM-ih-laze), which begins the digestive process by converting starch to sugar. It is manufactured mainly by three pairs of glands that function as accessory organs (see Fig. 17-4):

- The *parotid* (pah-ROT-id) *glands,* the largest of the group, are located below and in front of the ear.
- The *submandibular* (sub-man-DIB-u-lar), or *submaxillary* (sub-MAK-sih-ler-e), *glands* are located near the body of the lower jaw.
- The *sublingual* (sub-LING-gwal) *glands* are under the tongue.

All these glands empty by means of ducts into the oral cavity.

The Liver

The liver, often referred to by the word root *hepat,* is the largest glandular organ of the body (Fig. 17-8). It is located in the upper right portion of the abdominal cavity under the dome of the diaphragm. The lower edge of a normal-sized liver is level with the lower margin of the ribs. The human liver is the same reddish brown color as the animal liver seen in the supermarket. It has a large right lobe and a smaller left lobe; the right lobe includes two inferior smaller lobes. The liver is supplied with blood through two vessels: the portal vein and the hepatic artery. These vessels deliver about 1½ quarts of blood to the liver every minute. The hepatic artery carries oxygenated blood, whereas the portal system of veins carries blood that is rich in the end products of digestion. This most remarkable organ has so many functions that only some of its major activities can be listed here:

- The storage of glucose (simple sugar) in the form of *glycogen,* the animal equivalent of

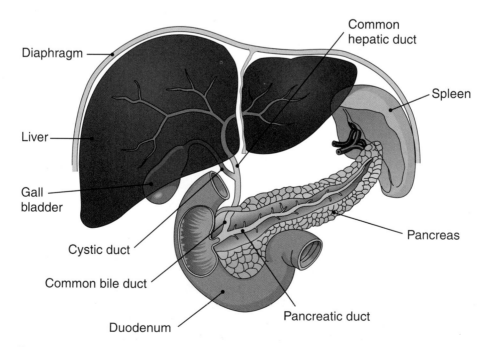

FIGURE **17•8**　Accessory organs of digestion.

the starch found in plants. When the blood sugar level falls below normal, liver cells convert glycogen to glucose, which is released into the bloodstream; this serves to restore the normal concentration of blood sugar.

- The formation of blood plasma proteins, such as albumin, globulins, and clotting factors
- The synthesis of **urea** (u-RE-ah), a waste product of protein metabolism. Urea is released into the blood and transported to the kidneys for elimination.
- The modification of fats, so that they can be used more efficiently by cells all over the body
- The manufacture of bile, a substance needed for the digestion of fats
- The destruction of old red blood cells and the recycling or elimination of their breakdown products. One byproduct, a pigment called **bilirubin** (BIL-ih-ru-bin), is eliminated in bile and gives the stool its characteristic dark color.
- The **detoxification** (de-tok-sih-fih-KA-shun) (removal of the poisonous properties) of harmful substances, such as alcohol and certain drugs
- The storage of some vitamins and iron

The main digestive function of the liver is the production of **bile.** The salts contained in bile act like a detergent to **emulsify** fat, that is, to break up fat into small droplets that can be acted on more effectively by digestive enzymes. Bile also aids in the absorption of fat from the small intestine.

Bile leaves the lobes of the liver by two ducts that merge to form the **common hepatic duct.** After collecting bile from the gallbladder, this duct, now called the **common bile duct,** delivers bile into the duodenum. These and the other accessory ducts are shown on Figure 17-8.

The Gallbladder

The gallbladder is a muscular sac on the inferior surface of the liver that serves as a storage pouch for bile. Although the liver may manufacture bile continuously, the body is likely to need

it only a few times a day. Consequently, bile from the liver flows into the hepatic ducts and then up through the **cystic** (SIS-tik) **duct** connected with the gallbladder. When chyme enters the duodenum, the gallbladder contracts, squeezing bile through the cystic duct and into the common bile duct leading to the duodenum.

The Pancreas

The pancreas is a long gland that extends from the duodenum to the spleen (see Fig. 17-8). The pancreas produces enzymes that digest fats, proteins, carbohydrates, and nucleic acids. The protein-digesting enzymes are produced in inactive forms, which must be converted to active forms in the small intestine by other enzymes.

The pancreas also produces large amounts of alkaline fluid, which neutralizes the chyme in the small intestine, thus protecting the lining of the digestive tract. These juices collect in a main duct that joins the common bile duct or empties into the duodenum near the common bile duct. Most people have an additional smaller duct that opens into the duodenum.

The pancreas also functions as an endocrine gland, producing the hormones insulin and glucagon that regulate sugar metabolism. These secretions of the islet cells are released directly into the blood.

> ✔ CHECKPOINT **8**:
>
>
> What are the names of the accessory organs of digestion?

THE PROCESS OF DIGESTION

Enzymes

Although the different organs of the digestive tract are specialized for digesting different types of food, the basic chemical process of digestion is the same for fats, proteins, and carbohydrates. In every case, this process requires enzymes. Enzymes are catalysts, substances that speed the rate of chemical reactions but that are not themselves changed or used up in the reaction.

17

All enzymes are proteins, and they are highly specific in their actions. In digestion, an enzyme acts only in a certain type of reaction involving a certain type of food molecule. For example, the carbohydrate-digesting enzyme amylase only splits starch into the disaccharide (double sugar) maltose. Another enzyme is required to split maltose into two molecules of the monosaccharide (simple sugar) glucose. Other enzymes split fats into their building blocks, glycerol and fatty acids, and still others split proteins into their building blocks, amino acids.

The Role of Water

Because water is added to nutrient molecules as they are split by enzymes, the process of digestion is referred to chemically as *hydrolysis* (hi-DROL-ih-sis), which means "splitting by means of water." You can now understand why a large amount of water is needed in digestion. Water not only is used to produce digestive juices and to dilute food, so that it can move more easily through the digestive tract, but also is used in the chemical process of digestion itself.

Digestion, Step-by-Step

Let us see what happens to a mass of food from the time it is taken into the mouth to the moment that it is ready to be absorbed.

In the mouth, the food is chewed and mixed with saliva, softening it so that it can be swallowed easily. Salivary amylase initiates the process of digestion by changing some of the starches into sugar (see Table 17-1).

Digestion in the Stomach

When the food reaches the stomach, it is acted on by gastric juice, which contains hydrochloric acid (HCl) and enzymes. The hydrochloric acid has the important function of breaking down proteins and preparing them for digestion. In addition, HCl activates the enzyme pepsin, which is secreted by the cells of the gastric lining in an inactive form. Once activated by hydrochloric acid, pepsin works to digest protein; this enzyme is the first to digest nearly every type of protein in the diet. The stomach also secretes a fat-digesting enzyme (lipase), but it is of little importance in adults.

The food, gastric juice, and mucus (which is also secreted by cells of the gastric lining) are mixed to form the semiliquid substance chyme. Chyme is moved from the stomach to the small intestine for further digestion.

Digestion in the Small Intestine

In the duodenum, the first part of the small intestine, chyme is mixed with the greenish yellow bile delivered from the liver and the gallbladder through the common bile duct. Bile does not contain enzymes; instead, it contains salts that emulsify (split) fats into smaller particles to allow the powerful pancreatic secretions to act on them most efficiently. The pancreatic juice contains a number of enzymes, including the following:

Table 17•1 **Summary of Digestion**			
ORGAN	ACTIVITY	NUTRIENTS DIGESTED	ACTIVE SECRETIONS
Mouth	Food chewed and mixed with saliva; formed into bolus for swallowing	Starch	Salivary amylase
Esophagus	Moves food by peristalsis into stomach	—	—
Stomach	Stores food; churns food and mixes it with digestive juices	Proteins	Hydrochloric acid; pepsin
Small intestine	Secretes enzymes; neutralizes acidity; receives secretions from pancreas and liver; absorbs food into bloodstream or lymph	Fats, proteins, carbohydrates, nucleic acids	Intestinal enzymes; pancreatic enzymes; bile from liver
Large intestine	Reabsorbs water; forms, stores, and eliminates stool	—	—

Lipase. After the physical division of fats into tiny particles by the action of bile, the highly active pancreatic enzyme lipase digests almost all of the fats. In this process, fats are usually broken down into two simpler compounds, glycerol (glycerin) and fatty acids, which are more readily absorbable. If pancreatic lipase is absent, fats are expelled with the feces in undigested form.

Amylase. This enzyme changes starch to sugar.

Trypsin (TRIP-sin). This enzyme splits proteins into amino acids, which are small enough to enter the bloodstream.

Nucleases (NU-kle-ases). These enzymes digest the nucleic acids DNA and RNA.

The intestinal juice contains a number of enzymes, including three that act on complex sugars to transform them into the simpler form in which they are absorbed. These are *maltase, sucrase,* and *lactase.* It must be emphasized that most of the chemical changes in foods occur in the intestinal tract because of the pancreatic juice, which has the ability to digest all types of foods. When pancreatic juice is absent, serious digestive disturbances always occur.

Table 17-2 summarizes the main substances used in digestion. Note that, except for HCl, sodium bicarbonate, and bile salts, all the substances listed are enzymes.

✔ CHECKPOINT **9**:

What organ produces the most complete digestive secretions?

ABSORPTION

The means by which the digested nutrients reach the blood is known as *absorption.* Most absorption takes place through the mucosa of the small intestine by means of the villi (see Fig. 17-1). Within each villus are a small artery and a small vein bridged with capillaries. Simple sugars, amino acids, some simple fatty acids, and water are absorbed into the blood through the capillary walls in the villi. From here, they pass by way of the portal system to the liver, to be stored or released and used as needed.

Absorption of Fats

Most fats have an alternative method of reaching the blood. Instead of entering the blood capillaries, they are absorbed by lymphatic capillaries in the villi that are called *lacteals.* The fat droplets give the lymph a milky appearance (the word *lacteal* means "like milk"). The mixture of lymph and fat globules that is drained

17

Table 17•2	Digestive Juices Produced by the Organs of the Digestive Tract and the Accessory Organs	
ORGAN	**MAIN DIGESTIVE JUICES SECRETED**	**ACTION**
Salivary glands	Salivary amylase*	Begins starch digestion
Stomach	Hydrochloric acid (HCl)	Breaks down proteins
	Pepsin*	Begins protein digestion
Small intestine	Peptidases*	Digest proteins to amino acids
	Lactase, maltase, sucrase*	Digest disaccharides to monosaccharides
Pancreas	Sodium bicarbonate	Neutralizes HCl
	Amylase*	Digests starch
	Trypsin*	Digests protein to amino acids
	Lipases*	Digest fats to fatty acids and glycerol
	Nucleases*	Digest nucleic acids
Liver	Bile salts	Emulsify fats

*Enzymes.

from the small intestine after a quantity of fat has been digested is called **chyle** (kile). It circulates in the lymph and eventually enters the bloodstream near the heart.

Absorption of Vitamins and Minerals

Minerals and vitamins taken in with food are also absorbed from the small intestine. The minerals and some of the vitamins dissolve in water and are absorbed directly into the blood. Other vitamins are incorporated in fats and are absorbed along with the fats. Some B vitamins and vitamin K are produced by the action of bacteria in the colon and are absorbed from the large intestine.

CONTROL OF DIGESTION

As food moves through the digestive tract, its rate of movement and the activity of each organ it passes through must be carefully regulated. If food moves too slowly or digestive secretions are inadequate, the body will not get enough nourishment. If food moves too rapidly or excess secretions are produced, digestion may be incomplete or the lining of the digestive tract may be damaged.

There are two types of control over digestion: nervous and hormonal. Both illustrate the principles of feedback control.

The nerves that control digestive activity are located in the submucosa and between the muscle layers of the organ walls. Instructions for action come from the autonomic (visceral) nervous system. In general, parasympathetic stimulation increases activity, and sympathetic stimulation decreases activity. Excess sympathetic stimulation, as in stress, can block the movement of food through the digestive tract and inhibit secretion of the mucus that is so important in protecting the lining of the digestive tract.

The digestive organs themselves produce the hormones involved in regulation of digestion. Let us look at some examples of these controls (Table 17-3).

The sight, smell, thought, taste, or feel of food in the mouth stimulates, through the nervous system, the secretion of saliva and the release of gastric juice. Once in the stomach, food stimulates the release into the blood of the hormone **gastrin,** which promotes stomach secretions and movement.

When chyme enters the duodenum, nerve impulses inhibit movement of the stomach, so that food will not move too rapidly into the small intestine. This action is a good example of negative feedback. At the same time, hormones released from the duodenum feed back to the stomach to reduce its activity. One of these hormones, **secretin** (se-KRE-tin), also stimulates the pancreas to release water and bicarbonate to dilute and neutralize the chyme. Another hormone, **cholecystokinin** (ko-le-sis-to-KI-nin) **(CCK),** stimulates the release of enzymes from the pancreas and causes the gallbladder to release bile.

✔ CHECKPOINT **10**:

What are the two types of control over the digestive process?

Hunger and Appetite

Hunger is the desire for food and can be satisfied by the ingestion of a filling meal. Hunger is regulated by centers in the hypothalamus that

Table 17•3	Hormones Active in Digestion	
HORMONE	SOURCE	ACTION
Gastrin	Stomach	Stimulates release of gastric juice
Gastric-inhibitory peptide (GIP)	Small intestine	Inhibits release of gastric juice
Secretin	Duodenum	Stimulates release of water and bicarbonate from pancreas; stimulates release of bile from liver; inhibits the stomach
Cholecystokinin (CCK)	Duodenum	Stimulates release of digestive enzymes from pancreas; stimulates release of bile from gallbladder; inhibits the stomach

respond to the levels of nutrients in the blood. When these levels are low, the hypothalamus stimulates a sensation of hunger. Strong, mildly painful contractions of the empty stomach may stimulate a feeling of hunger. Messages received by the hypothalamus reduce hunger as food is chewed and swallowed and begins to fill the stomach. The short-term regulation of food intake works to keep the amount of food taken in within the limits of what can be processed by the intestine. The long-term regulation of food intake maintains appropriate blood levels of certain nutrients.

Appetite differs from hunger in that, although it is basically a desire for food, it often has no relationship to the need for food. Even after an adequate meal that has relieved hunger, a person may still have an appetite for additional food.

A variety of factors, such as emotional state, cultural influences, habit, and memories of past food intake, can affect appetite. The regulation of appetite is not well understood.

✔ CHECKPOINT **11**:

What is the difference between hunger and appetite?

AGING AND THE DIGESTIVE SYSTEM

With age, receptors for taste and smell deteriorate, leading to a loss of appetite and decreased enjoyment of food. A decrease in saliva and poor gag reflex make swallowing more difficult. Loss of teeth or poorly fitting dentures may make chewing food more difficult.

Activity of the digestive organs decreases. These changes can be seen in poor absorption of certain vitamins and poor digestion of protein foods. Slowing of peristalsis in the large intestine and increased consumption of easily chewed, refined foods contribute to the common occurrence of constipation.

The tissues of the digestive system require constant replacement. Slowing of this process contributes to a variety of digestive disorders.

17

I. Function and design of the digestive system
1. Functions—digestion and absorption
2. Two groups of organs—digestive tract and accessory organs
A. The wall of the digestive tract—mucous membrane (mucosa), submucosa, smooth muscle, serosa
B. The peritoneum—serous membrane that lines the abdominal cavity and folds over organs

II. Organs of the digestive tract
A. Mouth
1. Functions
a. Ingest food
b. Prepare food for digestion
c. Begin digestion of starch with salivary amylase
2. Structures
a. Tongue—aids chewing (mastication) and swallowing; has taste buds
b. Teeth
(1) Deciduous (baby) teeth—20 (incisors, canines, molars)
(2) Permanent teeth—32 (incisors, canines, premolars, molars)
B. Pharynx (throat)—moves portion of

food (bolus) into esophagus by reflex swallowing (deglutition)

C. Esophagus—long muscular tube that carries food to stomach by peristalsis

D. Stomach
   1. Functions
      a. Storage of food
      b. Breakdown of food by churning
      c. Liquefaction of food with hydrochloric acid (HCl) to form chyme
      d. Digestion of protein with enzyme pepsin

E. Small intestine
   1. Functions
      a. Digestion of food
      b. Absorption of food through villi (small projections of intestinal lining)
   2. Divisions—duodenum, jejunum, ileum

F. Large intestine
   1. Functions
      a. Storage and elimination of waste (defecation)
      b. Reabsorption of water
   2. Divisions—cecum; ascending, transverse, descending, and sigmoid colons; rectum; anus

III. **Accessory organs**
   A. Salivary glands
      1. Functions of saliva
         a. Moistening food—aids chewing and swallowing
         b. Cleaning of mouth and teeth
         c. Digestion of starch with amylase
      2. Three pairs—parotid, submandibular, sublingual
   B. Liver
      1. Functions
         a. Storage of glucose
         b. Formation of blood plasma proteins
         c. Synthesis of urea
         d. Modification of fats
         e. Manufacture of bile
         f. Destruction of old red blood cells

g. Detoxification of harmful substances
h. Storage of vitamins and iron

C. Gallbladder
   1. Function—storage of bile until needed for digestion

D. Pancreas
   1. Secretes powerful digestive juice
   2. Secretes neutralizing fluid

IV. **The process of digestion**
   A. Enzymes—catalysts that speed reactions
      1. Products
         a. Simple sugars (monosaccharides) from carbohydrates
         b. Amino acids from proteins
         c. Glycerol and fatty acids from fats
   B. The role of water
      1. Used to split foods (hydrolysis)
      2. Lubricates and dilutes food
   C. Digestion, step by step
      1. Mouth—starch
      2. Stomach—protein
      3. Small intestine—remainder of food

V. **Absorption**—movement of nutrients into the circulation

VI. **Control of digestion**
   1. Nervous control
      a. Parasympathetic system—generally increases activity
      b. Sympathetic system—generally decreases activity
   2. Hormonal control
      a. Stimulation of digestive activity
      b. Feedback to inhibit stomach activity
      c. Examples—gastrin, secretin, CCK
   A. Hunger and appetite

VII. **Aging and the digestive system**

Questions for Study and Review

1. Describe the layers of the digestive tract wall.
2. Trace the path of a mouthful of food through the digestive tract.
3. What is the peritoneum? Name the two layers and the location of each. Name and locate four subdivisions of the peritoneum.
4. Differentiate between deciduous and permanent teeth with respect to kinds and numbers.
5. What is the pharynx and what are its three subdivisions?
6. What is peristalsis? Name some structures in which it occurs.
7. Name the purposes of the acid in gastric juice.
8. Define an enzyme and give several examples of enzymes.
9. Where does absorption occur, and what structures are needed for absorption?
10. What types of digested materials are absorbed into the blood?
11. What types of digested materials are absorbed into the lymph?
12. Name the accessory organs of digestion and the functions of each.
13. Name five functions of the liver.
14. Give examples of negative feedback in the control of digestion.
15. Name several hormones that regulate digestion.
16. How is hunger regulated?

✔ ANSWERS TO CHECKPOINTS

1. Food must be broken down by digestion into particles small enough to pass through the plasma membrane.
2. Most of the organs of the digestive tract have a wall composed of a mucous membrane, a submucosa, smooth muscle, and a serous membrane.
3. The peritoneum is the large serous membrane that lines the abdominopelvic cavity and covers the organs it contains.
4. There are 20 baby teeth, which are also called deciduous teeth.
5. Proteins are digested in the stomach.
6. Most digestion takes place in the small intestine under the effects of digestive juices from the small intestine and the accessory organs. Most absorption of digested food also occurs in the small intestine.
7. The large intestine serves to reabsorb water and to store, form, and eliminate the stool. It also houses bacteria that provide some vitamins.
8. The accessory organs of digestion are the salivary glands, liver, gallbladder, and pancreas.
9. The pancreas produces the most complete digestive secretions.
10. The two types of control over the digestive process are nervous control and hormonal control.
11. Hunger is the desire for food that can be satisfied by the ingestion of a filling meal. Appetite is a desire for food that is unrelated to a need for food.

17

Metabolism, Nutrition, and Body Temperature

Chapter

18

SELECTED KEY TERMS

The following terms are defined in the Glossary:

anabolism
catabolism
glucose
glycogen
kilocalorie
malnutrition
metabolic rate
mineral
oxidation
vitamin

BEHAVIORAL OBJECTIVES

After careful study of this chapter, you should be able to:

1. Differentiate between catabolism and anabolism
2. Differentiate between the anaerobic and aerobic phases of cellular respiration and give the end products and the relative amount of energy released from each
3. Define *metabolic rate*
4. Name several factors that affect the metabolic rate
5. Explain the role of glucose in metabolism
6. Compare the energy contents of fats, proteins, and carbohydrates
7. Define *essential amino acid*
8. Explain the roles of minerals and vitamins in nutrition and give examples of each
9. List the recommended percentages of fats, carbohydrates, and protein in the diet
10. List some adverse effects of alcohol consumption
11. Explain how heat is produced in the body
12. List the ways in which heat is lost from the body
13. Describe the role of the hypothalamus in regulating body temperature

METABOLISM

The end products of digestion are used for all the cellular activities of the body, which together make up *metabolism.* These activities fall into two categories:

- *Catabolism,* which is the breakdown of complex compounds into simpler compounds. Catabolism includes the digestion of food into small molecules and the release of energy from these molecules within the cell.
- *Anabolism,* which is the building of simple compounds into substances needed for cellular activities and the growth and repair of tissues.

Through the steps of catabolism and anabolism, there is a constant turnover of body materials as energy is consumed, cells function and grow, and waste products are generated.

✔ CHECKPOINT **1**:

What are the two phases of metabolism?

How Cells Obtain Energy From Food

Cellular Respiration
Energy is released from nutrients in a series of reactions called **cellular respiration** (Table 18-1). Early studies on cellular respiration were done with *glucose* as the starting compound. Glucose is a simple sugar that is the main energy source for the body.

The Anaerobic Phase
The first steps in the breakdown of glucose do not require oxygen; that is, they are *anaerobic.* This phase of catabolism, known as glycolysis (gli-KOL-ih-sis), occurs in the cytoplasm of the cell. It yields a small amount of energy, which is used to make ATP (adenosine triphosphate), the energy compound of the cells.

The anaerobic breakdown of glucose is incomplete and ends with formation of an organic product called *pyruvic* (pi-RU-vik) *acid.* This end product is further metabolized in the next phase of cellular respiration. In muscle cells operating briefly under anaerobic conditions, pyruvic acid is converted to lactic acid, which accumulates while the cells build up an oxygen debt, as described in Chapter 7. The body must soon rest, so that cells can restore their oxygen supplies and continue with cellular respiration.

The Aerobic Phase
To generate enough energy for survival, the body's cells must break glucose down completely. Further oxygen-requiring, or *aerobic,* reactions occur within the mitochondria of the cell, and these reactions transfer much of the energy remaining in the nutrients to ATP.

18

18

Table 18•1	Capsule Summary of Cellular Respiration of Glucose		
PHASE	LOCATION IN CELL	END PRODUCT(S)	ENERGY YIELD/GLUCOSE
Anaerobic (glycolysis)	Cytoplasm	Pyruvic acid	2 ATP
Aerobic	Mitochondria	Carbon dioxide and water	34–36 ATP

In the course of the aerobic steps of cellular respiration, carbon dioxide is released and must be transported to the lungs for elimination. In addition, water is formed by the combination of oxygen with hydrogen obtained from nutrient molecules. Because of the type of chemical reactions involved, and because oxygen is used in the final steps, cellular respiration is described as an **oxidation** of nutrients. Note that enzymes are required as catalysts in all the reactions of cellular respiration. Many of the vitamins and minerals described later in this chapter are parts of these enzymes.

Although the oxidation of food is often compared to the burning of fuel, this comparison is inaccurate. Burning results in a sudden and often wasteful release of energy in the form of heat and light. In contrast, metabolic oxidation occurs in steps, and much of the energy released is stored as ATP for later use by the cells; some of the energy is released as heat, which is used to maintain body temperature, as discussed later in this chapter.

For those who know how to read chemical equations, the net balanced equation for cellular respiration, starting with glucose, is as follows:

$$C_6H_{12}O_6 \ + \ 6O_2 \ \rightarrow \ 6CO_2 \ + \ 6H_2O$$
$$\text{(glucose)} \quad \text{(oxygen)} \quad \text{(carbon dioxide)} \quad \text{(water)}$$

✔ CHECKPOINT **2**:

What name is given to the series of reactions that releases energy from nutrients?

Metabolic Rate

Metabolic rate refers to the rate at which energy is released from nutrients in the cells. It is affected by a person's size, body fat, sex, age, activity, and hormones, especially thyroid hormone (thyroxine).

Basal metabolism is the amount of energy needed to maintain life functions while the body is at rest. Metabolic rate is high in children and adolescents and decreases with age. See Estimation of Daily Energy Needs for an explanation of how to calculate basal energy needs and

Estimation of Daily Energy Needs

Basal energy requirements for a day can be estimated with a simple formula.

An average female requires 0.9 kcal/kg/hour (1.0 kcal/kg/hour for a male). By multiplying 0.9 by your weight in kilograms,* by 24 (or 1.0 x kg x 24 for a male), you get your daily basal energy requirement. For example, for a female weighing 132 pounds; the equation would be as follows:

132 pounds ÷ 2.2 = 60 kg

0.9 × 60 kg = 54 kcal/hour

54 × 24 = 1296 kcal/day

To estimate your total energy needs for a day, basal requirements must be multiplied by a factor based on your activity level—couch potato to serious athlete. For a female with moderate activity levels, basal energy requirements are multiplied by 1.6; for a male by 1.7. Following the example given above, the following equation applies:

1296 × 1.6 = 2073.6
(about 2075 kcal/day)

*To convert pounds to kilograms, divide weight in pounds by 2.2

total energy needs for an individual who exercises moderately.

The unit used to measure the energy in food is the **kilocalorie** (kcal), which is the amount of heat needed to raise 1 kilogram of water 1°C.

The Use of Nutrients for Energy

As noted, the main source of energy in the body is glucose. Most of the carbohydrates in the diet are converted to glucose in the course of metabolism. Glucose circulates in the blood to provide energy for all the cells. Reserves of glucose are stored in liver and muscle cells as **glycogen** (GLI-ko-jen), a compound built from glucose molecules. When glucose is needed for energy, glycogen is broken down to yield glucose.

Glycerol and fatty acids (from fat digestion) and amino acids (from protein digestion) can also be used for energy, but they enter the breakdown process at different points.

Fat in the diet yields more than twice as much energy as protein or carbohydrate (it is more "fattening"); fat yields 9 kcal of energy per gram, whereas protein and carbohydrate each yield 4 kcal per gram. Food that is ingested in excess of need is converted to fat and stored in adipose tissue.

Before they are oxidized for energy, amino acids must have their nitrogen (amine) groups removed. This removal, called *deamination,* occurs in the liver, where the nitrogen groups are then formed into urea by combination with carbon dioxide. The bloodstream transports the urea to the kidneys to be eliminated.

> ✔ CHECKPOINT **3**:
>
> What is the main energy source for the cells?

Anabolism

Nutrient molecules are built into body materials by anabolic steps, all of which are catalyzed by enzymes.

Essential Amino Acids
Eleven of the 20 amino acids needed to build proteins can be manufactured internally by

metabolic reactions. These 11 amino acids are described as *nonessential* because they need not be taken in with food. The remaining 9 amino acids cannot be made by the body and therefore must be taken in with the diet; these are the **essential amino acids.** Most animal proteins supply all of the essential amino acids and are described as **complete proteins.** Vegetables may be lacking in one or more of the essential amino acids. People on strict vegetarian diets must learn to combine foods, such as beans with rice or wheat, to obtain all the essential amino acids each day.

Essential Fatty Acids
There are also two essential fatty acids that must be taken in with food. These are easily obtained through a healthful, balanced diet.

> ✔ CHECKPOINT **4**:
>
> What is meant when an amino acid or a fatty acid is described as essential?

Minerals and Vitamins

In addition to needing fats, proteins, and carbohydrates, the human body requires minerals and vitamins.

Minerals are chemical elements needed for body structure, fluid balance, and such activities as muscle contraction, nerve impulse conduction, and blood clotting. Some minerals are components of vitamins. A list of the main minerals needed in a proper diet is given in Table 18-2. Some additional minerals not listed are also required for good health. Minerals needed in extremely small amounts are referred to as **trace elements.**

Vitamins are complex organic substances needed in very small quantities. Vitamins are parts of enzymes or other substances essential for metabolism, and vitamin deficiencies lead to a variety of nutritional diseases.

The water-soluble vitamins are the B vitamins and vitamin C. These are not stored in the body and must be taken in regularly with food. The fat-soluble vitamins are A, D, E, and K. These vitamins are kept in reserve in fatty tissue. Excess intake of the fat-soluble vitamins

Table 18•2   Minerals

MINERAL	FUNCTIONS	SOURCES	RESULTS OF DEFICIENCIES
Calcium (Ca)	Formation of bones and teeth, blood clotting, nerve conduction, muscle contraction	Dairy products, eggs, green vegetables, legumes (peas and beans)	Rickets, tetany, osteoporosis
Phosphorus (P)	Formation of bones and teeth; found in ATP, nucleic acids	Meat, fish, poultry, egg yolk, dairy products	Osteoporosis, abnormal metabolism
Sodium (Na)	Fluid balance; nerve impulse conduction, muscle contraction	Most foods, especially processed foods, table salt	Weakness, cramps, diarrhea, dehydration
Potassium (K)	Fluid balance, nerve and muscle activity	Fruits, meats, seafood, milk, vegetables, grains	Muscular and neurologic disorders
Chloride (Cl)	Fluid balance, hydrochloric acid in stomach	Meat, milk, eggs, processed foods, table salt	Rarely occur
Iron (Fe)	Oxygen carrier (hemoglobin, myoglobin)	Meat, eggs, fortified cereals, legumes, dried fruit	Anemia, dry skin, indigestion
Iodine (I)	Thyroid hormones	Seafood, iodized salt	Hypothyroidism, goiter
Magnesium (Mg)	Catalyst for enzyme reactions, carbohydrate metabolism	Green vegetables, grains, nuts, legumes	Spasticity, arrhythmia, vasodilation
Manganese (Mn)	Catalyst in actions of calcium and phosphorus; facilitator of many cell processes	Many foods	Possible reproductive disorders
Copper (Cu)	Necessary for absorption and use of iron in formation of hemoglobin; part of some enzymes	Meat, water	Anemia
Chromium (Cr)	Works with insulin to regulate blood glucose levels	Meat, unrefined food, fats and oils	Inability to use glucose
Cobalt (Co)	Part of vitamin B_{12}	Animal products	Pernicious anemia
Zinc (Zn)	Promotes carbon dioxide transport and energy metabolism; found in enzymes	Meat, fish, poultry, grains, vegetables	Alopecia (baldness); possibly related to diabetes
Fluoride (F)	Prevents tooth decay	Fluoridated water, tea, seafood	Dental caries

can lead to toxicity. A list of vitamins is given in Table 18-3.

✔ CHECKPOINT **5**:

Both vitamins and minerals are needed in metabolism. What is the difference between vitamins and minerals?

NUTRITION GUIDELINES

Good nutrition is absolutely essential for the maintenance of health (see Food as Good Medicine). If any vital food material is missing from the diet, the body will suffer from ***malnutrition.*** One commonly thinks of a malnourished person as one who does not have enough to eat, but malnutrition can also occur from eating too much of the wrong foods.

The simplest and perhaps best advice for maintaining a healthful diet is to eat a wide variety of fresh, wholesome foods daily. The U.S. Department of Agriculture (USDA) presently recommends a distribution of food in the diet as shown in Figure 18-1. The "Food Guide Pyramid" emphasizes grains, fruits, and vegetables with limited intake of fats, oils, and sugars.

Carbohydrates, Fats, and Proteins

Because proteins, unlike carbohydrates and fats, are not stored, protein foods should be taken in on a regular basis. The average U.S.

Table 18•3 Vitamins

VITAMINS	FUNCTIONS	SOURCES	RESULTS OF DEFICIENCIES
A (retinol)	Required for healthy epithelial tissue and for eye pigments; involved in reproduction and immunity	Orange fruits and vegetables, liver, eggs, dairy products, dark green vegetables	Night blindness; dry, scaly skin; decreased immunity
B_1 (thiamin)	Required for enzymes involved in oxidation of nutrients; nerve function	Pork, cereal, grains, meats, legumes, nuts	Beriberi, a disease of nerves
B_2 (riboflavin)	In enzymes required for oxidation of nutrients	Milk, eggs, liver, green leafy vegetables, grains	Skin and tongue disorders
B_3 (niacin, nicotinic acid)	Involved in oxidation of nutrients	Yeast, meat, liver, grains, legumes, nuts	Pellagra with dermatitis, diarrhea, mental disorders
B_6 (pyridoxine)	Amino acid and fatty acid metabolism; formation of niacin; manufacture of red blood cells	Meat, fish, poultry, fruit, grains, legumes, vegetables	Anemia, irritability, convulsions, muscle twitching, skin disorders
Pantothenic acid	Essential for normal growth; energy metabolism	Yeast, liver, eggs, and many other foods	Sleep disturbances, digestive upset
B_{12} (cyanocobalamin)	Production of cells; maintenance of nerve cells; fatty acid and amino acid metabolism	Animal products	Pernicious anemia
Biotin	Involved in fat and glycogen formation, amino acid metabolism	Peanuts, liver, tomatoes, eggs, and many other foods	Lack of coordination, dermatitis, fatigue
Folate (folic acid)	Required for amino acid metabolism, DNA synthesis, maturation of red blood cells	Vegetables, liver, legumes, seeds	Anemia, digestive disorders, neural tube defects in the embryo
C (ascorbic acid)	Maintains healthy skin and mucous membranes; involved in synthesis of collagen; antioxidant	Citrus fruits, green vegetables, potatoes, orange fruits	Scurvy, poor wound healing, anemia, weak bones
D (calciferol)	Aids in absorption of calcium and phosphorus from intestinal tract	Fatty fish, liver, eggs, fortified milk	Rickets, bone deformities
E (tocopherol)	Protects cell membranes; antioxidant	Seeds, green vegetables, nuts, grains, oils, eggs	Anemia, muscle and liver degeneration, pain
K	Synthesis of blood clotting factors, bone formation	Bacteria in digestive tract, liver, cabbage, and leafy green vegetables	Hemorrhage

diet, however, contains more than enough protein and too much fat, especially animal fat. It is currently recommended that calories from the three types of food be distributed as follows:

- Carbohydrate: 58%
- Fat: 30%
- Protein: 12%

The carbohydrates should be mainly complex, naturally occurring carbohydrates, and refined sugars should be kept to a minimum.

Fats are subdivided into saturated and unsaturated forms. Most **saturated fats** are from an-imal sources and are solid at room temperature, such as butter and lard. Also included in this group are the so-called "tropical oils": coconut oil and palm oil. **Unsaturated fats** are derived from plants. They are liquid at room temperature and are generally referred to as *oils*.

No more than one third of the fats in the diet should be saturated fats. Diets high in saturated fats are associated with a higher than normal incidence of cancer, heart disease, and cardiovascular problems, although the relation between these factors is not fully understood.

Many commercial products contain fats that are artificially saturated to prevent rancidity

18

Food as Good Medicine

Does an apple a day keep the doctor away? This adage reflects what people have long known—that the foods we eat have a profound effect on our health. The apple has fiber, which is known to reduce the risk of colon cancer by diluting carcinogens in the bowel and reducing their contact with the bowel wall. It is also lacking in fats, which should be controlled in the diet, especially saturated fats. People with diets rich in fruits and vegetables have lower incidences of diabetes, cardiovascular disease, and several types of cancer. Vegetables in the mustard family, such as broccoli, cabbage, and kale, appear to contain compounds that inhibit the growth of cancer cells. Studies are now underway to identify which components of the various vegetables may provide this protection.

and provide a more solid consistency. These are listed on food labels as partially hydrogenated vegetable oils and are found in baked goods, peanut butter, vegetable shortening, and solid margarine. Evidence shows that components of hydrogenated fats, known as *trans-fatty acids,* may be just as harmful, if not more so, than natural saturated fats and should be avoided.

A weight loss diet should follow the same guidelines as given above with a reduction in portion sizes. Exercise is also recommended.

Vitamin and Mineral Supplements

The need for mineral and vitamin supplements to the diet is a subject of controversy. Some researchers maintain that adequate amounts of these substances can be obtained from a varied, healthful diet; others hold that pollution, depletion of the soils, and the storage, refining, and processing of foods make supplementation beneficial. Most agree, however, that children, elderly people, pregnant and lactating women, and teenagers, who often do not get enough of the proper foods, would profit from additional minerals and vitamins.

When required, supplements should be selected by a physician or nutritionist to fit the particular needs of the individual. Megavitamin dosages may cause unpleasant reactions and in some cases are hazardous. Vitamins A and D have both been found to cause serious toxic effects when taken in excess.

Food Allergies

The subject of allergies has received much attention. Some individuals develop clear allergic (hypersensitive) symptoms if they eat certain foods. The most common food allergens are wheat, yeast, milk, and eggs, but almost any food might cause an allergic reaction in a given individual. Although food allergies may be responsible for symptoms with no other known cause, most people can probably eat all types of foods.

Alcohol

Alcohol yields energy, in the amount of 7 kcal per gram, but it is not considered a nutrient because it does not yield useful end products. In fact, alcohol interferes with metabolism and contributes to a variety of disorders.

The body can metabolize about one half ounce of pure alcohol (ethanol) per hour. This amount translates into one glass of wine, one can of beer, or one shot of hard liquor. Consumed at a more rapid rate, alcohol enters the bloodstream and affects many cells, notably in the brain.

Alcohol is rapidly absorbed through the stomach and small intestine and is detoxified by the liver. When delivered in excess to the liver, alcohol can lead to the accumulation of fat and to cirrhosis. Metabolism of alcohol ties up enzymes needed for oxidation of nutrients and also results in byproducts that acidify body fluids. Other affects of alcoholism include obesity, malnutrition, cancer, ulcers, and fetal alcohol syndrome. Pregnant women are advised not to drink any alcohol. In addition, alcohol impairs judgment and leads to increased involvement in accidents.

Although consumption of alcohol is compatible with good health and may even have a beneficial effect on the cardiovascular system, alcohol should be consumed only in moderation.

Fats, oils, sweets
Use sparingly

Milk, yogurt
and cheese
2 to 3 servings

Meat, poultry,
fish, dry beans,
eggs and nuts
2 to 3 servings

Vegetables
3 to 5 servings

Fruits
2 to 4 servings

Bread, cereal,
grains and pasta
6 to 11 servings

FIGURE **18•1**   Guide to daily food choices. (Taylor C, Lillis C, LeMone P: Fundamentals of Nursing: The Art and Science of Nursing Care, 2nd ed, p. 805. Philadelphia, JB Lippincott, 1993)

Nutrition and Aging

With age, a person may find it difficult to maintain a balanced diet. Often, the elderly lose interest in buying and preparing food or are unable to do so. Because metabolism generally slows, and less food is required to meet energy needs, nutritional deficiencies may develop. Medications may interfere with appetite and with the absorption and use of specific nutrients.

It is important for older people to seek out foods that are "nutrient dense," that is, foods that have a high proportion of nutrients in comparison to the number of calories they provide. Exercise helps to boost appetite and maintains muscle tissue, which is more active metabolically.

BODY TEMPERATURE

Heat is an important byproduct of the many chemical activities constantly going on in tissues all over the body. Heat is always being lost through a variety of outlets. Because of a num-

18

ber of regulatory devices, however, under normal conditions, body temperature remains constant within quite narrow limits. Maintenance of a constant temperature despite both internal and external influences is one phase of homeostasis, the tendency of all body processes to maintain a normal state despite forces that tend to alter them.

Heat Production

Heat is produced when nutrients are oxidized in the cells. Thus, heat is a byproduct of the cellular reactions that generate energy. The amount of heat produced by a given organ varies with the kind of tissue and its activity.

Sources of Heat

Tissues vary in the amount of heat they generate at rest and during activity. While at rest, muscles may produce as little as 25% of total body heat, but when muscles contract, heat production is greatly multiplied, owing to the increase in metabolic rate. Under basal conditions (at rest), the liver and other abdominal organs produce about 50% of total body heat. The brain produces only 15% of body heat at rest, and an increase in nervous tissue activity produces little increase in heat production.

Although it would seem from this description that some parts of the body would tend to become much warmer than others, the circulating blood distributes the heat fairly evenly.

Factors Affecting Heat Production

The rate at which heat is produced is affected by a number of factors, including exercise, hormone production, food intake, and age.

Hormones, such as thyroxine from the thyroid gland and epinephrine (adrenaline) from the medulla of the adrenal gland, increase the rate of heat production.

The intake of food is also accompanied by increased heat production. The nutrients that enter the blood after digestion are available for increased cellular metabolism. In addition, the glands and muscles of the digestive system generate heat as they set to work. These responses do not account for all the increase, however, nor do they account for the much greater increase

in metabolism after a meal containing a large amount of protein. Although the reasons are not entirely clear, the intake of food definitely increases metabolism and thus adds to heat production.

✔ CHECKPOINT **6**:

What are some factors that affect heat production in the body?

Heat Loss

More than 80% of heat loss occurs through the skin. The remaining 15% to 20% is dissipated by the respiratory system and with the urine and feces.

Heat Loss Through the Skin

Networks of blood vessels in the dermis (deeper part) of the skin can bring considerable quantities of blood near the surface, so that heat can be dissipated to the outside. This can occur in several ways.

- Heat can be transferred to the surrounding air by means of the process of **conduction.**
- Heat also travels from its source in the form of heat waves or rays, a process termed **radiation.**
- If the air is moving, so that the layer of heated air next to the body is constantly being carried away and replaced with cooler air (as by an electric fan), the process is known as **convection.**
- Finally, heat loss may be produced by **evaporation,** the process by which liquid changes to the vapor state.

To illustrate evaporation, rub some alcohol on your skin; it evaporates rapidly, using so much heat from the skin that your arm feels cold. Perspiration does the same thing, although not as quickly. The rate of heat loss through evaporation depends on the humidity of the surrounding air. When this exceeds 60% or so, perspiration does not evaporate so readily, making one feel generally miserable unless one can resort to some other means of heat loss, such as convection caused by a fan.

Prevention of Heat Loss

Factors that play a part in heat loss through the skin include the volume of tissue compared with the amount of skin surface. A child loses heat more rapidly than does an adult. Such parts as fingers and toes are affected most by exposure to cold because they have a great amount of skin compared with total tissue volume.

If the temperature of the surrounding air is lower than that of the body, excessive heat loss is prevented by both natural and artificial means.

Clothing checks heat loss by trapping "dead air" in both its material and its layers. This noncirculating air is a good insulator.

An effective natural insulation against cold is the layer of fat under the skin. Even when skin temperature is low, this fatty tissue prevents the deeper tissues from losing much heat. On the average, this layer is slightly thicker in females than in males. Naturally, there are individual variations, but as a rule, the degree of insulation depends on the thickness of this layer of subcutaneous fat.

Temperature Regulation

Given that body temperature remains almost constant despite wide variations in the rate of heat production or loss, there must be internal mechanisms for regulating temperature.

The Role of the Hypothalamus

Many areas of the body take part in this heat-regulating process, but the most important center is the area inside the brain, located just above the pituitary gland, the ***hypothalamus.***

Some of the cells in the hypothalamus control the production of heat in the body tissues, whereas another group of cells controls heat loss. This control comes about in response to the temperature of the blood circulating through the brain as well as in response to nerve impulses from temperature receptors in the skin.

Conservation of Heat

If these two factors indicate that too much heat is being lost, impulses are sent quickly from the hypothalamus to the autonomic (involuntary) nervous system, which in turn causes constriction of the skin blood vessels to reduce heat loss. Other impulses are sent to the muscles to cause shivering, a rhythmic contraction of many body muscles, which results in increased heat production. Furthermore, the output of epinephrine may be increased if necessary. Epinephrine increases cell metabolism for a short period, and this in turn increases heat production.

Release of Heat

If there is danger of overheating, the hypothalamus transmits impulses that stimulate the sweat glands to increase their activity and dilate the blood vessels in the skin, so that increased blood flow results in greater loss of heat. The hypothalamus may also encourage the relaxation of muscles and thus minimize the production of heat in these organs.

The Role of Muscles

Muscles are especially important in temperature regulation because variations in the amount of activity in these large masses of tissue can readily increase or decrease the total amount of heat produced. Because muscles form roughly one third of the bulk of the body, either an involuntary or a purposeful increase in the activity of this big group of organs can form enough heat to offset a considerable decrease in the temperature of the environment.

 CHECKPOINT **7**:

What part of the brain is responsible for regulating body temperature?

Age Factors

Very young and very old people are limited in their ability to regulate body temperature when exposed to extremes in environment. The body temperature of a newborn infant decreases if the infant is exposed to a cool environment for a long period. Elderly people also are not able to produce enough heat to maintain body temperature in a cool environment.

With regard to overheating in these age groups, heat loss mechanisms are not fully developed in the newborn. The elderly do not lose

18

as much heat from their skin. Both groups should be protected from extreme temperatures.

Normal Body Temperature

The normal temperature range obtained by either a mercury or an electronic thermometer may extend from 36.2°C to 37.6°C (97°F to 100°F). Body temperature varies with the time of day. Usually, it is lowest in the early morning because the muscles have been relaxed and no food has been taken in for several hours. Temperature tends to be higher in the late afternoon and evening because of physical activity and consumption of food.

Normal temperature also varies in different parts of the body. Skin temperature obtained in the axilla (armpit) is lower than mouth temperature, and mouth temperature is a degree or so lower than rectal temperature. It is believed

that, if it were possible to place a thermometer inside the liver, it would register a degree or more higher than rectal temperature. The temperature within a muscle might be even higher during its activity.

Although the Fahrenheit scale is used in the United States, in most parts of the world, temperature is measured with the *Celsius* (SEL-se-us) thermometer. On this scale, the ice point is at 0° and the normal boiling point of water is at 100°, the interval between these two points being divided into 100 equal units. The Celsius scale is also called the *centigrade scale* (think of 100 cents in a dollar). See Appendix 2 for a comparison of the Celsius and Fahrenheit scales and formulas for converting from one to the other.

✔ CHECKPOINT **8**:

What is normal body temperature?

Summary

18

I. **Metabolism**—life-sustaining reactions that occur in the living cell
    1. Catabolism—breakdown of complex compounds into simpler compounds
    2. Anabolism—building of simple compounds into substances needed for cellular activities, growth, and repair
  A. How cells obtain energy from food
    1. Cellular respiration—a series of reactions in which food is oxidized for energy
      a. Anaerobic phase—does not require oxygen
        (1) Location—cytoplasm
        (2) Yield—small amount of energy
        (3) End product—organic (*i.e.,* pyruvic acid)

      b. Aerobic phase-requires oxygen
        (1) Location—mitochondria
        (2) Yield—almost all remaining energy in food
        (3) End products—carbon dioxide and water
    2. Metabolic rate—rate at which energy is released from food in the cells
      a. Basal metabolism—amount of energy needed to maintain life functions while at rest
  B. Use of nutrients for energy
    1. Glucose—main energy source
    2. Fats—highest energy yield
    3. Proteins—can be used for energy after removal of nitrogen
  C. Anabolism
    1. Essential amino acids and fatty acids must be taken in with food
      a. Complete proteins contain all the essential amino acids
  D. Minerals and vitamins
    1. Minerals—elements needed for body structure and cell activities

a. Trace elements—elements needed in extremely small amounts

2. Vitamins—organic substances needed in small amounts

II. Nutrition guidelines

1. Malnutrition—too little food or inadequate amounts of specific foods
2. Components of healthy diet
   a. USDA Food Guide Pyramid
   b. Less than 10% of total daily calories in form of saturated fats
A. Carbohydrates, fats, and proteins
B. Vitamin and mineral supplements
C. Food allergies
D. Alcohol
E. Nutrition and aging

III. Body temperature

A. Heat production
   1. Most heat produced in muscles and glands
   2. Distributed by the circulation
   3. Affected by exercise, hormones, food, age

B. Heat loss
   1. Avenues—skin, urine, feces, respiratory system
   2. Mechanisms—conduction, radiation, convection, evaporation
C. Temperature regulation
   1. Hypothalamus—main temperature-regulating center; responds to temperature of blood and temperature receptors in skin
   2. Responses to decrease in body temperature
      a. Constriction of blood vessels in skin
      b. Shivering
      c. Increased release of epinephrine
   3. Responses to increase in body temperature
      a. Dilation of skin vessels
      b. Sweating
      c. Relaxation of muscles
D. Normal body temperature—ranges from 36.2°C to 37.6°C; varies with time of day and location measured

18

Questions for Study and Review

1. Define *cellular respiration.*
2. In what part of the cell does anaerobic respiration occur? What are its end products?
3. In what part of the cell does aerobic respiration occur? What are its end products?
4. Define *metabolic rate.* What factors affect the metabolic rate?
5. What is the definition of *basal metabolism?*
6. About how many kilocalories are released from a gram of butter? a gram of egg white? a gram of sugar?
7. Gelatin is not a complete protein. What are the dangers of eating flavored gelatin as a sole source of protein?
8. Name the foods that are emphasized in the USDA Food Guide Pyramid; which are to be eaten sparingly?
9. If you eat 2000 kcal a day, how many kilocalories should come from carbohydrates? from fats? from proteins?
10. What organ metabolizes alcohol?
11. How is heat produced in the body? What structures produce the most heat during increased activity?
12. Name four factors that affect heat production.
13. How is heat lost from the body?
14. Name four ways in which heat escapes to the environment.

15. In what ways is heat kept in the body?
16. Name the main temperature regulator and describe what it does when the body is too hot and when it is too cold. What parts do muscles play?
17. What is the normal body temperature range? How does it vary with respect to the time of day and the part of the body?
18. Differentiate between the terms in each of the following pairs:
    a. *catabolism* and *anabolism*
    b. *aerobic* and *anaerobic*
    c. *mineral* and *vitamin*
    d. *saturated fats* and *unsaturated fats*

✔ ANSWERS TO CHECKPOINTS

1. The two phases of metabolism are catabolism, the breakdown phase of metabolism, and anabolism, the building phase of metabolism.
2. Cellular respiration is the series of reactions that releases energy from nutrients in the cell.
3. Glucose is the main energy source for the cells.
4. An essential amino acid or fatty acid cannot be made metabolically and must be taken in with the diet.
5. Minerals are chemical elements, and vitamins are complex organic substances.
6. Some factors that affect heat production are exercise, hormone production, food intake, and age.
7. The hypothalamus of the brain is responsible for regulating body temperature.
8. Normal body temperature is 36.2°C to 37.6°C (97°F to 100°F).

18

The Urinary System and Body Fluids

Chapter

19

SELECTED KEY TERMS

The following terms are defined in the Glossary:

angiotensin

antidiuretic hormone (ADH)

buffer

electrolyte

erythropoietin

excretion

extracellular

glomerular filtrate

glomerulus

interstitial

intracellular

kidney

micturition

nephron

pH

renin

urea

ureter

urethra

urinary bladder

urine

BEHAVIORAL OBJECTIVES

After careful study of this chapter, you should be able to:

1. List the systems that eliminate waste and name the substances eliminated by each

2. Describe the parts of the urinary system and give the functions of each

3. Trace the path of a drop of blood as it flows through the kidney

4. Describe a nephron

5. Describe the components and the functions of the juxtaglomerular apparatus

6. Name the four processes involved in urine formation and describe how each functions

7. Identify the role of ADH in urine formation

8. Describe the process of micturition

9. Name three normal constituents of urine

10. Compare intracellular and extracellular fluids

11. List four types of extracellular fluids

12. Name the systems that are involved in water balance

13. Define *electrolytes* and describe some of their functions

14. Describe the role of hormones in electrolyte balance

15. Describe three methods for regulating the pH of body fluids

The urinary system is also called the *excretory system* because one of its main functions is to remove waste products from the blood and eliminate them from the body. It has many other functions as well, including regulation of the volume, acid–base balance (pH), and electrolyte composition of body fluids.

EXCRETION

Although the focus of this chapter is the urinary system, certain aspects of other systems are also discussed because body systems work interdependently to maintain homeostasis (balance). The systems active in excretion and some of the substances that they eliminate are the following:

- The *urinary system* excretes water, waste products containing nitrogen, and salts. These are all constituents of the urine.
- The *digestive system* eliminates water, some salts, bile, and the residue of digestion, all of which are contained in the feces. The liver is important in eliminating the products of red blood cell destruction and in breaking down certain drugs and toxins.
- The *respiratory system* eliminates carbon dioxide and water. The latter appears as vapor, as can be demonstrated by breathing on a windowpane.

- The skin, or *integumentary system,* excretes water, salts, and very small quantities of nitrogenous wastes. These all appear in perspiration, although evaporation of water from the skin may go on most of the time without our being conscious of it.

✔ CHECKPOINT **1**:

The main function of the urinary system is to eliminate waste. What are some other systems that eliminate waste?

ORGANS OF THE URINARY SYSTEM

The main parts of the urinary system, shown in Figure 19-1, are as follows:

- Two *kidneys.* These organs extract wastes from the blood, balance body fluids, and form urine.
- Two *ureters* (U-re-ters). These tubes conduct urine from the kidneys to the urinary bladder.
- A single *urinary bladder.* This reservoir receives and stores the urine brought to it by the two ureters.
- A single *urethra* (u-RE-thrah). This tube

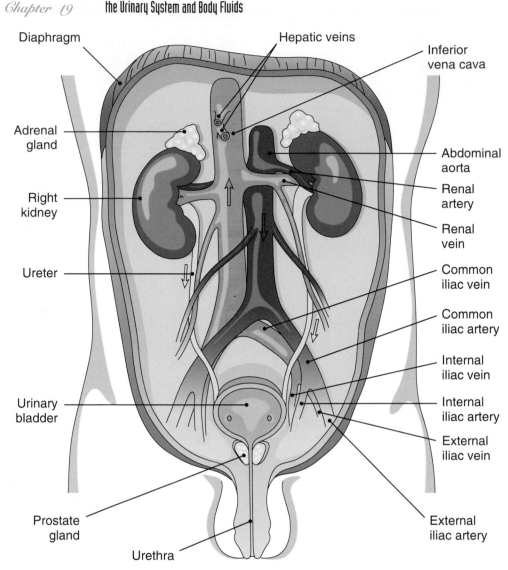

FIGURE **19•1** Urinary system, with blood vessels.

conducts urine from the bladder to the out-side of the body for elimination.

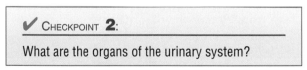

✔ CHECKPOINT **2**:

What are the organs of the urinary system?

THE KIDNEYS

Location of the Kidneys

The two kidneys lie against the muscles of the back in the upper abdomen. They are up under the dome of the diaphragm and are protected by the lower ribs and the rib (costal) cartilages. Each kidney is enclosed in a membranous cap-sule that is made of fibrous connective tissue; this capsule adheres loosely to the kidney itself. In addition, there is a crescent of fat called the *adipose capsule* around the organ. An outer layer of fascia (connective tissue) anchors the kidney to the peritoneum and abdominal wall. The kidneys, as well as the ureters, lie behind the peritoneum. Thus, they are not in the peri-toneal cavity but rather in an area known as the ***retroperitoneal*** (ret-ro-per-ih-to-NE-al) ***space.***

Blood Supply to the Kidney

The blood supply to the kidney is illustrated in Figure 19-2. Blood is brought to the kidney by a short branch of the abdominal aorta called the **renal artery.** After entering the kidney, the renal artery subdivides into smaller and smaller branches, which eventually make contact with the functional units of the kidney, the **nephrons** (NEF-ronz) (Figs. 19-3 and 19-4). Blood leaves the kidney by vessels that finally merge to form the **renal vein,** which carries blood into the inferior vena cava for return to the heart.

✔ CHECKPOINT **3**:

The kidneys are located in the retroperitoneal space. Where is this space?

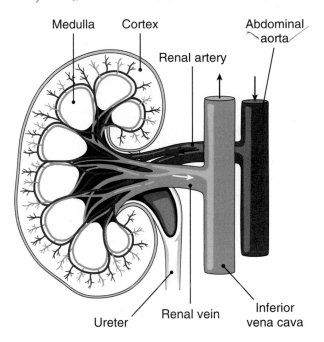

FIGURE **19•2** Blood supply and circulation of the kidney.

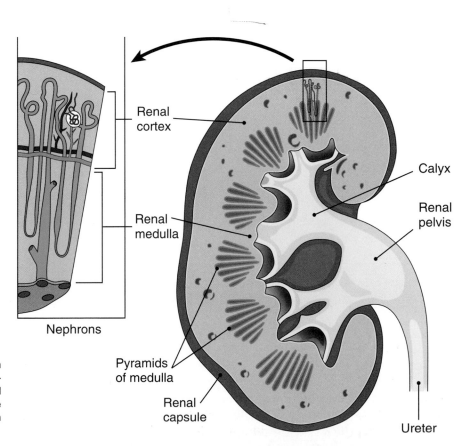

FIGURE **19•3** Longitudinal section through the kidney showing its internal structure and an enlarged diagram of nephrons. There are more than 1 million nephrons in each kidney.

Proximal
convoluted
tubule

Distal
convoluted
tubule

Efferent
arteriole

Afferent
arteriole

Bowman's
capsule

Glomerulus

Peritubular
capillaries

Loop of
Henle

From renal
artery

To
renal vein

Collecting
duct

Calyx

FIGURE **19•4** A nephron and its blood supply.

✔ CHECKPOINT **4**:

What vessel supplies blood to the kidney and what vessel drains blood from the kidney?

Structure of the Kidney

The kidney is a somewhat flattened organ about 10 cm (4 inches) long, 5 cm (2 inches) wide, and 2.5 cm (1 inch) thick. On the inner, or medial, border there is a notch called the **hilus**, at which region the renal artery, the renal vein, and the ureter connect with the kidney. The outer, or lateral, border is convex (curved outward), giving the entire organ a bean-shaped appearance.

The kidney is divided into two regions: the renal cortex and the renal medulla (see Fig. 19-3). The **renal cortex** is the outer portion of the kidney. The **renal medulla** contains the tubes in which urine is formed and collected. These tubes form a number of cone-shaped structures called **renal pyramids.** The tips of the pyramids point toward the **renal pelvis,** a funnel-shaped basin that forms the upper end of the ureter. Cuplike extensions of the renal pelvis surround the tips of the pyramids and collect urine; these extensions are called **calyces** (KA-lih-seze) (sing., **calyx** [KA-liks]). The urine that collects in the pelvis then passes down the ureters to the bladder.

The Nephron

As is the case with most organs, the most fascinating aspect of the kidney is too small to be seen with the naked eye. This basic unit of the kidney, where the kidney's work is actually done, is the **nephron** (see Fig. 19-4). The nephron is essentially a tiny coiled tube with a bulb at one end. This bulb, known as **Bowman's capsule,** surrounds a cluster of capillaries called the **glomerulus** (glo-MER-u-lus) (pl., *glomeruli* [glo-MER-u-li]). Each kidney contains about 1 million nephrons; if all these coiled tubes were separated, straightened out, and laid end to end, they would span some 120 kilometers (75 miles)! Figure 19-5 is a microscopic view of kidney tissue showing several glomeruli, each surrounded by a Bowman's capsule. It also shows sections through the tubular portions of the nephrons.

A small blood vessel, called the **afferent arteriole,** supplies the glomerulus with blood; another small vessel, called the **efferent arteriole,** carries blood from the glomerulus. When blood leaves the glomerulus, it does not head immediately back toward the heart. Instead, it flows into a capillary network that surrounds the tubular portion of the nephron. These small vessels, **peritubular capillaries,** are named for their location around the nephron.

The tubular part of the nephron consists of several portions. The coiled portion leading from Bowman's capsule is called the **proximal convoluted** (KON-vo-lu-ted) **tubule (PCT).** The tubule then uncoils to form a hairpin-shaped segment called the **loop of Henle.** Continuing from the loop, the tubule coils once again into the **distal convoluted tubule (DCT),** so called because it is farther along the tubule from Bowman's capsule than is the PCT. The distal end of each tubule empties into a collecting duct, which then continues through the medulla toward the renal pelvis.

The glomerulus, Bowman's capsule, and the proximal and distal convoluted tubules of the nephrons are within the renal cortex. The loops of Henle and collecting ducts extend into the medulla (see Fig. 19-3).

The Juxtaglomerular Apparatus

The first portion of the DCT curves back toward the glomerulus to pass between the afferent and efferent arterioles (Fig. 19-6). At the point where the DCT makes contact with the afferent arteriole, there are specialized cells in each that together make up the **juxtaglomerular** (juks-tah-glo-MER-u-lar) **(JG) apparatus.** The name means "near the glomerulus," which describes the location of this structure. The JG apparatus helps to regulate kidney function. When blood pressure falls, cells in the wall of the afferent arteriole secrete the enzyme **renin** (RE-nin), which raises blood pressure by a mechanism described later.

glomerulus

renal tubules

Bowman's capsule

FIGURE **19•5** Microscopic view of the kidney. (Courtesy of Dana Morse Bittus and B. J. Cohen)

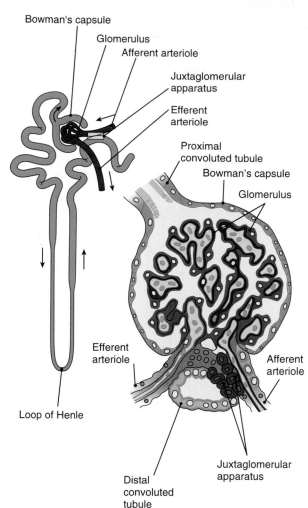

Bowman's capsule
Glomerulus
Afferent arteriole
Juxtaglomerular apparatus
Efferent arteriole
Proximal convoluted tubule
Bowman's capsule
Glomerulus
Efferent arteriole
Afferent arteriole
Loop of Henle
Juxtaglomerular apparatus
Distal convoluted tubule

FIGURE **19•6** Structure of the juxtaglomerular apparatus. Note how the distal convoluted tubule contacts the afferent arteriole.

✔ CHECKPOINT **5**:

What is the functional unit of the kidney called?

Functions of the Kidney

The kidneys are involved in the following processes:

- Excretion of unwanted substances, such as waste products from cell metabolism, excess salts, and toxins. One product of amino acid metabolism is nitrogen-containing waste material, a chief form of which is

urea (u-RE-ah). Urea is produced in the liver and transported in the bloodstream to the kidneys for elimination. The kidneys provide a specialized mechanism for the elimination of urea and other nitrogenous (ni-TROJ-en-us) wastes.

- Maintenance of water balance. Although the amount of water consumed in a day can vary tremendously, the kidneys can adapt to these variations, so that the volume of body water remains remarkably stable from day to day. Water is constantly lost in many ways: from the skin, from the respiratory system during exhalation, and from the intestinal tract. Normally, the amount of water taken in or produced (intake) is about equal to the amount lost (output).

- Regulation of the acid–base balance of body fluids. Acids are constantly being produced by cell metabolism, and certain foods can cause acids or bases to be formed in the body. Bases in the form of antacids, such as baking soda, may also be ingested. However, if the body is to function normally, a certain critical proportion of acids and bases must be maintained at all times.

- Regulation of blood pressure. If blood pressure falls too low for effective filtration through the glomerulus, the cells of the JG apparatus release the enzyme renin. In the blood, renin activates a protein called *angiotensin* (an-je-o-TEN-sin) that causes blood vessels to constrict, thus raising blood pressure.

- Regulation of red blood cell production. When the kidneys do not get enough oxygen, they produce the hormone *erythropoietin* (eh-rith-ro-POY-eh-tin) *(EPO),* which stimulates the production of red blood cells in the red bone marrow. EPO made by genetic engineering is now available to reduce severe anemia, such as occurs in the end stage of kidney failure.

✔ CHECKPOINT **6**:

What substance is produced by the JG apparatus and under what conditions is it produced?

Formation of Urine

Glomerular Filtration

The process of urine formation begins with the glomerulus in Bowman's capsule. The membranes that form the walls of the glomerular capillaries are sievelike and permit the free flow of water and soluble materials through them. Like other capillary walls, however, they are impermeable (im-PER-me-abl) to blood cells and large protein molecules, and these components remain in the blood (Fig. 19-7).

Because the diameter of the afferent arteriole is slightly larger than the diameter of the efferent arteriole (see Fig. 19-7), blood can enter the glomerulus more easily than it can leave. Thus, the pressure of the blood in the glomerulus is about three to four times as high as it is in other body capillaries. To understand this effect, think of placing your thumb over the end of a garden hose as water comes through. Because the diameter of the opening is made smaller, water is forced out under higher pressure. As a result of this increased pressure in the glomerulus, materials are constantly being pushed out of the blood and into Bowman's capsule of the nephron. This movement of materials under pressure from the blood into Bowman's capsule is known as ***glomerular filtration.***

The fluid that enters Bowman's capsule, called the ***glomerular filtrate,*** begins its journey along the tubular system of the nephron. In addition to water and the normal soluble substances in the blood, other substances, such as drugs, may also be filtered and become part of the glomerular filtrate.

> ✔ CHECKPOINT **7**:
> The first step in urine formation is glomerular filtration. What is glomerular filtration?

Tubular Reabsorption

About 160 to 180 liters of filtrate are formed each day in the kidneys. However, only 1 to 1.5 liters of urine are eliminated daily. Clearly, most of the water that enters the nephron is not excreted with the urine but rather is returned to the circulation. In addition to water, many substances that are needed by the body, such as nutrients and ions, also pass into the nephron as part of the filtrate. These must be returned to the body as well. Therefore, the process of filtration that occurs in Bowman's capsule is followed by a process of ***tubular reabsorption.*** As the filtrate travels through the tubular system of the nephron, water and other needed substances leave the tubule by diffusion and active transport and enter the surrounding tissue fluids. They then enter the blood in the peritubular capillaries and return to the circulation. In contrast, most of the urea and other nitrogenous waste materials are kept within the tubule to be eliminated with the urine (see The Transport Maximum).

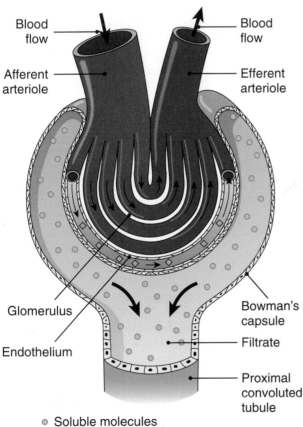

FIGURE **19•7** Diagram showing the process of filtration in the formation of urine. Blood pressure inside the glomerulus forces water and dissolved substances into Bowman's capsule. Blood cells and proteins remain behind in the blood. The smaller caliber of the efferent arteriole as compared with that of the afferent arteriole maintains pressure.

The Transport Maximum

The kidney works very efficiently to return valuable substances to the blood after glomerular filtration. However, the carriers that are needed for active transport of these substances can become overloaded. There is a limit to the amount of each substance that can be reabsorbed in a given time period. The limit of this rate of reabsorption is called the **transport maximum (Tm)** for that substance, and it is measured in milligrams (mg) per minute.

If a substance is present in excess in the blood, it may exceed its transport maximum and then, because it cannot be totally reabsorbed, some will be excreted in the urine. For example, if the concentration of glucose in the blood exceeds 180 mg/dL, glucose will begin to appear in the urine, a condition called **glucosuria** (glu-ko-SU-re-ah). The most common cause of glucosuria is uncontrolled diabetes mellitus.

Tubular Secretion

Before the filtrate leaves the body as urine, final adjustments in composition are made by the process of **tubular secretion.** In this process, some substances are actively moved from the blood into the nephron. Notably, potassium ions are moved into the urine by this process. Also, by the active secretion of hydrogen ions, the kidneys regulate the acid–base (pH) balance of body fluids.

Concentration of the Urine

The amount of water that is eliminated with the urine is regulated by a complex mechanism within the nephron that is influenced by **antidiuretic hormone (ADH),** a hormone released from the posterior portion of the pituitary gland. The process is called the **countercurrent mechanism** because it involves fluid traveling in opposite directions within the loop of Henle. The countercurrent mechanism is illustrated in Figure 19-8. Its essentials are described as follows.

As the filtrate passes through the loop of Henle, salts, especially sodium, are actively pumped out by the cells of the nephron, with the result that the interstitial fluid of the medulla becomes increasingly concentrated. Because the nephron is not very permeable to water at this point, the fluid within the nephron becomes increasingly dilute. As the fluid passes through the more permeable DCT and through the collecting duct, water is drawn out by the concentrated fluids around the nephron and returned to the blood. (Remember, according to the laws of diffusion, water follows salt.) In this manner, the urine becomes more concentrated, and its volume is reduced.

ADH

The role of ADH is to make the walls of the DCT and collecting tubule more permeable to water, so that more water will be reabsorbed and less will be excreted with the urine. The release of ADH from the pituitary is regulated by a feedback system. As the blood becomes more concentrated, the hypothalamus causes more ADH to be released from the posterior pituitary; as the blood becomes more dilute, less ADH is released. In the disease diabetes insipidus, there is inadequate secretion of ADH from the hypothalamus. This results in the elimination of large amounts of dilute urine accompanied by excessive thirst.

Summary of Urine Formation

The processes involved in urine formation are summarized below and illustrated in Figure 19-9.

- Glomerular filtration allows all diffusible materials to pass from the blood into the nephron.
- Tubular reabsorption moves useful substances back into the blood while keeping waste products in the nephron to be eliminated in the urine.
- Tubular secretion moves additional substances from the blood into the nephron for elimination. Movement of hydrogen ions is one means by which the pH of body fluids is balanced.
- The countercurrent mechanism concentrates the urine and reduces the volume excreted. The pituitary hormone ADH allows more water to be reabsorbed from the nephron.

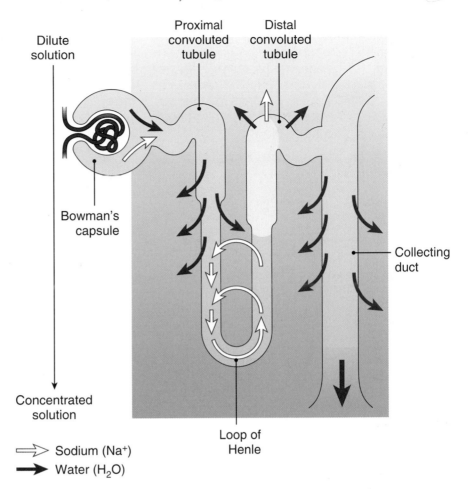

FIGURE **19•8** Loop of Henle, where the proportions of waste and water in urine are regulated according to the body's constantly changing needs. The concentration of urine is determined by means of intricate exchanges of water and salt, constituting the counter-current mechnism.

$\Longrightarrow$ Sodium (Na⁺)

$\longrightarrow$ Water (H₂O)

19

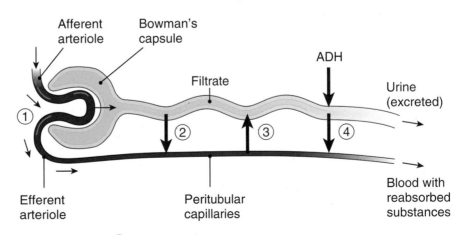

① Filtration from blood into nephron
② Reabsorption from filtrate into blood
③ Tubular secretion from blood into filtrate
④ Reabsorption of water under effects of ADH

FIGURE **19•9** Summary of urine formation in nephron.

Although this story seems complex, and there appears to be a great deal of back-and-forth exchanges, these processes together allow the kidney to "fine tune" body fluids. As the filtrate makes its slow journey through the twists and turns of the nephron, there is ample time for exchanges to take place between the kidney tubules and the circulating blood.

✔ CHECKPOINT **8**:

What are the four processes involved in the formation of urine?

STORAGE AND TRANSPORT OF URINE

The Ureters

The two ureters are long, slender, muscular tubes that extend from the kidney down to and through the lower part of the urinary bladder (see Fig. 19-1). The ureters are entirely extraperitoneal, being located behind and, at the lower part, below the peritoneum. Their length naturally varies with the size of the individual, and they may be anywhere from 25 cm to 32 cm (10–13 inches) long. Nearly 2.5 cm (1 inch) of the lower part of the ureter enters the bladder by passing obliquely (at an angle) through the bladder wall. Because of the oblique direction taken by the ureter through the lower bladder wall, a full bladder compresses the ureter and prevents the backflow of urine.

The wall of the ureter includes a lining of epithelial cells, a relatively thick layer of involuntary muscle, and finally an outer coat of fibrous connective tissue. The lining of the ureter is continuous with that of the renal pelvis and the bladder. The muscles of the ureters are capable of the same rhythmic contraction (peristalsis) found in the digestive system. Urine is moved along the ureter from the kidneys to the bladder by gravity and by peristalsis at frequent intervals.

The Urinary Bladder

When it is empty, the urinary bladder (Fig. 19-10) is located below the parietal peritoneum and behind the pubic joint. When it is filled, it pushes the peritoneum upward and may extend well into the abdominal cavity proper. The urinary bladder is a temporary reservoir for urine, just as the gallbladder is a storage sac for bile.

The bladder wall has many layers. It is lined with mucous membrane; the lining of the bladder, like that of the stomach, is thrown into folds called *rugae* when the organ is empty. Beneath the mucosa is a layer of connective tissue. Then follows a three-layered coat of involuntary muscle tissue that is capable of great stretching. Finally, there is an incomplete coat of peritoneum that covers only the upper portion of the bladder.

When the bladder is empty, the muscular wall becomes thick, and the entire organ feels firm. As the bladder fills, the muscular wall becomes thinner, and the organ may increase from a length of 5 cm (2 inches) up to as much as 12.5 cm (5 inches) or even more. A moderately full bladder holds about 470 mL (1 pint) of urine.

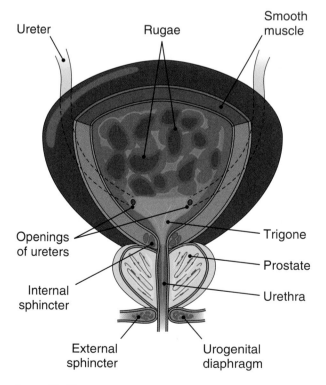

FIGURE **19•10** Interior of the urinary bladder, shown in the male. The trigone is a triangle in the floor of the bladder marked by the openings of the ureters and the urethra.

Labels: Ureter, Rugae, Smooth muscle, Openings of ureters, Internal sphincter, External sphincter, Urogenital diaphragm, Trigone, Prostate, Urethra

In the floor of the bladder is the ***trigone*** (TRI-gone), a triangle formed by the openings of the two ureters and the urethra (see Fig. 19-10). As the bladder fills with urine, it expands upward, leaving the trigone at the base stationary. This stability prevents stretching of the ureteral openings and the possible back flow of urine into the ureters.

The Urethra

The ***urethra*** is the tube that extends from the bladder to the outside (see Fig. 19-1) and is the means by which the bladder is emptied. The urethra differs in men and women; in the male, it is part of both the reproductive system and the urinary system, and it is much longer than is the female urethra.

The male urethra is about 20 cm (8 inches) in length. Early in its course, it passes through the prostate gland, where it is joined by the two ducts carrying the male sex cells. From, here it leads through the ***penis*** (PE-nis), the male organ of copulation, to the outside. The male urethra serves the dual purpose of conveying the sex cells and draining the bladder.

The urethra in the female is a thin-walled tube about 4 cm (1.5 inches) long. It is located behind the pubic joint and is embedded in the muscle of the front wall of the vagina. The external opening, called the ***urinary meatus,*** is located just in front of the vaginal opening between the labia minora. The female urethra drains the bladder only and is entirely separate from the reproductive system.

Urination

The process of expelling (voiding) urine from the bladder is called ***urination*** or ***micturition*** (mik-tu-RISH-un). This process is controlled both voluntarily and involuntarily with the aid of two rings of muscle (sphincters) that surround the urethra (see Fig. 19-10). Near the outlet of the bladder is an involuntary ***internal urethral sphincter*** formed by a continuation of the smooth muscle of the bladder wall. Below this muscle is a voluntary ***external urethral sphincter*** formed by the muscles of the pelvic

floor. By learning to control the voluntary sphincter, one can gain control over emptying of the bladder.

As the bladder fills with urine, stretch receptors in its wall send impulses to a center in the lower part of the spinal cord. Motor impulses from this center stimulate contraction of the bladder wall, forcing urine outward as both the internal and external sphincters are made to relax. In the infant, this emptying occurs automatically as a simple reflex. Early in life, a person learns to control urination from higher centers in the brain until the time is appropriate, a process known as *toilet training*. The impulse to urinate will override conscious controls if the bladder becomes too full.

The bladder can be emptied voluntarily by relaxing the muscles of the pelvic floor and increasing the pressure in the abdomen. The resulting increased pressure in the bladder triggers the spinal reflex that leads to urination.

✔ CHECKPOINT **9**:

What is the name of the tube that carries urine from the kidney to the bladder?

✔ CHECKPOINT **10**:

What is the name of the tube that carries urine from the bladder to the outside?

THE EFFECTS OF AGING ON THE URINARY SYSTEM

Aging causes the kidneys to lose some of their ability to concentrate urine. With aging, progressively more water is needed to excrete the same amount of waste. Older people find it necessary to drink more water than young people, and they eliminate larger amounts of urine (polyuria), even at night (nocturia).

Beginning at about 40 years of age, there is a decrease in the number and size of the nephrons. Often, more than half of them are lost before the age of 80 years. There may be an increase in blood urea nitrogen (BUN) without serious symptoms. Elderly people are more susceptible than are young people to infections of the urinary system. Childbearing may cause damage to the musculature of the pelvic floor, resulting in urinary tract problems in later years.

Enlargement of the prostate, common in older men, may cause obstruction and a back pressure in the ureters and kidneys. If this condition is untreated, it will cause permanent damage to the kidneys. Age changes may predispose to but do not cause incontinence. Most elderly people (60% in nursing homes and up to 90% living independently) have no incontinence.

THE URINE

Urine is a yellowish liquid that is about 95% water and 5% dissolved solids and gases. The pH (acidity) of freshly collected urine averages 6.0, with a range of 4.5 to 8.0. Diet may cause considerable variation in pH.

The amount of dissolved substances in urine is indicated by its *specific gravity.* The specific gravity of pure water, used as a standard, is 1.000. Because of the dissolved materials it contains, urine has a specific gravity that normally varies from 1.002 (very dilute urine) to 1.040 (very concentrated urine). When the kidneys are diseased, they lose the ability to concentrate urine, and the specific gravity no longer varies as it does when the kidneys function normally.

Normal Constituents

Some of the dissolved substances normally found in the urine are the following:

- *Nitrogenous waste products,* including urea, uric acid, and *creatinine* (kre-AT-ih-nin)
- *Electrolytes,* including sodium chloride (as in common table salt) and different kinds of sulfates and phosphates. Electrolytes are excreted in appropriate amounts to keep their blood concentration constant.
- *Yellow pigment,* which is derived from certain bile compounds. Pigments from

foods and drugs also may appear in the urine.

BODY FLUIDS

The Importance of Water

Water is important to living cells as a solvent, as a transport medium, and as a participant in metabolic reactions. The normal proportion of body water varies from 50% to 70% of a person's weight. It is highest in the young and in thin, muscular individuals. As the amount of fat increases, and as a person ages, the percentage of water in the body decreases.

Various electrolytes (salts), nutrients, gases, waste, and special substances, such as enzymes and hormones, are dissolved or suspended in body water. The composition of body fluids is an important factor in homeostasis. Whenever the volume or chemical makeup of these fluids deviates even slightly from normal, disease results. The constancy of body fluids is maintained in the following ways:

- The thirst mechanism, which maintains the volume of water at a constant level
- Kidney activity, which regulates the volume and composition of body fluids
- Hormones, which serve to regulate fluid volume and electrolytes
- Regulators of pH (acidity), including buffers, respiration, and kidney function

Fluid Compartments

Although body fluids have much in common no matter where they are located, there are some important differences between fluid inside and fluid outside cells. Accordingly, fluids are grouped into two main compartments:

- *Intracellular fluid* is contained within the cells. About two thirds to three fourths of all body fluids are in this category.
- *Extracellular fluid* includes all body fluids outside of cells. In this group are included the following:

- ○ **Blood plasma,** which constitutes about 4% of a person's body weight
- ○ **Interstitial** (in-ter-STISH-al) **fluid,** or more simply, tissue fluid. This fluid is located in the spaces between the cells in tissues all over the body. It is estimated that tissue fluid constitutes about 15% of body weight.
- ○ **Lymph,** the fluid that drains from the tissues into the lymphatic system
- ○ **Fluid in special compartments,** such as cerebrospinal fluid, the aqueous and vitreous humors of the eye, serous fluid, and synovial fluid. Together, these make up about 1% to 3% of total body fluids.

Fluids are not locked into one compartment. There is a constant interchange between compartments as fluids are transferred across semi-permeable cell membranes by diffusion and osmosis (Fig. 19-11).

> ✔ CHECKPOINT **11**:
>
> What are the two main compartments into which body fluids are grouped?

Water Balance

In a person whose health is normal, the quantity of water taken in (intake) is about equal to the quantity lost (output). The quantity of water consumed in a day varies considerably. The average adult in a comfortable environment takes in about 2500 mL of water (about 2½ quarts) daily (see How Much to Drink). About half of this quantity comes from drinking water and other

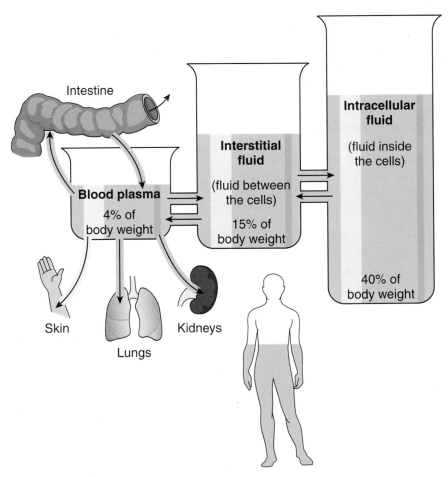

FIGURE **19•11** Main fluid compartments showing the relative percentage of body fluid in each.

How Much to Drink

Most people engaging in routine activities drink 6 to 8 cups of fluid daily to meet their needs. This may be in the form of water, juices, or milk. Beverages containing alcohol or caffeine should not be included in this total because they act as diuretics and increase water loss. The thirst center of the brain should stimulate enough drinking to balance fluids, but this is not always the case. When exercising vigorously, especially in hot weather, the body can dehydrate rapidly. People may not drink enough to replace needed fluids. In addition, if plain water is consumed, the dilution of body fluids may depress the thirst center. Athletes exercising very strenuously may need to drink beverages with some carbohydrates for energy and also some electrolytes to keep fluids in balance.

beverages, and about half comes from foods—fruits, vegetables, and soups.

Water is constantly being lost from the body by the following routes:

- The **skin.** Although sebum and keratin help prevent dehydration, water is constantly evaporating from the surface of the skin. Larger amounts of water are lost from the skin in the form of sweat when it is necessary to cool the body.
- The **lungs** expel water along with carbon dioxide.
- The **intestinal tract** eliminates water along with the feces.
- The **kidneys** excrete the largest quantity of water lost each day. About 1 to 1.5 liters of water are eliminated daily in the urine.

> ✔ CHECKPOINT **12**:
>
> What are three routes for water loss from the body?

Sense of Thirst

The control center for the sense of thirst is located in the hypothalamus of the brain. This center plays a major role in the regulation of total fluid volume. A decrease in fluid volume or an increase in the concentration of body fluids stimulates the thirst center and thus causes an individual to drink water or other fluids containing large amounts of water. Dryness of the mouth also causes a sensation of thirst. Excessive thirst, such as that caused by excessive urine loss in cases of diabetes, is called **polydipsia** (pol-e-DIP-se-ah).

> ✔ CHECKPOINT **13**:
>
> Where is the control center for the sense of thirst located?

Electrolytes and Their Functions

Electrolytes are important constituents of body fluids. These are compounds that separate in solution into positively and negatively charged ions. Positively charged ions are called *cations;* negatively charged ions are called *anions.* Electrolytes are so-named because they conduct an electrical current in solution. A few of the most important ions are reviewed next:

- Positive ions (cations)
  - **Sodium** is chiefly responsible for maintaining osmotic balance and body fluid volume. It is the main positive ion in extracellular fluids. Sodium is required for nerve impulse conduction and is important in maintaining acid–base balance.
  - **Potassium** is also important in the transmission of nerve impulses and is a major positive ion in intracellular fluids. Potassium is involved in cellular enzyme activities, and it helps regulate the chemical reactions by which carbohydrate is converted to energy and amino acids are converted to protein.
  - **Calcium** is required for bone formation, muscle contraction, nerve impulse transmission, and blood clotting.
- Negative ions (anions)
  - **Phosphate** is essential in the metabolism of carbohydrates, bone formation, and acid–base balance. Phosphates are found in the cell membrane and in the nucleic acids (DNA and RNA).

○ ***Chloride*** is essential for the formation of the hydrochloric acid in the gastric juice.

 CHECKPOINT **14**:

What is the main cation in extracellular fluid? In intracellular fluid?

Electrolyte Balance

Electrolytes must be kept in the proper concentration in both intracellular and extracellular fluids. The maintenance of water and electrolyte balance is one of the most difficult problems for health workers in caring for patients. Although some electrolytes are lost in the feces and through the skin as sweat, the job of balancing electrolytes is left mainly to the kidneys, as described earlier in this chapter.

The Role of Hormones

Several hormones are involved in balancing electrolytes. Aldosterone, produced by the adrenal cortex, promotes the reabsorption of sodium (and water) and the elimination of potassium.

When the blood concentration of sodium rises above the normal range, the pituitary secretes more antidiuretic hormone (ADH). This hormone increases the reabsorption of water in the kidney to dilute the excess sodium.

Hormones from the parathyroid and thyroid glands regulate calcium and phosphate levels. Parathyroid hormone increases blood calcium levels by causing the bones to release calcium and by causing the kidneys to reabsorb calcium. The thyroid hormone calcitonin lowers blood calcium by causing calcium to be deposited in the bones.

✔ CHECKPOINT **15**:

What are some mechanisms for regulating electrolytes in body fluids?

Acid–Base Balance

The pH scale is a measure of how acidic or basic (alkaline) a solution is. Body fluids are slightly alkaline at about pH 7.4. These fluids must be kept within a narrow range of pH, or damage, even death, will result.

Regulation of pH

Several systems act together to maintain acid–base balance. These are as follows:

Buffer systems. Buffers are substances that prevent sharp changes in hydrogen ion (H^+) concentration and thus maintain a relatively constant pH. Buffers work by accepting or releasing these ions as needed to keep the pH steady. The main buffer systems in the body are bicarbonate buffers, phosphate buffers, and proteins, such as hemoglobin in red blood cells and plasma proteins.

Respiration. The role of respiration in controlling pH was described in Chapter 16. Recall that the release of carbon dioxide from the lungs acts to make the blood more alkaline by reducing the amount of carbonic acid formed. In contrast, retention of carbon dioxide makes the blood more acidic. Respiratory rate can adjust pH for short-term regulation.

Kidney function. The kidneys serve to regulate pH by reabsorbing or eliminating hydrogen ions as needed. The kidneys are responsible for the long-term regulation of pH.

✔ CHECKPOINT **16**:

What are three mechanisms for maintaining the acid–base balance of body fluids?

19

Summary

I. Excretion—removal and elimination of waste materials from blood
1. Systems that eliminate waste
   a. Urinary system
   b. Digestive system—eliminates undigested food, water, salts, bile
   c. Respiratory system—eliminates carbon dioxide, water
   d. Skin—eliminates water, salts, nitrogen waste
   A. Organs of the urinary system
   1. Kidneys (2)
   2. Ureters (2)
   3. Urinary bladder (1)
   4. Urethra (1)

II. Kidneys
   A. Location of the kidneys
   1. In upper abdomen against the back
   2. In retroperitoneal space (behind the peritoneum)
   3. Blood supply
      a. Renal artery—carries blood to kidney from aorta
      b. Renal vein—carries blood from kidney to inferior vena cava
   B. Structure of the kidney
   1. Cortex—outer portion
   2. Medulla—inner portion
   3. Pelvis
      a. Upper end of ureter
      b. Calyces—cuplike extensions that receive urine
   4. Nephron
      a. Functional unit of kidney
      b. Parts
         (1) Bowman's capsule—around glomerulus
         (2) Proximal convoluted tubule
         (3) Henle's loop
         (4) Distal convoluted tubule
   5. Blood supply to nephron
      a. Afferent arteriole—enters Bowman's capsule
      b. Glomerulus—coil of capillaries in Bowman's capsule
      c. Efferent arteriole—leaves Bowman's capsule
      d. Peritubular capillaries—surround nephron
   6. Juxtaglomerular apparatus
      a. Consists of cells in afferent arteriole and distal convoluted tubule
      b. Releases renin to regulate blood pressure
   C. Functions of the kidney
   1. Excretion of waste, excess salts, toxins
   2. Water balance
   3. Acid–base balance (pH)
   4. Regulation of blood pressure
   5. Regulation of red blood cells
      a. Releases erythropoietin (EPO)—hormone that stimulates red blood cell production
   D. Formation of urine
   1. Glomerular filtration—driven by blood pressure in glomerulus
      a. Water and soluble substances forced out of blood and into Bowman's capsule
      b. Blood cells and proteins remain in blood
      c. Glomerular filtrate—material that leaves blood and enters the nephron
   2. Tubular reabsorption
      a. Most of filtrate leaves nephron by diffusion and active transport
      b. Returns to blood through peritubular capillaries
   3. Tubular secretion—materials moved from blood into nephron for excretion
   4. Concentration of urine
      a. Countercurrent mechanism—method for concentrating urine based on movement of ions out of nephron
      b. ADH
         (1) Hormone from posterior pituitary
         (2) Promotes reabsorption of water

III. Storage and transport of urine
  A. The ureters—carry urine from the kidneys to the bladder
  B. The urinary bladder
    1. Stores urine until it is eliminated
    2. Trigone—triangle in base of bladder; remains stable as bladder fills
  C. Urethra—carries urine out of body
    1. Male urethra—20 cm long; carries both urine and semen
    2. Female urethra—4 cm long; opens in front of vagina
  D. Urination (micturition)
    1. Both voluntary and involuntary
    2. Sphincters
      a. Internal urethral sphincter—involuntary (smooth muscle)
      b. External urethral sphincter—voluntary (skeletal muscle)
    3. Stretch receptors in bladder wall signal reflex emptying
    4. Can be controlled through higher brain centers

IV. Effects of aging
    1. Polyuria—increased elimination of urine
    2. Nocturia—urination at night
    3. Incontinence
    4. Increased blood urea nitrogen (BUN)
    5. Prostate enlargement

V. Urine
    1. pH averages 6.0
    2. Specific gravity—measures dissolved substances
  A. Normal constituents—water, nitrogenous waste, electrolytes, pigments

VI. Body fluids
    1. Water
      a. Functions
        (1) Solvent
        (2) Transport medium
        (3) Participant in metabolic reactions
      b. 50% to 70% of body
      c. Carries electrolytes, nutrients, gases, wastes, hormones, and other substances
      d. Important in homeostasis
  A. Fluid compartments
    1. Intracellular fluid—contained within the cells
    2. Extracellular fluid—outside the cells
      a. Blood plasma
      b. Interstitial (tissue) fluid
      c. Lymph
      d. Fluid in special compartments
  B. Water balance
    1. Output—through skin, lungs, intestinal tract, kidneys
    2. Intake—through beverages, food, intravenous fluid
      a. Sense of thirst—control center in hypothalamus
  C. Electrolytes and their functions
    1. Electrolytes release ions in solution
      a. Positive ions (cations)—sodium, potassium, calcium
      b. Negative ions (anions)—phosphate, chloride
  D. Electrolyte balance
    1. Kidneys—main regulators
    2. Role of hormones
      a. Aldosterone (from adrenal cortex)
        (1) Promotes reabsorption of sodium
        (2) Promotes excretion of potassium
      b. ADH (from pituitary)
        (1) Causes kidney to retain water
      c. Parathyroid hormone (from parathyroid glands)
        (1) Increases blood calcium level
      d. Calcitonin (from thyroid)
        (1) Decreases blood calcium level
  E. Acid–base balance
    1. Normal pH is 7.4
    2. Regulation of pH
      a. Buffers—maintain constant pH
      b. Respiration—release of carbon dioxide increases alkalinity; retention of carbon dioxide increases acidity
      c. Kidney—regulates amount of hydrogen ion excreted

Questions for Study and Review

1. Name the body systems that have excretory functions.
2. Name the organs of the urinary system.
3. Where are the kidneys located?
4. Describe the internal structure of the kidney.
5. Describe the structure of a nephron.
6. Name and locate the blood vessels associated with the nephron.
7. Compare the afferent arteriole and the efferent arteriole in structure and function.
8. What happens to the glomerular filtrate as it passes through the nephron?
9. What is the function of the JG apparatus?
10. How does ADH affect kidney function?
11. What structures empty into the kidney pelvis and what drains the pelvis?
12. What is micturition? How is it controlled?
13. Describe the female urethra and tell how it differs from the male urethra in structure and function.
14. What are some of the effects of aging on the urinary system?
15. What is urea? Where is it formed and how is it eliminated?
16. List four types of extracellular fluid.
17. In a healthy person, what is the ratio of fluid intake to output?
18. Explain the role of the hypothalamus in water balance.
19. Name five common ions in the body. How is each used?
20. Name three hormones involved in electrolyte balance and explain what each does.
21. Define *buffer* and name the three main buffer systems in the body.
22. How does the respiratory system help regulate pH?

19

✔ ANSWERS TO CHECKPOINTS

1. Systems other than the urinary system that eliminate waste include the digestive, respiratory, and integumentary systems.
2. The urinary system consists of two kidneys, two ureters, the bladder, and the urethra.
3. The retroperitoneal space is behind the peritoneum.
4. The renal artery supplies blood to the kidney, and the renal vein drains the kidney.
5. The functional unit of the kidney is the nephron.
6. The JG apparatus produces renin when blood pressure falls too low for effective filtration.
7. Glomerular filtration is the movement of materials under pressure from the blood into Bowman's capsule of the nephron.
8. The four processes involved in the formation of urine are glomerular filtration, tubular reabsorption, tubular secretion, and the countercurrent mechanism for concentrating the urine.
9. The ureter carries urine from the kidney to the bladder.
10. The urethra carries urine from the bladder to the outside.
11. Body fluids are grouped into intracellular fluid and extracellular fluid.
12. Water is lost from the body through the skin, the lungs, the intestinal tract, and the kidneys.
13. The control center for the sense of thirst is located in the hypothalamus of the brain.
14. Sodium is the main cation in extracellular fluid. Potassium is the main cation in intracellular fluid.
15. Some electrolytes are lost through the feces and through sweat. The kidneys have the main job of balancing electrolytes. Several hormones, such as aldosterone, parathyroid hormone, and calcitonin, are also involved.
16. The acid–base balance of body fluids is maintained by buffer systems, respiration, and kidney function.

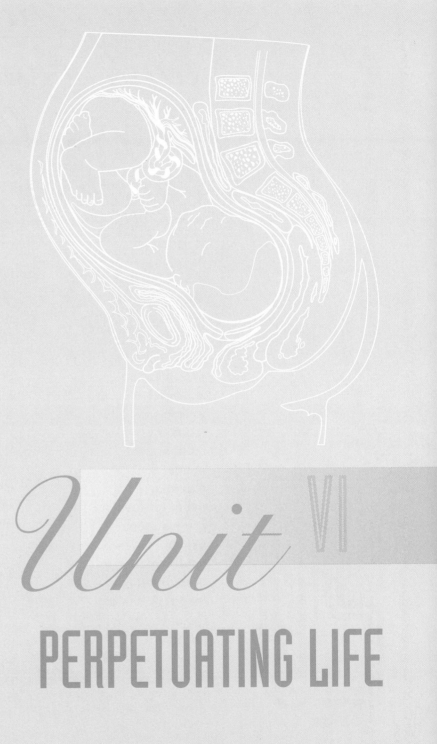

The last unit includes two chapters on the structures and functions related to reproduction and inheritance. The reproductive system is not necessary for the continuation of the life of the individual but rather is needed for the continuation of the human species. The germ cells and their genes have been studied intensively during recent years as part of the rapidly advancing science of genetics.

Unit VI

PERPETUATING LIFE

The Male and Female Reproductive Systems

SELECTED KEY TERMS

The following terms are defined in the Glossary:

contraception

corpus luteum

endometrium

estrogen

follicle

gamete

menopause

ovary

ovulation

ovum (pl., ova)

progesterone

semen

spermatozoon (pl., spermatozoa)

testis (pl., testes)

testosterone

uterus

BEHAVIORAL OBJECTIVES

After careful study of this chapter, you should be able to:

1. Name the male and female gonads and describe the function of each

2. State the purpose of meiosis

3. List the accessory organs of the male and female reproductive tracts and cite the function of each

4. Describe the composition and function of semen

5. Draw and label a spermatozoon

6. List in the correct order the hormones produced during the menstrual cycle and cite the source of each

7. Describe the functions of the main male and female sex hormones

8. Explain how negative feedback regulates reproductive function in both males and females

9. Describe the changes that occur during and after menopause

10. Define *contraception* and cite the main methods of contraception in use

REPRODUCTION

The chapters in this unit deal with what is certainly one of the most interesting and mysterious attributes of life: the ability to reproduce. The simplest forms of life, one-celled organisms, usually need no partner to reproduce; they simply divide by themselves. This form of reproduction is known as *asexual* (nonsexual) reproduction.

In most animals, however, reproduction is *sexual,* meaning that there are two kinds of individuals, males and females, each of which has specialized cells designed specifically for the perpetuation of the species. These specialized sex cells are known as *germ cells,* or *gametes* (GAM-etes). In the male, they are called *spermatozoa* (sper-mah-to-ZO-ah), or simply sperm cells, and in the female, they are called *ova* (O-vah) or egg cells.

Meiosis

Germ cells are characterized by having half as many chromosomes as are found in any other cell in the body. During their formation, they go through a special process of cell division, called *meiosis* (mi-O-sis), that halves the number of chromosomes. In humans, meiosis reduces the chromosome number in a cell from 46 to 23.

Divisions of the Reproductive System

Although the male and female reproductive systems are different, the organs of both may be divided into two groups: primary and accessory.

- The primary organs are the *gonads* (GO-nads), or sex glands; they produce the germ cells and manufacture hormones. The male gonads are the *testes* (TES-teze), and the female gonads are the *ovaries* (O-vah-reze).
- The *accessory organs* include a series of ducts that provide for the transport of germ cells as well as various exocrine glands.

✔ CHECKPOINT **1**:

What is the process of cell division that halves the chromosome number in a cell to produce a gamete?

THE MALE REPRODUCTIVE SYSTEM

The Testes

The testes (male gonads) are located outside the body proper, suspended between the thighs in a sac called the *scrotum* (SKRO-tum) (Fig. 20-1).

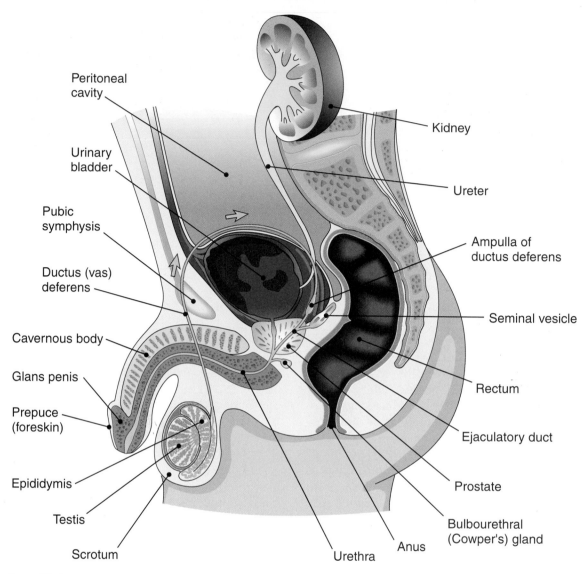

FIGURE **20•1**   Male genitourinary system. The arrows indicate the course of sperm cells through the duct system.

The testes are oval organs measuring about 3.7 to 5 cm (1.5 to 2 inches) in length and about 2.5 cm (1 inch) in each of the other two dimensions. During embryonic life, each testis develops from tissue near the kidney.

A month or two before birth, the testis normally descends (moves downward) through the ***inguinal*** (ING-gwih-nal) ***canal*** in the abdominal wall into the scrotum. Each testis then remains suspended by a ***spermatic cord*** (Fig. 20-2) that extends through the inguinal canal. This cord contains blood vessels, lym-

phatic vessels, nerves, and the tube (ductus deferens) that transports spermatozoa away from the testis. The gland must descend completely if it is to function normally; to produce spermatozoa, the testes must be kept at the temperature of the scrotum, which is several degrees lower than that of the abdominal cavity.

Internal Structure

Most of the specialized tissue of the testis consists of tiny coiled ***seminiferous*** (seh-mih-NIF-

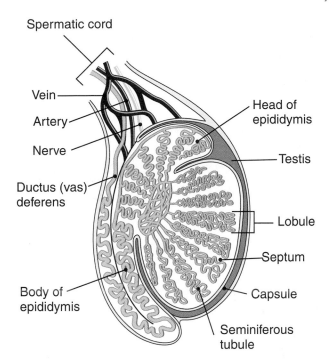

Spermatic cord

Vein

Artery

Nerve

Ductus (vas)
deferens

Body of
epididymis

Head of
epididymis

Testis

Lobule

Septum

Capsule

Seminiferous
tubule

FIGURE **20•2** Structure of the testis, also showing the epididymis and spermatic cord.

er-us) *tubules.* Cells in the walls of these tubules produce spermatozoa. Between the tubules are specialized *interstitial* (in-ter-STISH-al) *cells* that secrete the male sex hormone *testosterone* (tes-TOS-teh-rone). Figure 20-3 is a microscopic view of the testis in cross-section, showing the seminiferous tubules, interstitial cells, and developing spermatozoa.

Testosterone

After being secreted by the testis, testosterone is absorbed directly into the bloodstream. This hormone has two functions:

- Maintenance of the reproductive structures, including development of the spermatozoa
- Development of *secondary sex characteristics,* traits that characterize males and females but are not directly concerned with reproduction. In males, these traits include a deeper voice, broader shoulders, narrower hips, a greater percentage of muscle tissue, and more body hair than are found in females.

✔ CHECKPOINT **2**:

What is the male gonad?

✔ CHECKPOINT **3**:

What is the main male sex hormone?

The Ducts

The tubes that carry the spermatozoa begin with tubules inside the testis itself. From these tubes, the cells are collected by a greatly coiled tube called the *epididymis* (ep-ih-DID-ih-mis), which is 6 meters (20 feet) long and is located

primitive
spermatozoa

mature
spermatozoa

seminiferous
tubule

interstitial
cells

FIGURE **20•3** Microscopic view of the testis. (Courtesy of Dana Morse Bittus and B. J. Cohen) inside the scrotal sac (see Fig. 20-2). While they are temporarily stored in the epididymis, the sperm cells mature and become motile, that is, able to move, or "swim," by themselves.

The epididymis finally extends upward as the **ductus deferens** (DEF-er-enz), also called the **vas deferens.** The ductus deferens, contained in the spermatic cord, continues through the inguinal canal into the abdominal cavity. Here, it separates from the remainder of the spermatic cord and curves behind the urinary bladder. The ductus deferens then joins with the duct of the **seminal vesicle** (VES-ih-kl) on the same side to form the **ejaculatory** (e-JAK-u-lah-to-re) **duct.** The two ejaculatory ducts travel through the body of the prostate gland and then empty into the urethra.

✔ CHECKPOINT **4**:

What is the order in which sperm cells travel through the ducts of the male reproductive system?

Formation of Semen

Semen (SE-men) is the mixture of sperm cells and various secretions that is expelled from the body. The secretions serve several functions:

- Nourish the spermatozoa
- Transport the spermatozoa
- Neutralize the acidity of the vaginal tract
- Lubricate the reproductive tract during sexual intercourse

The glands discussed next contribute secretions to the semen (see Fig. 20-1).

The Seminal Vesicles

The seminal vesicles are twisted muscular tubes with many small outpouchings. They are about 7.5 cm (3 inches) long and are attached to the connective tissue at the back of the urinary bladder. The glandular lining produces a thick, yellow, alkaline secretion containing large quantities of simple sugar and other substances that provide nourishment for the sperm. The seminal fluid forms a large part of the volume of the semen.

The Prostate Gland

The prostate gland lies immediately below the urinary bladder, where it surrounds the first part of the urethra. Ducts from the prostate carry its secretions into the urethra. The thin, alkaline prostatic secretion helps neutralize the acidity of the vaginal tract and enhance the motility of the spermatozoa. The prostate gland is also supplied with muscular tissue, which, upon signal from the nervous system, contracts to aid in the expulsion of the semen from the body.

Bulbourethral Glands

The **bulbourethral** (bul-bo-u-RE-thral), **glands,** also called **Cowper's glands,** are a pair of pea-sized organs located in the pelvic floor just below the prostate gland. They secrete mucus to lubricate the urethra and tip of the penis during sexual stimulation. The ducts of these glands extend about 2.5 cm (1 inch) from each side and empty into the urethra before it extends into the penis.

Other very small glands secrete mucus into the urethra as it passes through the penis.

✔ CHECKPOINT **5**:

What glands, aside from the testis, contribute secretions to semen?

The Urethra and Penis

The male urethra, as discussed in Chapter 19, serves the dual purpose of conveying urine from the bladder and carrying the reproductive cells and their accompanying secretions to the outside. The ejection of semen into the receiving canal (vagina) of the female is made possible by the **erection,** or stiffening and enlargement, of the penis, through which the longest part of the urethra extends. The penis is made of spongy tissue containing many blood spaces that are relatively empty when the organ is flaccid but fill with blood and distend when the penis is erect. This tissue is subdivided into three segments, each called a **corpus** (meaning "body") (Fig. 20-4). A single, ventrally located **corpus spongiosum** contains the urethra. On either side is a larger **corpus cavernosum** (pl., *corpora cavernosa*). At the distal end of the penis,

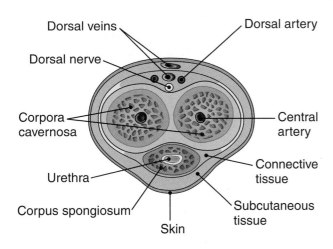

FIGURE **20•4** Cross section of the penis.

the corpus spongiosum enlarges to form the **glans** penis. This enlargement is covered with a loose fold of skin, the **prepuce** (PRE-puse), commonly called the *foreskin*. It is the foreskin that is removed in a circumcision.

The penis and scrotum together are referred to as the *external genitalia* of the male.

Ejaculation

Ejaculation (e-jak-u-LA-shun) is the forceful expulsion of semen through the urethra to the outside. The process is initiated by reflex centers in the spinal cord that stimulate contraction of smooth muscle tissue in the prostate. This is followed by contraction of skeletal muscle in the pelvic floor, which provides the force needed for expulsion. During ejaculation, the involuntary sphincter at the base of the bladder closes to prevent the release of urine.

The Spermatozoa

Spermatozoa are tiny individual cells (Fig. 20-5). They are so small that at least 200 million are contained in the average ejaculation. Sperm cells are manufactured continuously in the testes. As they develop within the seminiferous tubules, they are nourished and protected by special cells called **Sertoli,** or "nurse," *cells.*

The individual sperm cell has an oval head that is largely a nucleus containing chromosomes. Covering the head like a cap is the **acrosome** (AK-ro-some), which contains enzymes that help the sperm cell to penetrate the ovum.

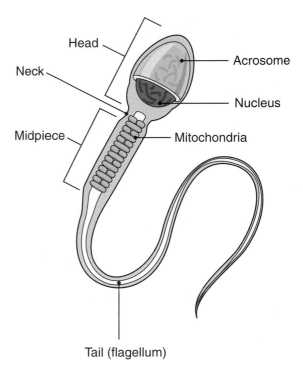

FIGURE **20•5** Diagram of a human spermatozoon showing major structural features.

Whiplike movements of the tail (flagellum) propel the sperm through the female reproductive system to the ovum. A middle region (midpiece) of the cell contains many mitochondria that provide energy for movement.

Out of the millions of spermatozoa in an ejaculation, only one, if any, fertilizes the ovum. The remainder of the cells live from only a few hours up to a maximum of 3 days.

✔ CHECKPOINT **6**:

What are the main subdivisions of a spermatozoon?

HORMONAL CONTROL OF MALE REPRODUCTION

The activities of the testes are under the control of two hormones produced by the anterior pituitary gland (hypophysis). These hormones are named for their activity in female reproduction, although they are chemically the same in both males and females.

- *Follicle-stimulating hormone (FSH)* stimulates the Sertoli cells and promotes the formation of spermatozoa.
- *Luteinizing hormone (LH),* called *interstitial cell–stimulating hormone (ICSH)* in males, stimulates the interstitial cells to produce testosterone, which is also needed for sperm cell development.

The pituitary gland is regulated by a region of the brain located just above it, the hypothalamus. Starting at puberty, the hypothalamus begins to secrete hormones that trigger the release of FSH and LH. These hormones are secreted continuously in the male.

The activity of the hypothalamus is in turn regulated by a negative feedback mechanism involving testosterone. As the level of testosterone in the blood increases, the hypothalamus secretes less releasing hormone; as the level of testosterone decreases, the hypothalamus secretes more releasing hormone (see Fig. 11-2 in Chap. 11).

✔ CHECKPOINT **7**:

What two pituitary hormones regulate both male and female reproduction?

The Effects of Aging on Male Reproduction

A gradual decrease in the production of testosterone and spermatozoa begins as early as 20 years of age and continues throughout life. Secretions from the prostate and seminal vesicles decrease in amount and become less viscous. In a few men (less than 10%), sperm cells remain late in life, even to 80 years of age.

THE FEMALE REPRODUCTIVE SYSTEM

The Ovaries

In the female, the counterparts of the testes are the two *ovaries,* where the female sex cells, or *ova,* are formed (Fig. 20-6). The ovary is a small,

somewhat flattened oval body measuring about 4 cm (1.6 inches) in length, 2 cm (0.8 inch) in width, and 1 cm (0.4 inch) in depth. Like the testes, the ovaries descend, but only as far as the pelvic portion of the abdomen. Here, each is held in place by ligaments, including the broad ligament, the ovarian ligament, and others, that attach them to the uterus and the body wall.

The Egg Cell and Ovulation

The outer layer of the ovary is made of a single layer of epithelium. Beneath this layer, the ova (egg cells) are produced. The ovaries of a newborn female contain a large number of potential ova. Each month during the reproductive years, several ripen, but usually only one is released. The complicated process of maturation, or "ripening," of an ovum takes place in a small fluid-filled cluster of cells called the *ovarian follicle* (o-VA-re-an FOL-ih-kls) or *graafian* (GRAF-e-an) *follicle* (Fig. 20-7). As the ovum develops, the cells of the ovarian follicle wall secrete the hormone estrogen, which stimulates growth of the uterine lining. When an ovum has ripened, the ovarian follicle may rupture and discharge the egg cell from the surface of the ovary. The rupture of a follicle allowing the escape of an ovum is called *ovulation* (ov-u-LA-shun). Any developing ova that are not released simply degenerate.

After it is released, the egg cell makes its way to the nearest *oviduct* (O-vih-dukt). The oviduct is a tube that arches over the ovary and leads to the uterus.

The Corpus Luteum

After the ovum has been expelled, the remaining follicle is transformed into a solid glandular mass called the *corpus luteum* (LU-te-um), a name that means "yellow body." This structure secretes both estrogen and progesterone, another hormone needed in the reproductive cycle. Commonly, the corpus luteum shrinks and is replaced by scar tissue. When a pregnancy occurs, however, this structure remains active. (See In Vitro Fertilization.)

Sometimes, as a result of normal ovulation, the corpus luteum persists and forms a small ovarian cyst (fluid-filled sac). This condition usually resolves without treatment.

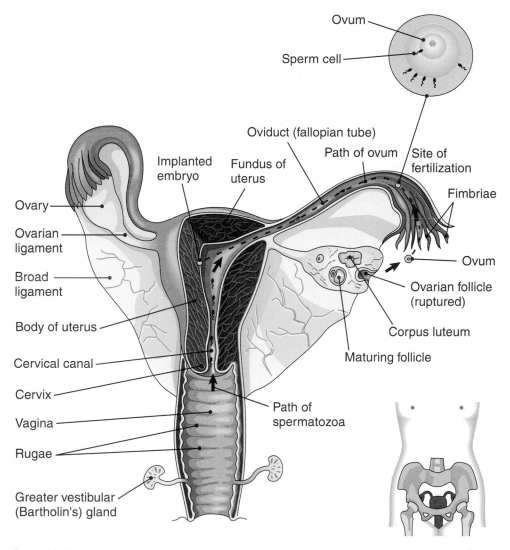

FIGURE **20•6**   Female reproductive system.

20

✔ CHECKPOINT **8**:

What is the process of releasing an egg cell from the ovary called?

The Oviducts

The tubes that transport the ova in the female reproductive system, the oviducts, are also known as *uterine* (U-ter-in) *tubes,* or *fallopian* (fah-LO-pe-an) *tubes.* Each is a small, muscular structure, nearly 12.5 cm (5 inches) long, extend-

ing from a point near the ovary to the uterus (womb). There is no direct connection between the ovary and this tube. The ovum is swept into the oviduct by a current in the peritoneal fluid produced by the small, fringelike extensions called *fimbriae* (FIM-bre-e) that are located at the edge of the abdominal opening of the tubes.

Unlike the sperm cell, the ovum cannot move by itself. Its progress through the oviduct toward the uterus depends on the sweeping action of cilia in the lining of the tube and on peristalsis of the tube. It takes about 5 days for an ovum to reach the uterus from the ovary.

ovum

ovarian
(Graafian)
follicle

FIGURE **20•7** Microscopic view of the ovary showing egg cells developing within ovarian follicles.
(Courtesy of Dana Morse Bittus and B. J. Cohen)

The Uterus

The organ to which the oviducts lead is the
uterus (U-ter-us), and it is within this structure
that the developing fetus grows to maturity.

In Vitro Fertilization

The term *in vitro* literally means "in glass." It is
used to describe tests or procedures done in the
laboratory. In vitro fertilization (IVF) refers to fertilization of an egg cell outside the mother's
body in a laboratory dish. The first such procedure was done successfully in 1978.

The woman participating in IVF must be
given hormones to cause ovulation of several
eggs. These are then withdrawn with a needle
and fertilized with the father's sperm. After a
few divisions, the fertilized egg is placed in the
uterus for development. Additional fertilized
eggs can be frozen to repeat the procedure in
case of failure or for later pregnancies. Other
possibilities for IVF include using donor eggs,
donor sperm cells, or both, or using a surro-
gate mother for gestation.

Because of a lack of guidelines or restric-
tions in the United States in the field of as-
sisted reproductive technology, some problems have arisen. These issues concern the
use of stored embryos and gametes, the use
of embryos without consent, and improper
screening for disease among donors. In addition, the implantation of more than one fertilized egg has resulted in a high incidence of
multiple births, even up to seven or eight offspring in a single pregnancy, a situation that
imperils the survival and health of the babies.

Structure of the Uterus

The uterus is a pear-shaped, muscular organ
about 7.5 cm (3 inches) long, 5 cm (2 inches)
wide, and 2.5 cm (1 inch) deep. The upper portion rests on the upper surface of the urinary
bladder; the lower portion is embedded in the
pelvic floor between the bladder and the rectum. The wider upper portion is called the **corpus,** or body; the lower, narrower part is the
cervix (SER-viks), or neck. The small, rounded
part above the level of the tubal entrances
is known as the **fundus** (FUN-dus) (see Fig.
20-6).

The cavity inside the uterus is shaped somewhat like a capital T, but it is capable of changing shape and dilating as a fetus develops. The
cervix leads to the **vagina** (vah-JI-nah), the
lower part of the birth canal, which opens to the
outside of the body.

The lining of the uterus is a specialized epithelium known as **endometrium** (en-do-ME-
tre-um), and it is this layer that is involved in
menstruation.

Supporting Tissues

The **broad ligaments** support the uterus,
extending from each side of the organ to the
lateral body wall. Along with the uterus,
these two portions of peritoneum form a partition dividing the female pelvis into anterior and posterior areas. The ovaries are suspended from the broad ligaments, and the
oviducts lie within the upper borders. Blood
vessels that supply these organs are found between the layers of the broad ligament (see Fig.
20-6).

> ✔ CHECKPOINT **9**:
>
> In what organ does a fetus develop?

The Vagina

The vagina is a muscular tube about 7.5 cm (3 inches) long connecting the uterine cavity with the outside. At the top, it receives the cervix, which dips into the upper vagina in such a way that a circular recess, known as the **fornix** (FOR-niks), is formed. The deepest area of the fornix, located behind the cervix, is the **posterior fornix** (FOR-niks) (Fig. 20-8). This recess in the posterior vagina lies adjacent to the lowest part of the peritoneal cavity, a narrow passage between the uterus and the rectum named the **cul-de-sac** (from a French term meaning "bottom of the sack"). This area is also known as the *rectouterine pouch* or the *pouch of Douglas*. A rather thin layer of tissue separates the posterior fornix from this region, so that abscesses or tumor cells in the peritoneal cavity can sometimes be detected by vaginal examination.

The lining of the vagina is a wrinkled mucous membrane something like that found in the stomach. The folds (rugae) permit enlargement so that childbirth usually does not tear the lining. In addition to being a part of the birth canal, the vagina is the organ that receives the penis during sexual intercourse. A fold of membrane called the **hymen** may sometimes be

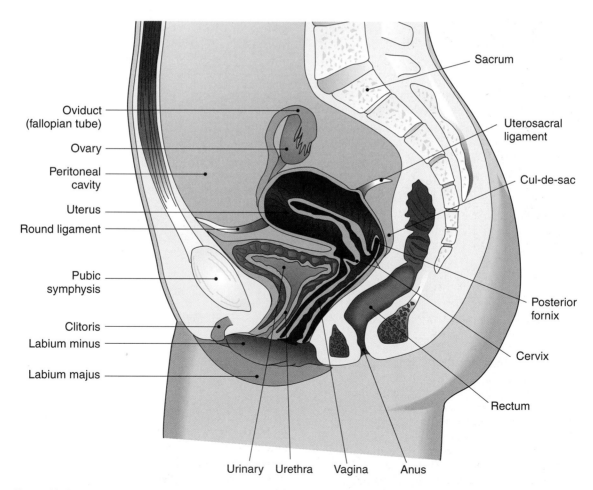

FIGURE **20•8** Female reproductive system, as seen in sagittal section.

found at or near the vaginal (VAJ-ih-nal) canal opening.

The Greater Vestibular Glands

Just above and to each side of the vaginal opening are the mucus-producing **greater vestibular** (ves-TIB-u-lar), or **Bartholin's, glands**. These glands secrete into an area near the vaginal opening known as the **vestibule**. The glands may become infected, leading to painful swelling and abscess, in which case a surgical incision to promote drainage may be required.

The Vulva and the Perineum

The external parts of the female reproductive system form the **vulva** (VUL-vah), which includes two pairs of lips, or **labia** (LA-be-ah); the **clitoris** (KLIT-o-ris), which is a small organ of great sensitivity; and related structures (Fig. 20-9). Although the entire pelvic floor in both the male and female is properly called the **perineum** (per-ih-NE-um) (see Fig. 7-11 in Chap. 7), those who care for pregnant women usually refer to the limited area between the vaginal opening and the anus as the perineum.

THE MENSTRUAL CYCLE

In the female, as in the male, reproductive function is controlled by hormones from the pituitary gland as regulated by the hypothalamus. Female activity differs, however, in that it is cyclic, that is, shows regular patterns of increases and decreases in hormone levels. These changes are regulated by hormonal feedback.

The length of the menstrual cycle varies between 22 and 45 days in normal women, but 28 days is taken as an average, with the first day of menstrual flow being considered the first day of the cycle (Fig. 20-10).

Beginning of the Cycle

At the start of each cycle, under the influence of FSH produced by the pituitary, a follicle begins to develop in the ovary. This follicle produces increasing amounts of **estrogen** as the ovum matures. (*Estrogen* is the term used for a group of related hormones, the most active of which is estradiol.) The estrogen is carried in the bloodstream to the uterus, where it starts preparing the endometrium for a possible pregnancy. This

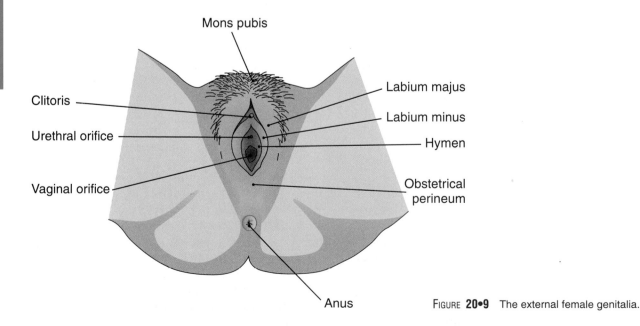

Mons pubis

Clitoris

Urethral orifice

Vaginal orifice

Labium majus

Labium minus

Hymen

Obstetrical perineum

Anus

FIGURE **20•9** The external female genitalia.

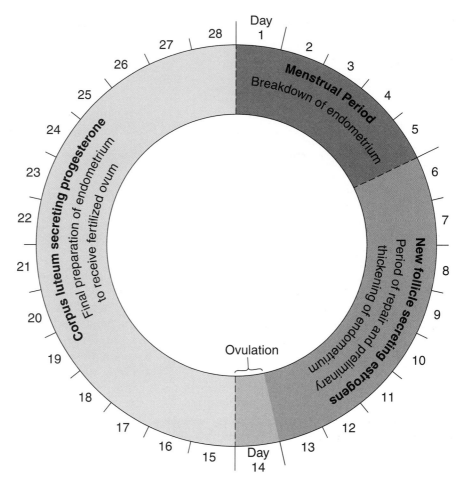

Day
1
2
3
4
5
6
7
8
9
10
11
12
13
Day
14
15
16
17
18
19
20
21
22
23
24
25
26
27
28

Menstrual Period
Breakdown of endometrium

New follicle secreting estrogens
Period of repair and preliminary thickening of endometrium

Ovulation

Corpus luteum secreting progesterone
Final preparation of endometrium to receive fertilized ovum

FIGURE **23•10** Summary of events in an average 28-day menstrual cycle.

preparation includes thickening of the endometrium and elongation of the glands that produce the uterine secretion. Estrogen in the blood also acts as a feedback messenger to inhibit the release of FSH and stimulate the release of LH from the pituitary (see Fig. 11-2 in Chap. 11).

Ovulation

About 1 day before ovulation, there is an ***LH surge,*** a sharp rise in LH. This hormone causes ovulation and transforms the ruptured follicle into the corpus luteum. The corpus luteum produces some estrogen and large amounts of ***progesterone.*** Under the influence of these hormones, the endometrium continues to thicken, and the glands and blood vessels increase in size. The rising levels of estrogen and progesterone

feed back to inhibit the release of FSH and LH from the pituitary (Fig. 20-11). During this time, the ovum makes its journey to the uterus by way of the oviduct. If the ovum is not fertilized while passing through the uterine tube, it dies within 2 to 3 days and then disintegrates.

Menstrual Flow

If fertilization does not occur, the corpus luteum degenerates, and the levels of estrogen and progesterone decrease. Without the hormones to support growth, the endometrium degenerates. Small hemorrhages appear in this lining, producing the bleeding known as ***menstrual flow,*** or ***menses*** (MEN-seze). Bits of endometrium break away and accompany the flow of blood. The average duration of this discharge is 2 to 6 days.

20

FIGURE **20•11** Hormones in the menstrual cycle. (Redrawn from Djerassi C.: Fertility awareness: Jet-age rhythm method? Science 1990;248: 1061)

Before the flow ceases, the endometrium begins to repair itself through the growth of new cells. The low levels of estrogen and progesterone allow the release of FSH from the anterior pituitary. FSH causes a new ovum to begin to ripen within the ovaries, and the cycle begins anew.

The activity of ovarian hormones as negative feedback messengers is the basis of hormonal methods of contraception (birth control). Estrogen and progesterone act to inhibit the release of FSH and LH from the pituitary, resulting in a menstrual period but no ovulation.

 CHECKPOINT **10**:

What are the two hormones produced in the ovaries?

MENOPAUSE

Menopause (MEN-o-pawz) is the period during which menstruation ceases altogether. It ordinarily occurs between the ages of 45 and 55 years and is caused by a normal decline in ovarian function. The ovary becomes chiefly scar tissue and no longer produces ova or appreciable amounts of estrogen. Eventually, the uterus, oviducts, vagina, and vulva all become somewhat atrophied.

Menopause is an entirely normal condition, but its onset sometimes brings about effects that are temporarily disturbing. The decrease in estrogen levels can cause such nervous symptoms as irritability, "hot flashes," and dizzy spells.

Hormone Replacement Therapy

Although still a subject of controversy, the use of estrogen replacement therapy generally is considered to be of overall benefit for menopausal and postmenopausal women. Estrogen therapy, also called hormone replacement therapy (HRT), has proved effective in alleviating hot flashes and the sensitivity of a thinning vaginal mucosa. Some women may require hormone therapy to prevent or halt osteoporosis (bone weakening). It has also been found to reduce the risk of heart attacks, which increase among women after menopause.

Risks of HRT

Hormone replacement therapy has some potential side effects, and each woman should weigh the pros and cons with her physician before beginning treatment. Cancer of the uterine lining (endometrial cancer) is one possible risk, and the longer the duration of hormone treatment, the greater the risk. Reducing the dosages and the duration of the therapy lessens this danger, as does giving the estrogen in combination with progesterone (progestin) to prevent overgrowth of the endometrium.

Other factors that must be considered involve the risk for thrombosis and embolism, which is highest among women who smoke. Some studies have also shown an increased risk for breast cancer in the wake of long-term estrogen therapy. A woman who has a family history of cancer of the breast or of the uterus should avoid such treatment.

 CHECKPOINT **11**:

What is the definition of menopause?

CONTRACEPTION

Contraception is defined as the use of artificial methods to prevent fertilization of the ovum or implantation of the fertilized ovum. Table 20-1 presents a brief description of the main contraceptive methods currently in use along with some advantages and disadvantages of each. The list is given in rough order of decreasing effectiveness.

The spread of AIDS and other sexually transmitted diseases has stimulated interest in the development of better condoms, including a female condom, because these not only prevent conception but also reduce the chances of infection. See Preventing STDs.

Most other advances involve new methods for administering birth control hormones. Capsules of synthetic progesterone implanted under the skin are effective for 5 years and avoid the side effects of estrogen. This same drug may be given by injection at 3-month intervals.

Although not strictly a contraceptive, the drug ***RU 486*** is taken after conception to terminate an early pregnancy. It blocks the action of progesterone, causing the uterus to shed its lining and release the fertilized egg. It must be combined with administration of prostaglandins to expel the uterine tissue.

Table 20•1   **Main Methods of Contraception Currently in Use**

METHOD	DESCRIPTION	ADVANTAGES	DISADVANTAGES
Surgical			
Vasectomy/tubal ligation	Cutting and tying of tubes carrying gametes	Nearly 100% effective; involves no chemical or mechanical devices	Not usually reversible: rare surgical complications
Hormonal			
Birth control pills	Estrogen and progesterone or progesterone alone taken orally to prevent ovulation	Highly effective; requires no last-minute preparation	Alters physiology; possible serious side effects
Birth control shot	Injection of synthetic progesterone every 3 months to prevent ovulation	Highly effective; lasts for 3 to 4 months	Alters physiology; possible side effects include menstrual irregularity, amenorrhea
Birth control implants	Devices containing synthetic progesterone implanted under skin to prevent ovulation	Highly effective; lasts for 5 years	Alters physiology; possible side effects include menstrual irregularity, amenorrhea; expensive
Barrier			
Male condom	Sheath that fits over erect penis and prevents release of semen	Easily available; does not affect physiology; protects against sexually transmitted disease (STD)	Must be applied just before intercourse; may slip or tear
Female condom	Sheath that fits in vagina, held in place with rings	Easily available; protects against STD	More expensive than male condom; must be applied before intercourse
Diaphragm (with spermicide)	Rubber cap that fits over cervix and prevents entrance of sperm	Does not affect physiology; some protection against STD	Must be inserted before intercourse; requires fitting by physician
Other			
Spermicide	Chemicals used to kill sperm; best when used in combination with a barrier method	Easily available; does not affect physiology; some protection against STD	Local irritation; must be used just before intercourse
Fertility awareness	Abstinence during fertile part of cycle as determined by menstrual history, basal body temperature, or quality of cervical mucus	Does not affect physiology; accepted by certain religions	High failure rate; requires careful record keeping

20

Other drugs for producing medical abortions are also being tested.

✔ CHECKPOINT **12**:

What is the definition of contraception?

Preventing STDs

Sexually transmitted disease (STD), formerly known as venereal disease (VD), is infection spread through intimate sexual contact. Examples are gonorrhea, syphilis, human papillomavirus (HPV), genital herpes, hepatitis B, and chlamydia. These diseases can lead to sterility, cancer of the cervix, and increased susceptibility to AIDS. A trend toward participation in sex at earlier ages exposes people to more sexual contacts and an increased risk of infection.

The following techniques can prevent many cases of STD:

- Use a barrier, such as the male or female condom. The effectiveness of barriers is enhanced when a contraceptive foam or cream is used at the same time.
- Limit sexual activities when either partner suspects an infection. Do not engage in intimate relations until an infection has been adequately treated. Reinfection is always possible unless both partners are treated.
- Follow after-sex hygiene measures, which include cleaning the genitals after intercourse and urinating to reduce the possible ascent of organisms in the reproductive tract.

Women are more likely to contract STDs than are men. The same mechanisms that transport sperm cells through the female reproductive tract also move infectious organisms. Also, symptoms in women may be less apparent than in men.

Drugs to kill STD-causing organisms are effective in many cases. A vaccine is available for some diseases transmitted sexually, such as hepatitis B, and immunizations for other STDs are under study.

Summary

20

I. Reproduction
A. Meiosis—reduces chromosome number from 46 to 23
1. Gametes (sex cells)
   a. Spermatozoa—male
   b. Ova—female
B. Divisions of the reproductive system
1. Gonads
   a. Testes—male
   b. Ovaries—female
2. Accessory organs
   a. Ducts
   b. Exocrine glands

II. Male reproductive system
A. Testes

1. Scrotum—sac that holds the testes
2. Inguinal canal—channel through which testis descends
3. Internal structure
   a. Seminiferous tubules—tubes in which sperm cells are produced
   b. Interstitial cells—secrete hormones
      (1) Testosterone
         (a) Maintains reproductive structures
         (b) Promotes development of secondary sex characteristics
B. Ducts
1. Epididymis—stores spermatozoa until ejaculation
2. Ductus (vas) deferens—conducts sperm cells through spermatic cord
3. Ejaculatory duct—empties into urethra

C. Formation of semen
  1. Functions of semen
     a. Nourish spermatozoa
     b. Transport spermatozoa
     c. Neutralize vaginal tract
     d. Lubricate reproductive tract during intercourse
  2. Glands
     a. Seminal vesicles
     b. Prostate—around first portion of urethra
     c. Bulbourethral (Cowper's) glands
D. Urethra and penis
  1. Urethra
     a. Conveys urine and semen through penis
  2. Penis
     a. Structure
        (1) Corpus spongiosum—central
        (2) Corpora cavernosa—lateral
        (3) Glans—distal enlargement of corpus spongiosum
        (4) Prepuce—foreskin
     b. Erection—stiffening and enlargement of penis
     c. Ejaculation—forceful expulsion of semen
E. Spermatozoa (sperm cells)
  1. Sertoli (nurse) cells—nourish and protect spermatozoa
  2. Parts of sperm cell
     a. Head—contains chromosomes
     b. Acrosome—covers head; has enzymes to help penetration of ovum
     c. Midpiece—contains mitochondria
     d. Tail (flagellum)—propels sperm

III. **Hormonal control of male reproduction**
  1. Pituitary hormones
     a. FSH (follicle stimulating hormone)
        (1) Stimulates Sertoli cells
        (2) Promotes formation of spermatozoa
     b. LH (luteinizing hormone)
        (1) Also called ICSH (interstitial cell–stimulating hormone)
        (2) Stimulates interstitial cells to produce testosterone
A. Effects of aging on male reproduction
  1. Decline in testosterone, spermatozoa, and semen

IV. **Female reproductive system**
  A. Ovaries—glands in which ova (egg cells) form
     1. Egg cell and ovulation
        a. Egg ripens in graafian follicle
        b. Ovulation—release of ovum from ovary
     2. Corpus luteum
        a. Remainder of follicle in ovary
        b. Continues to function if egg fertilized
        c. Disintegrates if egg not fertilized
  B. Oviducts (uterine tubes, fallopian tubes)
     1. Fimbriae—fringelike extensions that sweep egg into oviduct
  C. Uterus
     1. Holds developing fetus
     2. Endometrium—lining of uterus
     3. Cervix—narrow, lower part
  D. Vagina
     1. Tube connecting uterus to outside
     2. Hymen—fold of membrane over vaginal opening
     3. Greater vestibular glands- secrete mucus
  E. Vulva and perineum
     1. Vulva—external genitalia
        a. Labia—two sets of folds (major, minor)
        b. Clitoris—organ of great sensitivity
     2. Perineum—pelvic floor
        a. In obstetrics—area between vagina and anus

V. **Menstrual cycle**—average 28 days
  A. Beginning of the cycle
     1. FSH stimulates follicle
     2. Follicle secretes estrogen
     3. Estrogen thickens lining of uterus
  B. Ovulation
     1. LH surge 1 day before
     2. Corpus luteum produces progesterone

20

3. Progesterone continues growth of endometrium
4. Ovum disintegrates if not fertilized
C. Menstrual flow (menses)
   1. If egg not fertilized, corpus luteum degenerates
   2. Lining of uterus breaks down

VI. Menopause—period during which menstruation stops
   A. Hormone replacement therapy (HRT)
      1. Reduces symptoms of menopause; other beneficial effects
         a. Risks—endometrial cancer, thrombosis, embolism, breast cancer

VII. Contraception—use of artificial methods to prevent fertilization

Questions for Study and Review

1. In what fundamental respect does reproduction in some single-celled animals, such as the ameba, differ from that in most animals?
2. Name the sex cells of both the male and the female.
3. Name all the parts of the male reproductive system and describe the function of each.
4. List the functions of semen.
5. Name and locate the glands that contribute to semen.
6. Draw and label the parts of a sperm cell.
7. Name the hormones that regulate male reproductive activity.
8. What changes occur in the male reproductive system with age?
9. Name the principal parts of the female reproductive system and describe the function of each.
10. Beginning with the first day of the menstrual flow, describe the events of one complete cycle, including the role of the various hormones.
11. Describe the process of ovulation.
12. What is menopause? What causes it? What are some of the changes that take place in the body as a result?
13. What are the values of hormone replacement therapy after menopause? What are some of the dangers of such therapy?
14. Define *contraception.* Describe methods of contraception that involve (1) barriers; (2) chemicals; (3) hormones; (4) prevention of implantation.

20

✔ ANSWERS TO CHECKPOINTS

1. Meiosis is the process of cell division that halves the chromosome number in a cell to produce a gamete.
2. The testis is the male gonad.
3. Testosterone is the main male sex hormone.
4. Sperm cells leave the ducts within the testis and then travel through the epididymis, ductus (vas) deferens, ejaculatory duct, and urethra.
5. Glands that contribute secretions to the semen are the seminal vesicles, prostate, and bulbourethral glands.
6. The main subdivisions of the sperm cell are the head, midpiece, and tail (flagellum).
7. Follicle-stimulating hormone (FSH) and luteinizing hormone (LH), also called ICSH, are the pituitary hormones that regulate male and female reproduction.
8. Ovulation is the process of releasing an egg cell from the ovary.
9. The fetus develops in the uterus.
10. The two hormones produced in the ovaries are estrogen and progesterone.
11. Menopause is the period during which menstruation ceases.
12. Contraception is the use of artificial methods to prevent fertilization of the ovum or implantation of the fertilized ovum.

Development and Heredity

Chapter

21

SELECTED KEY TERMS

The following terms are defined in the Glossary:

abortion

amniotic sac

carrier

chromosome

dominant

embryo

fertilization

fetus

gene

genetic

gestation

heredity

implantation

lactation

meiosis

mutation

parturition

placenta

progeny

recessive

sex-linked

umbilical cord

trait

zygote

BEHAVIORAL OBJECTIVES

After careful study of this chapter, you should be able to:

1. Describe fertilization and the early development of the fertilized egg

2. Describe the structure and function of the placenta

3. Briefly describe changes that occur in the fetus and the mother during pregnancy

4. Briefly describe the four stages of labor

5. Compare fraternal and identical twins

6. Cite the advantages of breastfeeding

7. Briefly describe the mechanism of gene function

8. Explain the difference between dominant and recessive genes

9. Describe what is meant by a *carrier* of a genetic trait

10. Define *meiosis* and explain the function of meiosis in reproduction

11. Explain how sex is determined in humans

12. Describe what is meant by the term *sex linked* and list several sex-linked traits

13. List several factors that may influence the expression of a gene

14. Define *mutation*

PREGNANCY

Pregnancy begins with fertilization of an ovum and ends with delivery of the fetus and after-birth. During this 38-week period of development, known as **gestation** (jes-TA-shun), all body tissues differentiate from a single fertilized egg. Along the way, many changes occur in both the mother and the growing offspring.

Fertilization and the Start of Pregnancy

When semen is deposited in the vagina, the many spermatozoa immediately wriggle about in all directions, some traveling into the uterus and oviducts (see Fig. 20-6 in Chap. 20). If an egg cell is present in the oviduct, many spermatozoa cluster around it. Using enzymes, they dissolve the coating around the ovum, so that eventually one sperm cell can penetrate the cell membrane of the egg. The nuclei of the sperm and egg then combine.

The result of this union is a single cell with the full human chromosome number of 46. This new cell, called a **zygote** (ZI-gote), can divide and grow into a new individual. The zygote divides rapidly into two cells and then four cells, and soon a ball of cells is formed. During this time, the cell cluster is traveling toward the uterine cavity, pushed along by cilia lining the

oviduct and by peristalsis (contractions) of the tube. After reaching the uterus, the little ball of cells burrows into the greatly thickened uterine lining, where it is soon completely covered and implanted.

> ✔ CHECKPOINT **1**:
>
> What structure is formed by the union of an ovum and a spermatozoon?

Development and Functions of the Placenta

After **implantation** in the lining of the uterus, a group of cells within the developing ball of cells becomes an **embryo** (EM-bre-o), the future offspring. The outer cells of the cluster form projections, called **villi,** that invade the uterine wall and maternal blood channels (venous sinuses). This tissue eventually forms the **placenta** (plah-SEN-tah), a flat, circular organ that consists of a spongy network of blood-filled lakes and capillary-containing villi (Fig. 21-1). The placenta serves as the organ of nutrition, respiration, and excretion for the embryo by means of exchanges that occur between the blood of the embryo and the blood of the mother through the capillaries of the placental villi.

21

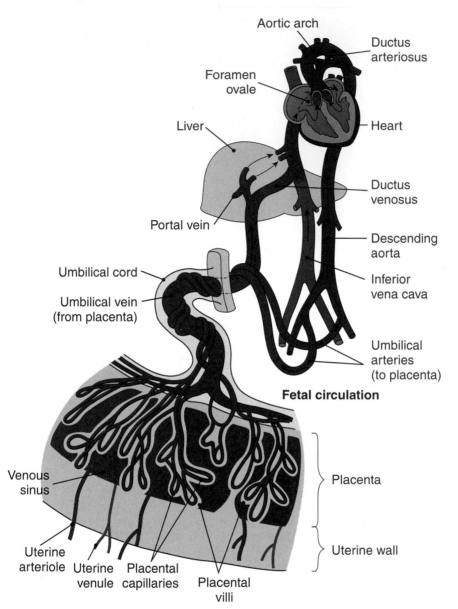

Aortic arch
Ductus arteriosus
Foramen ovale
Liver
Heart
Ductus venosus
Portal vein
Descending aorta
Umbilical cord
Inferior vena cava
Umbilical vein (from placenta)
Umbilical arteries (to placenta)
Fetal circulation
Placenta
Venous sinus
Uterine wall
Uterine arteriole   Uterine venule   Placental capillaries   Placental villi

FIGURE **21•1**   Fetal circulation and placenta. Color shows relative oxygen content of blood.

The Umbilical Cord

The embryo, later called the *fetus* (FE-tus), is connected to the developing placenta by a stalk of tissue that eventually becomes the *umbilical* (um-BIL-ih-kal) *cord.* This cord carries blood to and from the fetus. It encloses two arteries that carry blood from the fetus to the placenta and one vein that carries blood from the placenta to the fetus (see Fig. 21-1). The fetus has special features of the circulation to carry blood to and from the umbilical cord and to bypass the lungs (see Fetal Circulation).

Placental Hormones

In addition to maintaining the fetus, the placenta serves as an endocrine organ. Beginning soon after implantation, some of the embryonic cells produce a hormone called *human chorionic gonadotropin* (ko-re-ON-ik gon-ah-do-TRO-pin) *(hCG).* This hormone stimulates the corpus luteum of the ovary, prolonging its lifespan (to 11 or 12 weeks) and causing it to secrete increasing amounts of progesterone and estrogen.

Progesterone is essential for the maintenance

Fetal Circulation

The developing fetus has several adaptations in the cardiovascular system that change at birth. These adaptations serve to bypass the lungs, which are not functional. Fetal blood is oxygenated instead by the placenta (see Fig. 21-1).

Blood comes from the placenta to the fetus in the umbilical vein, which is contained in the umbilical cord. Most of this blood joins the inferior vena cava by way of a small vessel, the ductus venosus, and is carried to the heart. Once in the right atrium, a portion of the blood flows directly into the left atrium through a hole in the septum called the foramen ovale. This blood bypasses the pulmonary circuit.

Blood that does enter the right ventricle is pumped into the pulmonary artery. However, most of this blood shunts directly into the systemic circulation through a small vessel, the ductus arteriosus, that connects the pulmonary artery to the aorta. Blood returns to the placenta through two umbilical arteries.

Most of these adaptations close at birth, when the lungs begin to function. The foramen ovale seals to become a depression in the septum between the atria. The various vessels constrict into fibrous cords. Only the proximal parts of the umbilical arteries persist as arteries to the urinary bladder.

---

of pregnancy. It promotes endometrial secretion to nourish the embryo, and it decreases the ability of the uterine muscle to contract, thus preventing the embryo from being expelled from the body. During pregnancy, progesterone also helps prepare the breasts for the secretion of milk.

Estrogen promotes enlargement of the uterus and breasts. By the 11th or 12th week of pregnancy, the corpus luteum is no longer needed; by this time, the placenta itself can secrete adequate amounts of progesterone and estrogen, and the corpus luteum disintegrates. Miscarriages (loss of an embryo or fetus) frequently occur during this critical time when hormone secretion is shifting from the corpus luteum to the placenta.

> ✔ CHECKPOINT **2**:
>
> What organ nourishes the developing fetus?

> ✔ CHECKPOINT **3**:
>
> What is the function of the umbilical cord?

Development of the Embryo

For the first 8 weeks of life, the developing offspring is referred to as an *embryo* (Fig. 21-2). The beginnings of all body systems are established during this period. The heart and the brain are among the first organs to develop. A primitive nervous system begins to form in the third week. The heart and blood vessels originate during the second week, and the first heartbeat appears during week 4, at the same time that other muscles begin to develop.

By the end of the first month, the embryo is about 0.62 cm (0.25 inches) long, with four small swellings at the sides called *limb buds,* which will develop into the four extremities. At this time, the heart produces a prominent bulge at the front of the embryo.

By the end of the second month, the embryo takes on an appearance that is recognizably human. The study of embryonic development is *embryology* (em-bre-OL-o-je).

> ✔ CHECKPOINT **4**:
>
> All body systems originate during the early development of the embryo. At about what time in gestation does the heartbeat first appear?

The Fetus

The term *fetus* is used for the developing individual from the beginning of the third month until birth. During this period, the organ systems continue to grow and mature. For study, the period of development (gestation) may be divided into three equal segments or *trimesters.*

The most rapid growth of the fetus occurs

21

Umbilical
stalk

28 days

6 weeks

8 weeks

Umbilical cord

3 months

5 months

FIGURE **21•2** Development of an embryo into a fetus.

during the second trimester (months 4–6). By the end of the fourth month, the fetus is almost 15 cm (6 inches) long, and its external genitalia are sufficiently developed to reveal its sex. By the seventh month, the fetus is usually about 35 cm (14 inches) long and weighs about 1.1 kg (2.4 pounds). At the end of pregnancy, the normal length of the fetus is 45 to 56 cm (18–22.5 inches), and the weight varies from 2.7 to 4.5 kg (6–10 pounds).

The ***amniotic*** (am-ne-OT-ik) ***sac,*** which is filled with a clear liquid known as ***amniotic fluid,*** surrounds the fetus and serves as a protective cushion for it (Fig. 21-3). The amniotic sac ruptures at birth, an event marked by the common expression that the mother's "water broke."

During development, the skin of the fetus is protected by a layer of cheeselike material called ***vernix caseosa*** (VER-niks KA-se-o-sa).

✔ CHECKPOINT **5**:

What is the name of the fluid-filled sac that holds the fetus?

The Mother

The total period of pregnancy, from fertilization of the ovum to birth, is about 266 days, also given as 280 days or 40 weeks from the last menstrual period (LMP). During this time, the mother must supply all the food and oxygen for

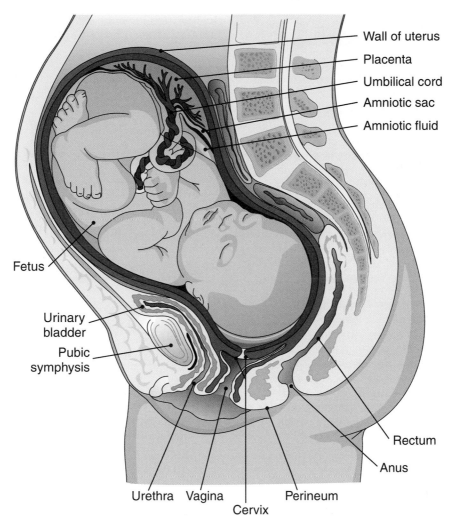

Wall of uterus
Placenta
Umbilical cord
Amniotic sac
Amniotic fluid

Fetus

Urinary bladder
Pubic symphysis

Rectum

Anus

Urethra Vagina Perineum
Cervix

FIGURE **21•3** Midsagittal section of a pregnant uterus with intact fetus.

the fetus and eliminate its waste materials. To support the additional demands of the growing fetus, the mother's metabolism changes markedly, with increased demands being made on several organ systems:

- The heart pumps more blood to supply the needs of the uterus and its contents.
- The lungs provide more oxygen to supply the fetus by increasing the rate and depth of respiration.
- The kidneys excrete nitrogenous wastes from the fetus and from the mother's body.
- Nutritional needs are increased to provide for the growth of maternal organs (uterus

and breasts) and growth of the fetus as well as for preparation for labor and the secretion of milk.

(See Start Being Healthy Before Pregnancy.)
Nausea and vomiting are common discomforts in early pregnancy. The specific cause of these symptoms is not known, but they may be due to the great changes in hormone levels that occur at this time. The nausea and vomiting usually last for only a few weeks.

Frequency of urination and constipation are often present during the early stages of pregnancy and then usually disappear. They may reappear late in pregnancy as the head of the

Start Being Healthy Before Pregnancy

The way that a woman cares for herself directly affects her health and the health of her unborn infant.

There are several ways to get a headstart on a healthy pregnancy.

- Get a complete physical examination. It is far easier to learn to manage disorders such as diabetes, high blood pressure, or anemia before adding the changes that a pregnancy brings. Make sure your immunizations are up to date.
- Have a gynecologist examine your reproductive structures. It is much easier to clear up a vaginal or urinary infection before than during pregnancy. An abnormality of the cervix is best treated when a woman is not pregnant.
- Include enough of the B vitamin folic acid in your diet before and during pregnancy. This vitamin plays an important role in the early formation of the central nervous system— the brain and spinal cord. Because folic acid is needed before a woman is aware of her pregnancy, it needs to be taken in adequate amounts even when pregnancy is anticipated.

fetus drops from the abdominal region down into the pelvis, pressing on the rectum and the urinary bladder.

The Use of Ultrasound in Obstetrics

Ultrasonography (ul-trah-son-OG-rah-fe) is a safe, painless, and noninvasive method for studying soft tissue. It has proved extremely valuable for monitoring pregnancies and deliveries.

An ultrasound image, called a *sonogram,* is made by sending high-frequency sound waves into the body. Each time a wave meets an interface between two tissues of different densities, an echo is produced. An instrument called a *transducer* converts the reflected sound waves into electrical energy, and a computer is used to generate an image on a viewing screen.

Ultrasound scans can be used in obstetrics to diagnose pregnancy, judge the age of the fetus, and determine the location of the placenta. The

technique can also show the presence of excess amniotic fluid and fetal abnormalities.

CHILDBIRTH

The mechanisms that trigger the beginning of uterine contractions for childbirth are still unknown. The uterine muscle becomes increasingly sensitive to the pituitary hormone oxytocin late in pregnancy. After labor begins, stimuli from the cervix and vagina produce reflex secretion of this hormone, which in turn increases the uterine contractions.

The Four Stages of Labor

The process by which the fetus is expelled from the uterus is known as *labor* and *delivery;* it also may be called *parturition* (par-tu-RISH-un). It is divided into four stages:

1. The *first stage* begins with the onset of regular contractions of the uterus. With each contraction, the cervix becomes thinner and the opening larger. Rupture of the amniotic sac may occur at any time, with a gush of fluid from the vagina.
2. The *second stage* begins when the cervix is completely dilated and ends with the delivery of the baby. This stage involves the passage of the fetus, usually head first, through the cervical canal and the vagina to the outside.
3. The *third stage* begins after the child is born and ends with the expulsion of the *afterbirth.* The afterbirth includes the placenta, the membranes of the amniotic sac, and the umbilical cord, except for a small portion remaining attached to the baby's *umbilicus* (um-BIL-ih-kus), or navel.
4. The *fourth stage* begins with the expulsion of the afterbirth and constitutes a period in which bleeding is controlled. Contraction of the uterine muscle acts to close off the blood vessels leading to the placental site.

To prevent the pelvic floor tissues from being torn during childbirth, as often happens, the physician may cut the mother's perineum just before her infant is born and then repair this clean cut immediately after childbirth; such an operation is called an *episiotomy* (eh-piz-e-OT-o-me). The area between the vagina and the anus that is cut in an episiotomy is referred to as the *surgical* or *obstetrical perineum* (see Fig. 20-9 in Chap. 20).

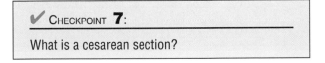

✔ CHECKPOINT **6**:

What is parturition?

Cesarean Section

A *cesarean* (se-ZAR-re-an) *section* (C section) is an incision made in the abdominal wall and in the wall of the uterus for delivery of a fetus. A cesarean section may be required for a variety of reasons, including abnormalities of the placenta, abnormal position of the fetus, disproportion between the head of the fetus and the mother's pelvis that makes vaginal delivery difficult or dangerous, and other problems that may arise during pregnancy and delivery.

✔ CHECKPOINT **7**:

What is a cesarean section?

Multiple Births

Until recently, statistics indicated that twins occurred in about 1 of every 80 to 90 births, varying somewhat in different countries. Triplets occurred much less frequently, usually once in several thousand births, whereas quadruplets occurred very rarely. The birth of quintuplets represented a historic event unless the mother had taken fertility drugs. Now these fertility drugs, usually gonadotropins, are given quite frequently, and the number of multiple births has increased significantly. Multiple fetuses tend to be born prematurely and therefore have a high death rate. However, better care of infants and newer treatments have resulted in more living multiple births than ever.

Twins originate in two different ways and on this basis are divided into two types:

- *Fraternal twins* are formed as a result of the fertilization of two different ova by two spermatozoa. Two completely different individuals, as distinct from each other as brothers and sisters of different ages, are produced. Each fetus has its own placenta and surrounding sac.
- *Identical twins* develop from a single zygote formed from a single ovum fertilized by a single spermatozoon. Obviously, they are always the same sex and carry the same inherited traits. Sometime during the early stages of development, the embryonic cells separate into two units. Usually, there is a single placenta, although there must be a separate umbilical cord for each fetus.

Other multiple births may be fraternal, identical, or combinations of these. The tendency to multiple births seems to be hereditary.

Termination of Pregnancy

A pregnancy may end before its full term has been completed. The term *live birth* is used if the baby breathes or shows any evidence of life such as heartbeat, pulsation of the umbilical cord, or movement of voluntary muscles. An *immature* or *premature* infant is one born before the organ systems are mature. Infants born before the 37th week of gestation or weighing less than 2500 grams (5.5 pounds) are considered *preterm.*

Loss of the fetus is classified according to the duration of the pregnancy:

- The term *abortion* refers to loss of the embryo or fetus before the 20th week or weight of about 500 grams (1.1 pound). This loss can be either spontaneous or induced.
  - *Spontaneous abortions* occur naturally with no interference. The most common causes are related to an abnormality of the embryo or fetus. Other causes include abnormality of the mother's reproductive organs, infections, or chronic

disorders, such as kidney disease or hypertension. ***Miscarriage*** is the lay term for spontaneous abortions.

○ ***Induced abortions*** occur as a result of artificial or mechanical interruption of pregnancy. ***Therapeutic abortions*** are abortions performed by physicians as a form of treatment for a variety of reasons. With more liberal use of this type of abortion, there has been a dramatic decline in the incidence of death related to illegal abortion.

● The term ***fetal death*** refers to loss of the fetus after the eighth week of pregnancy. ***Stillbirth*** refers to the delivery of an infant that is lifeless.

Immaturity is a leading cause of death in the newborn. After the 20th week of pregnancy, the fetus is considered ***viable,*** that is, able to live outside the uterus. A fetus expelled before the 28th week or before reaching a weight of 1000 grams (2.2 pounds) has a less than 50% chance of survival. One born at a point closer to the full 40 weeks stands a much better chance of living.

Increasing numbers of immature infants are being saved because of advances in neonatal intensive care.

THE MAMMARY GLANDS AND LACTATION

The ***mammary glands,*** or the breasts of the female, are accessories of the reproductive system. They are designed to provide nourishment for the baby after its birth, and the secretion of milk at this time is known as ***lactation*** (lak-TA-shun).

The mammary glands are constructed in much the same manner as the sweat glands. Each of these glands is divided into a number of lobes composed of glandular tissue and fat, and each lobe is further subdivided. The secretions from the lobes are conveyed through ***lactiferous*** (lak-TIF-er-us) ***ducts,*** all of which converge at the nipple (Fig. 21-4).

The mammary glands begin developing during puberty, but they do not become functional until the end of a pregnancy. The hormone ***pro-***

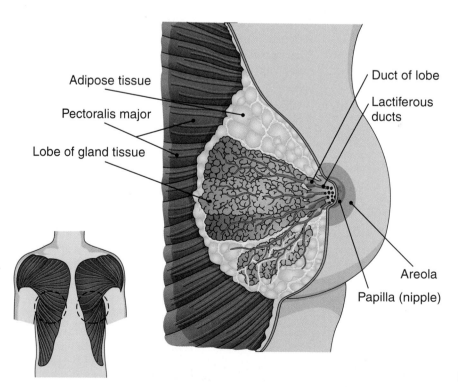

Adipose tissue

Pectoralis major

Lobe of gland tissue

Duct of lobe

Lactiferous ducts

Areola

Papilla (nipple)

FIGURE **21•4** Section of the breast.

lactin (PRL), produced by the anterior lobe of the pituitary, stimulates the secretory cells of the mammary glands.

The first mammary gland secretion is a thin liquid called **colostrum** (ko-LOS-trum). It is nutritious but has a somewhat different composition from milk. Secretion of milk begins within a few days and can continue for several months as long as milk is frequently removed by the suckling baby or by pumping. Stimulation of the breast by the suckling infant causes the release of *oxytocin* from the posterior pituitary gland. This hormone causes the milk ducts to contract, resulting in the ejection, or *letdown*, of milk.

The digestive tract of the newborn baby is not ready for the usual mixed diet of an adult. Mother's milk is more desirable for the young infant than milk from other animals for several reasons, some of which are listed below:

- Infections that may be transmitted by foods exposed to the outside air are avoided by nursing.
- Both breast milk and colostrum contain maternal antibodies that help protect the baby against pathogens.
- The proportions of various nutrients and other substances in human milk are perfectly suited to the human infant. Substitutes are not exact imitations of human milk. Nutrients are present in more desirable amounts if the mother's diet is well balanced.
- The psychological and emotional benefits of nursing are of infinite value to both the mother and the infant.

✔ CHECKPOINT **8**:

What is lactation?

HEREDITY

We are often struck by the resemblance of a baby to one or both of its parents, yet rarely do we stop to consider *how* various traits are transmitted from parents to offspring. This subject—heredity—has fascinated humans for thousands of years; the *Old Testament* contains numerous references to heredity (although, of course, the word was unknown in biblical times). It was not until the 19th century, however, that methodical investigation into heredity was begun. At that time, an Austrian monk, Gregor Mendel, discovered through his experiments with garden peas that there was a precise pattern in the appearance of differences among parents and their progeny. Mendel's most important contribution to the understanding of heredity was the demonstration that there are independent units of hereditary in the cells. Later, these independent units were given the name *genes*.

Genes and Chromosomes

Genes are actually segments of DNA (deoxyribonucleic acid) contained in the threadlike chromosomes within the nucleus of each cell. Genes act by controlling the manufacture of enzymes, which are necessary for all the chemical reactions that occur within the cell.

When body cells divide by the process of mitosis, the DNA that makes up the chromosomes is duplicated and distributed to the daughter cells, so that each daughter cell gets exactly the same kind and number of chromosomes as were in the original cell. Each chromosome (aside from the Y chromosome, which determines sex) may carry thousands of genes, and each gene carries the code for a specific trait (characteristic). These traits constitute the physical, biochemical, and physiologic makeup of every cell in the body.

In humans, every cell except the sex cells contains 46 chromosomes. These chromosomes exist in pairs. One member of each pair was received at the time of fertilization from the father of the offspring, and one was received from the mother. These paired chromosomes, except for the pair that determines sex, are alike in size and appearance and carry genes for the same traits. Thus, the genes for each trait exist in pairs.

✔ CHECKPOINT **9**:

What is a gene?

Dominant and Recessive Genes

Another of Mendel's discoveries was that genes can be either dominant or recessive. A **dominant** gene is one that expresses its effect in the cell regardless of whether the gene at the same site on the matching chromosome is the same as or different from the dominant gene. The gene need be received from only one parent to be expressed in the offspring.

The effect of a **recessive** gene is not evident unless the gene at that site in the matching chromosome of the pair is also recessive. Thus, a recessive trait appears only if the recessive genes for that trait are received from both parents. For example, genes for dark eyes are dominant, whereas genes for light eyes are recessive. Light eyes appear in the offspring only if genes for light eyes are received from both parents.

A recessive gene is not expressed if it is present in the cell together with a dominant gene. However, the recessive gene can be passed on to offspring and may thus appear in future generations. An individual who shows no evidence of a trait but has a recessive gene for that trait is described as a **carrier** of the gene.

> ✔ CHECKPOINT **10**:
>
> What is the difference between a dominant and a recessive gene?

Distribution of Chromosomes to Offspring

The reproductive cells (ova and spermatozoa) are produced by a special process of cell division called **meiosis** (mi-O-sis). This process divides the chromosome number in half, so that each reproductive cell has 23 chromosomes. Moreover, the division occurs in such a way that each cell receives one member of each chromosome pair that was present in the original cell. The separation occurs at random, meaning that either member of the original pair may be included in a given germ cell. Thus, the maternal and paternal sets of chromosomes get mixed up and redistributed at this time, leading to increased variety within the population.

> ✔ CHECKPOINT **11**:
>
> What is the process of cell division that forms the gametes?

Sex Determination

The two chromosomes that determine the sex of the offspring, unlike the other 22 pairs of chromosomes, are not matched in size and appearance. The female X chromosome is larger than most other chromosomes and carries genes for other characteristics in addition to that for sex. The male Y chromosome is smaller than other chromosomes and mainly determines sex. A female has two X chromosomes in each body cell; a male has one X and one Y.

By the process of meiosis, each male sperm cell receives either an X or a Y chromosome, whereas every egg cell receives only an X chromosome (Fig. 21-5). If a sperm cell with an X chromosome fertilizes an ovum, the resulting infant will be female; if a sperm with a Y chromosome fertilizes an ovum, the resulting infant will be male (see Fig. 21-5).

Sex-Linked Traits

Any trait that is carried on a sex chromosome is said to be **sex linked.** Because the Y chromosome carries few traits aside from sex determination, most sex-linked traits are carried on the X chromosome and are described as *X linked.* Examples are hemophilia, certain forms of baldness, and red-green color blindness.

Sex-linked traits appear almost exclusively in males. The reason for this is that most of these traits are recessive, and if a recessive gene is located on the X chromosome in a male it cannot be masked by a matching dominant gene. (Remember that the Y chromosome with which the X chromosome pairs is very small and carries few genes.) Thus, a male who has only one recessive gene for a trait will exhibit that characteristic, whereas a female must have two recessive genes to show the trait.

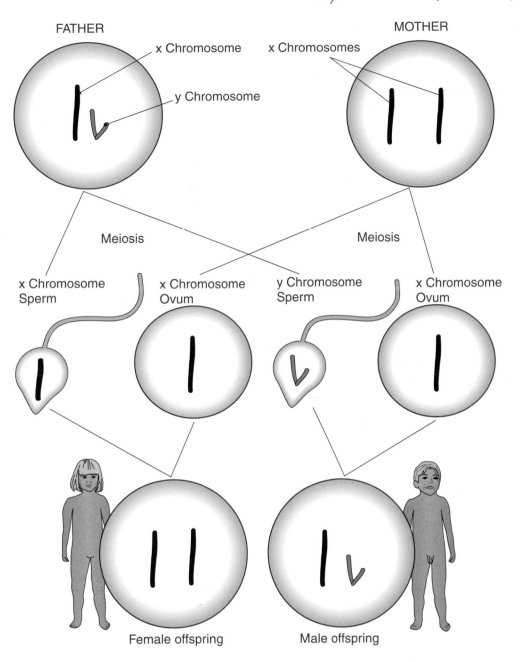

FIGURE **21•5**   If an X chromosome from a male unites with an X chromosome from a female, the child is female; if a Y chromosome from a male unites with an X chromosome from a female, the child is male.

✔ CHECKPOINT **12**:

What sex chromosome combination determines a female? a male?

✔ CHECKPOINT **13**:

What term is used to describe a trait carried on a sex chromosome?

HEREDITARY TRAITS

Some observable hereditary traits are skin, eye, and hair color and facial features. Also influenced by genetics are less clearly defined traits, such as weight, body build, life-span, and susceptibility to disease.

Some human traits, including the traits involved in many genetic diseases, are determined by a single pair of genes; most, however, are the result of two or more gene pairs acting together in what is termed ***multifactorial inheritance.*** This type of inheritance accounts for the wide range of variations within populations in such characteristics as coloration, height, and weight, all of which are determined by more than one pair of genes.

Gene Expression

The effect or expression of a gene may be influenced by a variety of factors, including the sex of the individual and the presence of other genes. For example, the genes for certain types of baldness and certain types of color blindness may be inherited by either males or females, but the traits appear mostly in males under the effects of male sex hormone.

Environment also plays a part in the expression of genes. One inherits a potential for a given size, for example, but one's actual size is additionally influenced by such factors as nutrition, development, and general state of health. The same is true of life-span and susceptibility to diseases.

Genetic Mutation

As a rule, chromosomes replicate exactly during cell division. Occasionally, however, for reasons not yet totally understood, the genes or chromosomes change. This change may involve a single gene or whole chromosomes. Alternatively, it may consist of chromosomal breakage, in which there is loss or rearrangement of gene fragments. Such changes are termed genetic ***mutations.*** Mutations may occur spontaneously or may be induced by some agent, such as ionizing radiation or chemicals, described as a ***mutagenic agent.***

If the mutation occurs in an ovum or a sperm cell involved in reproduction, the altered trait will be inherited by the offspring. The vast majority of harmful mutations never are expressed because the affected fetus dies and is spontaneously aborted. Most remaining mutations are so inconsequential that they have no visible effect. Beneficial mutations, on the other hand, tend to survive and increase as a population evolves.

✔ CHECKPOINT **14**:

What is a mutation?

Summary

I. **Pregnancy (gestation)**—lasts 38 weeks
  A. Fertilization and the start of pregnancy
    1. Fertilization occurs in oviduct
    2. Zygote (fertilized egg)—formed by fusion of egg and sperm nuclei
      a. Divides rapidly
      b. Travels to uterus
      c. Implants in lining
  B. Development and functions of the placenta
    1. Formed by cells around embryo and lining of uterus
    2. Umbilical cord—connects fetus to placenta
    3. Functions
      a. Provision of nourishment to embryo

21

b. Gas exchange with embryo

c. Removal of waste from embryo

d. Production of human chorionic gonadotropin (hCG)—maintains corpus luteum until 11 to 12 weeks of pregnancy

C. Development of the embryo

1. First 8 weeks

2. All body systems begin to develop

D. The fetus

1. Third month to birth

2. Amniotic sac

a. Surrounds fetus

b. Contains fluid to cushion and protect fetus

E. The mother

1. Increased demands on heart, lungs, kidneys

2. Increased nutritional needs

3. Ultrasound used to monitor pregnancy and delivery

II. Childbirth

A. Four stages of labor

1. Contractions

2. Delivery of baby

3. Expulsion of afterbirth

4. Contraction of uterus

B. Cesarean section

1. Incision to remove fetus

C. Multiple births

1. Fraternal twins formed from two different ova

2. Identical twins develop from a single zygote

3. Larger multiples follow either pattern or a combination

4. Increased by fertility drugs

D. Termination of pregnancy

1. Immature (premature) infant—born before organ system mature

2. Preterm—born before 37th week or weighing less than 2500 grams

3. Abortion—loss of fetus before 20th week or weighing less than 500 grams

4. Fetal death—loss of fetus after 8 weeks of pregnancy

III. Mammary glands and lactation

1. Lactation—secretion of milk

a. Colostrum—first mammary secretion

2. Hormones

a. Prolactin—stimulates secretory cells

b. Oxytocin—promotes letdown (ejection) of milk

3. Advantages of breastfeeding

a. Reduces infections

b. Transfers antibodies

c. Provides best form of nutrition

d. Emotional satisfaction

IV. Heredity

A. Genes and chromosomes

1. Genes

a. Hereditary units

b. Segments of DNA

c. Control manufacture of enzymes

2. Chromosomes

a. Threadlike bodies in nucleus

b. Composed of genes

c. Exist in matched pairs

d. Human cells (except sex cells) have 46

B. Dominant and recessive genes

1. Dominant gene—always expressed

2. Recessive gene—expressed only if gene received from both parents

a. Carrier—person with recessive gene that is not apparent but can be passed to offspring

C. Distribution of chromosomes to offspring

1. Meiosis

a. Cell division that forms sexcells

b. Divides chromosomes number in half (23)

c. Each cell receives one of each chromosome pair

D. Sex determination

1. Sex chromosomes not matched in size and appearance

2. X larger and carries other traits

3. Y smaller and carries mainly gene for sex determination

4. Female cells have XX; male cells have XY

E. Sex-linked traits

1. Traits carried on sex chromosome (usually X)

2. Sex-linked traits appear mostly in males
   a. Passed from mother to son on X chromosome
   b. If recessive, not masked by dominant gene on Y
   c. Examples—hemophilia, baldness, red-green color blindness

V. Hereditary traits
1. Genes determine physical, biochemical, and physiologic characteristics of every cell
2. Some traits determined by single gene pairs
3. Most determined by multifactorial inheritance
   a. Involves multiple gene pairs
   b. Produces a range of variations in a population
   c. Examples—height, weight, coloration, susceptibility to disease

A. Gene expression
1. Factors
   a. Sex
   b. Presence of other genes
   c. Environment

B. Genetic mutation
1. Change in genes or chromosomes
2. May be passed to offspring if occurs in germ cells
3. Mutagenic agents
   a. Factors causing mutation
   b. Examples—ionizing radiation, chemicals

Questions for Study and Review

1. Distinguish among the following: zygote, embryo, fetus.
2. Describe events between fertilization of an ovum and the start of its growth within the uterus.
3. List hormones specifically involved in pregnancy and cite the functions of each.
4. Explain the role of the placenta in fetal development.
5. Describe the amniotic sac and explain its role in development.
6. Is blood in the umbilical arteries relatively low or high in oxygen? in the umbilical vein?
7. Describe some of the changes that take place in the mother's body during pregnancy.
8. What is the major event of each of the four stages of labor and delivery?
9. What is an episiotomy? Why is it done?
10. Distinguish between fraternal and identical twins.
11. Define *abortion; premature infant; preterm infant.*
12. Name two hormones involved in lactation. Where do they originate and what do they do?
13. List some of the advantages associated with breastfeeding a baby.
14. Explain the relationship between genes and chromosomes.
15. How many chromosomes are there in a human body cell? in a human sex cell?
16. What process results in the distribution of chromosomes to the offspring?
17. Under what circumstances are dominant genes expressed? recessive genes?
18. What sex chromosomes are present in a male? in a female?
19. From which parent does a male child receive an X-linked gene?
20. Explain how two normal parents can give birth to a child with a recessive hereditary disease.
21. Explain the great variation in the color of skin, hair, and eyes in humans.
22. What is a mutation?
23. List several mutagenic agents.

✔ ANSWERS TO CHECKPOINTS

1. A zygote is formed by the union of an ovum and a spermatozoon.
2. The placenta nourishes the developing fetus.
3. The umbilical cord carries blood between the fetus and the placenta.
4. The heartbeat first appears during the fourth week of embryonic development.
5. The amniotic sac is the fluid-filled sac that holds the fetus.
6. Parturition is the process of labor and delivery.
7. A cesarean section is an incision made in the abdominal wall and the wall of the uterus for delivery of a fetus.
8. Lactation is the secretion of milk from the mammary glands.
9. A gene is an independent unit of heredity. Each is a segment of DNA contained in a chromosome.
10. A dominant gene is always expressed, regardless of the gene on the matching chromosome. A recessive gene is only expressed if the gene on the matching chromosome is also recessive.
11. Meiosis is the process of cell division that forms the gametes.
12. The sex chromosome combination that determines a female is XX; a male is XY.
13. A trait carried on a sex chromosome is described as sex linked.
14. A mutation is a change in the genetic material (a gene or chromosome) of a cell.

21

Suggestions for Further Study

Agur A: Grant's Atlas of Anatomy, 10th ed. Baltimore, Williams & Wilkins, 1999

Anne EA: Clinical Hematology, 2nd ed. Philadelphia, Lippincott-Raven, 1998

Bishop ML, et al: Clinical Chemistry: Principles, Procedures, Correlations, 3rd ed. Philadelphia, Lippincott-Raven, 1996

Clemente CD: Gray's Anatomy of the Human Body, 13th ed. Baltimore, Williams & Wilkins, 1985

Clinical Laboratory Tests, 2nd ed. Springhouse, PA, Springhouse Corp, 1995

Cormack DH: Clinically Integrated Histology. Philadelphia, Lippincott-Raven, 1998

DeMyer W: Neuroanatomy, 2nd ed. Baltimore, Williams & Wilkins, 1997

Dorland's Illustrated Medical Dictionary, 28th ed. Philadelphia, WB Saunders, 1994

Escott-Stump S: Nutrition and Diagnosis Related Care, 4th ed. Baltimore, Williams & Wilkins, 1997

Fischbach FT: Nurses' Quick Reference to Common Laboratory and Diagnostic Tests, 2nd ed. Philadelphia, Lippincott-Raven, 1997

Friedman JM: Genetics, 2nd ed. Baltimore, Williams & Wilkins, 1996

Ganong WF: Review of Medical Physiology, 18th ed. Stamford, CT, Appleton & Lange, 1997

Gartner LP, Hiatt JL: Color Atlas of Histology, 2nd ed. Baltimore, Williams & Wilkins, 1994

Guyton AC, Hall JE: Textbook of Medical Physiology, 9th ed. Philadelphia, WB Saunders, 1996

Innerarity SA: Fluids and Electrolytes, 3rd ed. Springhouse, PA, Springhouse Corp, 1997

Jean AT, et al: Bowes and Church's Food Values of Portions Commonly Used, 17th ed. Philadelphia, Lippincott-Raven, 1997

Junqueira LC, et al: Basic Histology, 9th ed. Englewood Cliffs, NJ, Prentice Hall, 1998

Martini F: Fundamentals of Anatomy and Physiology, 4th ed. Upper Saddle River, NJ, Prentice Hall, 1998

Moore KL: Clinically Oriented Anatomy, 4th ed. Baltimore, Williams & Wilkins, 1998

Moore KL, et al: Before We Are Born: Essentials of Embryology and Birth Defects, 5th ed. Philadelphia, WB Saunders, 1998

Schull PD: Assessment Made Incredibly Easy. Springhouse, PA, Springhouse Corp, 1997

Shier D, et al: Hole's Human Anatomy and Physiology, 7th ed. New York, McGraw-Hill, 1996

Shaw P: Fluids and Electrolytes. Springhouse, PA, Springhouse Corp, 1997

Tortora GJ, Grabowski SR: Principles of Anatomy and Physiology, 8th ed. Menlo Park, CA, Addison-Wesley, 1996

Whitney EN, Rolfes SR: Understanding Nutrition, 8th ed. Belmont, CA, West/Wadsworth, 1999

Willis MC: Medical Terminology. Baltimore, Williams & Wilkins, 1996

Glossary

Abduction (ab-DUK-shun) Movement away from the midline

Abortion (ah-BOR-shun) Loss of an embryo or fetus before the 20th week of pregnancy

Absorption (ab-SORP-shun) Transfer of digested nutrients from the digestive tract into the circulation

Accommodation (ah-kom-o-DA-shun) Coordinated changes in the eye that enable one to focus on near and far objects

Acetylcholine (as-e-til-KO-lene) **(ACh)** Neurotransmitter; released at synapses within the nervous system and at the neuromuscular junction

Acid (AH-sid) Substance that can donate a hydrogen ion to another substance

Acidosis (as-ih-DO-sis) Condition that results from a decrease in the pH of body fluids

Acquired immunodeficiency syndrome (AIDS) Viral disease that attacks the immune system, specifically the T-helper lymphocytes with CD4 receptors

Acrosome (AK-ro-some) Caplike structure over the head of the sperm cell that helps the sperm to penetrate the ovum

ACTH See Adrenocorticotropic hormone

Actin (AK-tin) One of the two contractile proteins in muscle cells, the other being myosin

Action potential Sudden change in the electric charge on a cell membrane, which then spreads along the membrane; nerve impulse

Active transport Movement of a substance into or out of a cell in a direction opposite that in which it would normally flow by diffusion

Adduction (ad-DUK-shun) Movement toward the midline

Adenosine triphosphate (ah-DEN-o-sene tri-FOS-fate) **(ATP)** Energy-storing compound found in all cells

ADH See Antidiuretic hormone

Adipose (AD-ih-pose) Referring to a type of connective tissue that stores fat

Adrenal (ah-DRE-nal) Endocrine gland located above the kidney; suprarenal gland

Adrenaline (ah-DREN-ah-lin) See Epinephrine

Adrenocorticotropic (ah-dre-no-kor-tih-ko-TRO-pik) **hormone (ACTH)** Hormone produced by the pituitary that stimulates the adrenal cortex

Aerobic (air-O-bik) Requiring oxygen

Afferent (AF-fer-ent) Carrying toward a given point, such as a sensory neuron that carries nerve impulses toward the central nervous system

Agglutination (ah-glu-tih-NA-shun) Clumping of cells due to an antigen–antibody reaction

AIDS See Acquired immunodeficiency syndrome

Albumin (al-BU-min) Protein in blood plasma and other body fluids; helps maintain the osmotic pressure of the blood

Aldosterone (al-DOS-ter-one) Hormone released by the adrenal cortex that promotes the reabsorption of sodium and water in the kidneys

Alkalosis (al-kah-LO-sis) Condition that results from an increase in the pH of body fluids

Allergy (AL-er-je) Tendency to react unfavorably to a substance that is normally harmless to most people; hypersensitivity

Alveolus (al-VE-o-lus) Small sac or pouch; usually a tiny air sac in the lungs through which gases are exchanged between the outside air and the blood; tooth socket; pl., alveoli

Amino (ah-ME-no) **acid** Building block of protein

Amniotic (am-ne-OT-ik) **sac** Fluid-filled sac that surrounds and cushions the developing fetus

Amphiarthrosis (am-fe-ar-THRO-sis) Slightly movable joint

Anabolism (ah-NAB-o-lizm) Metabolic building of simple compounds into more complex substances needed by the body

Anaerobic (an-air-O-bik) Not requiring oxygen

Anastomosis (ah-nas-to-MO-sis) Communication between two structures, such as blood vessels

Anatomy (ah-NAT-o-me) Study of body structure

Anemia (ah-NE-me-ah) Abnormally low level of hemoglobin or red cells in the blood, resulting in inadequate delivery of oxygen to the tissues

Angiotensin (an-je-o-TEN-sin) Substance formed in the blood by the action of the enzyme renin from the kidneys. It increases blood pressure by causing constriction of the blood vessels and stimulating the release of aldosterone from the adrenal cortex.

Anion (AN-i-on) Negatively charged particle (ion)

ANS See Autonomic nervous system

Antagonist (an-TAG-o-nist) Muscle that has an action opposite that of a given movement; substance that opposes the action of another substance

Anterior (an-TE-re-or) Toward the front or belly surface; ventral

Antibody (AN-te-bod-e) Substance produced in response to a specific antigen

Antidiuretic (an-ti-di-u-RET-ik) **hormone (ADH)** Hormone released from the posterior pituitary gland that increases the reabsorption of water in the kidneys, thus decreasing the volume of urine excreted

Antigen (AN-te-jen) **(Ag)** Foreign substance that produces an immune response

Antiserum (an-te-SE-rum) Serum containing antibodies; may be given for the purpose of providing passive immunity

Aorta (a-OR-tah) Large artery that carries blood out of the left ventricle of the heart

Apex (A-peks) The pointed region of a cone-shaped structure

Aponeurosis (ap-o-nu-RO-sis) Broad sheet of fibrous connective tissue that attaches muscle to bone or to other muscle

Appendicular (ap-en-DIK-u-lar) **skeleton** Part of the skeleton that includes the bones of the upper extremities, lower extremities, shoulder girdle, and hips

Arachnoid (ah-RAK-noyd) Middle layer of the meninges

Areolar (ah-RE-o-lar) Referring to loose connective tissue

Arteriole (ar-TE-re-ole) Vessel between a small artery and a capillary

Artery (AR-ter-e) Vessel that carries blood away from the heart

Atom (AT-om) Fundamental unit of a chemical element

ATP See Adenosine triphosphate

Atrioventricular (a-tre-o-ven-TRIK-u-lar) **(AV) node** Part of the conduction system of the heart

Atrium (A-tre-um) One of the two upper chambers of the heart; adj., atrial

Attenuated (ah-TEN-u-a-ted) Weakened

Autonomic (aw-to-NOM-ik) **nervous system (ANS)** The part of the nervous system that controls smooth muscle, cardiac muscle, and glands; motor portion of the visceral or involuntary nervous system

AV node See Atrioventricular node

Axial (AK-se-al) **skeleton** The part of the skeleton that includes the skull, spinal column, ribs, and sternum

Axilla (ak-SIL-ah) Hollow beneath the arm where it joins the body; armpit

Axon (AK-son) Fiber of a neuron that conducts impulses away from the cell body

Basal ganglia (BA-sal GANG-le-ah) Gray masses in the lower part of the forebrain that aid in muscle coordination

Base Substance that can accept a hydrogen ion (H^+); substance that donates a hydroxide ion (OH^-)

Basophil (BA-so-fil) Granular white blood cell that shows large, dark blue cytoplasmic granules when stained with basic stain

B cell Agranular white blood cell that produces antibodies in response to an antigen; B lymphocyte

Bile Substance produced in the liver that emulsifies fats

Blood urea nitrogen (BUN) Amount of nitrogen from urea in the blood; test to evaluate kidney function

Bradycardia (brad-e-KAR-de-ah) Heart rate of less than 60 beats per minute

Brain stem Portion of the brain that connects the cerebrum with the spinal cord; contains the midbrain, pons, and medulla oblongata

Bronchiole (BRONG-ke-ole) Microscopic terminal branch of a bronchus

Bronchus (BRONG-kus) Large air passageway in the lung; pl., bronchi (BRONG-ki)

Buffer (BUF-er) Substance that prevents sharp changes in the pH of a solution

BUN See Blood urea nitrogen

Bursa (BER-sah) Small, fluid-filled sac found in an area subject to stress around bones and joints; pl., bursae (BER-se)

Capillary (CAP-ih-lar-e) Microscopic vessel through which exchanges take place between the blood and the tissues

Carbohydrate (kar-bo-HI-drate) Simple sugar or compound made from simple sugars linked together, such as starch or glycogen

Carbon dioxide (di-OX-ide) (CO_2) The gaseous waste product of cellular metabolism

Carrier Individual who has a gene that is not expressed but that can be passed to offspring

Cartilage (KAR-tih-lij) Type of hard connective tissue

CAT See Computed tomography

Catabolism (kah-TAB-o-lizm) Metabolic breakdown of substances into simpler substances; includes the digestion of food and the oxidation of nutrient molecules for energy

Cation (KAT-i-on) Positively charged particle (ion)

Cecum (SE-kum) Small pouch at the beginning of the large intestine

Cell Basic unit of life

Cell membrane Outer covering of a cell; regulates what enters and leaves cell; plasma membrane

Cellular respiration Series of reactions by which nutrients are oxidized for energy within the cell

Central nervous system (CNS) Part of the nervous system that includes the brain and spinal cord

Centrifuge (SEN-trih-fuje) An instrument that separates materials in a mixture based on density

Centriole (SEN-tre-ole) Rod-shaped body near the nucleus of a cell; functions in cell division

Cerebellum (ser-eh-BEL-um) Small section of the brain located under the cerebral hemispheres; functions in coordination, balance, and muscle tone

Cerebral (SER-e-bral) **cortex** The very thin outer layer of gray matter on the surface of the cerebral hemispheres

Cerebrospinal (ser-e-bro-SPI-nal) **fluid (CSF)** Fluid that circulates in and around the brain and spinal cord

Cerebrum (SER-e-brum) Largest part of the brain; composed of the cerebral hemispheres

Cerumen (seh-RU-men) Earwax; adj., ceruminous (seh-RU-min-us)

Cervix (SER-vix) Constricted portion of an organ or part, such as the lower portion of the uterus; neck.; adj., cervical

Chemoreceptor (ke-mo-re-SEP-tor) Receptor that detects chemical changes

Cholesterol (ko-LES-ter-ol) An organic fatlike compound found in animal fat, bile, blood, myelin, liver, and other parts of the body

Choroid (KO-royd) Pigmented middle layer of the eye

Chromosome (KRO-mo-some) Dark-staining, threadlike body in the nucleus of a cell; contains genes that determine hereditary traits

Chyle (kile) Milky-appearing fluid absorbed into the lymphatic system from the small intestine. It consists of lymph and droplets of digested fat.

Chyme (kime) Mixture of partially digested food, water, and digestive juices that forms in the stomach

Cilia (SIL-e-ah) Hairs or hairlike processes, such as eyelashes or microscopic extensions from the surface of a cell; sing., cilium

Circumduction (ser-kum-DUK-shun) Circular movement at a joint

CNS See Central nervous system

Coagulation (ko-ag-u-LA-shun) Clotting, as of blood

Cochlea (KOK-le-ah) Coiled portion of the inner ear that contains the organ of hearing

Collagen (KOL-ah-jen) Flexible white protein that gives strength and resilience to connective tissue, such as bone and cartilage

Colloidal (kol-OYD-al) **suspension** Mixture in which suspended particles do not dissolve but remain distributed in the solvent because of their small size (*e.g.,* cytoplasm); colloid

Colon (KO-lon) Main portion of the large intestine

Complement (KOM-ple-ment) Group of blood proteins that helps antibodies to destroy foreign cells

Compliance (kom-PLI-ans) The ease with which the lungs and thorax can be expanded

Compound Substance composed of two or more chemical elements

Computed tomography (to-MOG-rah-fe) **(CT)** Imaging method in which multiple radiographic views taken from different angles are analyzed by computer to show a cross-section of an area; used to detect tumors and other abnormalities; also called computed axial tomography (CAT)

Congenital (con-JEN-ih-tal) Present at birth

Conjunctiva (kon-junk-TI-vah) Membrane that lines the eyelid and covers the anterior part of the sclera (white of the eye)

Contraception (con-trah-SEP-shun) Prevention of fertilization of an ovum or implantation of a fertilized ovum; birth control

Convergence (kon-VER-jens) The centering of both eyes on the same visual field

Cornea (KOR-ne-ah) Clear portion of the sclera that covers the front of the eye

Coronary (KOR-on-ar-e) Referring to the heart or to the arteries supplying blood to the heart

Corpus callosum (kal-O-sum) Thick bundle of myelinated nerve cell fibers, deep within the brain, that carries nerve impulses from one cerebral hemisphere to the other

Corpus luteum (LU-te-um) Yellow body formed from ovarian follicle after ovulation; produces progesterone

Cortex (KOR-tex) Outer layer of an organ, such as the brain, kidney, or adrenal gland

Covalent (KO-va-lent) **bond** Chemical bond formed by the sharing of electrons between atoms

CSF See Cerebrospinal fluid

CT See Computed tomography

Cutaneous (ku-TA-ne-us) Referring to the skin

Cytology (si-TOL-o-je) Study of cells

Cytoplasm (SI-to-plazm) Substance that fills the cell and holds the organelles

Defecation (def-e-KA-shun) Act of eliminating undigested waste from the digestive tract

Deglutition (deg-lu-TISH-un) Act of swallowing

Dehydration (de-hi-DRA-shun) Excessive loss of body fluid

Dendrite (DEN-drite) Fiber of a neuron that conducts impulses toward the cell body

Deoxyribonucleic (de-OK-se-ri-bo-nu-kle-ik) **acid (DNA)** Genetic material of the cell; makes up the chromosomes in the nucleus of the cell

Dermis (DER-mis) True skin; deeper part of the skin

Dextrose (DEK-strose) Glucose; simple sugar

Diabetes mellitus (di-ah-BE-teze mel-LI-tus) Disease of insufficient insulin in which excess glucose is found in blood and urine; characterized by abnormal metabolism of glucose, protein, and fat

Diagnosis (di-ag-NO-sis) Identification of an illness

Dialysis (di-AL-ih-sis) Method for separating molecules in solution based on differences in their ability to pass through a semipermeable membrane; method for removing nitrogen waste products from the body, as by hemodialysis or peritoneal dialysis

Diaphragm (DI-ah-fram) Dome-shaped muscle under the lungs that flattens during inhalation; separating membrane or structure

Diaphysis (di-AF-ih-sis) Shaft of a long bone

Diarthrosis (di-ar-THRO-sis) Freely movable joint; synovial joint

Diastole (di-AS-to-le) Relaxation phase of the cardiac cycle; adj., diastolic (di-as-TOL-ik)

Diencephalon (di-en-SEF-ah-lon) Region of the brain between the cerebral hemispheres and the midbrain; contains the thalamus, hypothalamus, and pituitary gland

Diffusion (dih-FU-zhun) Movement of molecules from a region where they are in higher concentration to a region where they are in lower concentration

Digestion (di-JEST-yun) Process of breaking down food into absorbable particles

Dilation (di-LA-shun) Widening of a part, such as the pupil of the eye, a blood vessel, or the uterine cervix; dilatation

Distal (DIS-tal) Farther from the origin of a structure or from a given reference point

DNA See Deoxyribonucleic acid

Dominant (DOM-ih-nant) Referring to a gene that is always expressed if present

Dorsal (DOR-sal) Toward the back; posterior

Duct Tube or vessel

Ductus deferens (DEF-er-enz) Tube that carries sperm cells from the testis to the urethra; vas deferens

Duodenum (du-o-DE-num) First portion of the small intestine

Dura mater (DU-rah MA-ter) Outermost layer of the meninges

ECG See Electrocardiograph

Echocardiograph (ek-o-KAR-de-o-graf) Instrument to study the heart by means of ultrasound; the record produced is an echocardiogram

EEG See Electroencephalograph

Effector (ef-FEK-tor) Muscle or gland that responds to a stimulus; effector organ

Efferent (EF-fer-ent) Carrying away from a given point, such as a motor neuron that carries nerve impulses away from the central nervous system

Ejaculation (e-jak-u-LA-shun) Expulsion of semen through the urethra

EKG See Electrocardiograph

Electrocardiograph (e-lek-tro-KAR-de-o-graf) **(ECG, EKG)** Instrument to study the electrical activity of the heart; record made is an electrocardiogram

Electroencephalograph (e-lek-tro-en-SEF-ah-lo-graf) **(EEG)** Instrument used to study electrical activity of the brain; record made is an electroencephalogram

Electrolyte (e-LEK-tro-lite) Compound that forms ions in solution; substance that conducts an electric current in solution

Electron (e-LEK-tron) Negatively charged particle located in an orbital outside the nucleus of an atom

Element (EL-eh-ment) One of the substances from which all matter is made; substance that cannot be decomposed into a simpler substance

Embryo (EM-bre-o) Developing offspring during the first 2 months of pregnancy

Emulsify (e-MUL-sih-fi) To break up fats into small particles; n., emulsification

Endocardium (en-do-KAR-de-um) Membrane that lines the heart chambers and covers the valves

Endocrine (EN-do-krin) Referring to a gland that secretes directly into the bloodstream

Endometrium (en-do-ME-tre-um) Lining of the uterus

Endoplasmic reticulum (en-do-PLAS-mik re-TIK-u-lum) **(ER)** Network of membranes in the cytoplasm of a cell

Endosteum (en-DOS-te-um) Thin membrane that lines the marrow cavity of a bone

Endothelium (en-do-THE-le-um) Epithelium that lines the heart, blood vessels, and lymphatic vessels

Enzyme (EN-zime) Organic catalyst; speeds the rate of a reaction but is not changed in the reaction

Eosinophil (e-o-SIN-o-fil) Granular white blood cell that shows beadlike, bright pink cytoplasmic granules when stained with acid stain; acidophil

Epicardium (ep-ih-KAR-de-um) Membrane that forms the outermost layer of the heart wall and is continuous with the lining of the pericardium; visceral pericardium

Epidermis (ep-ih-DER-mis) Outermost layer of the skin

Epiglottis (ep-e-GLOT-is) Leaf-shaped cartilage that covers the larynx during swallowing

Epimysium (ep-ih-MIS-e-um) Sheath of fibrous connective tissue that encloses a muscle

Epinephrine (ep-ih-NEF-rin) Neurotransmitter and hormone; released from neurons of the sympathetic nervous system and from the adrenal medulla; adrenaline

Epiphysis (eh-PIF-ih-sis) End of a long bone

Episiotomy (eh-piz-e-OT-o-me) Cutting of the perineum between the vaginal opening and the anus to reduce the tearing of tissue in childbirth

Epithelium (ep-ih-THE-le-um) One of the four main types of tissue; forms glands, covers surfaces, and lines cavities; adj., epithelial

ER See Endoplasmic reticulum

Erythrocyte (eh-RITH-ro-site) Red blood cell

Erythropoietin (EPO) (eh-rith-ro-POY-eh-tin) Hormone released from the kidney that stimulates the production of red blood cells in the bone marrow

Esophagus (eh-SOF-ah-gus) Tube that carries food from the throat to the stomach

Estrogen (ES-tro-jen) Group of female sex hormones that promotes development of the uterine lining and maintains secondary sex characteristics

Eustachian (u-STA-shun) **tube** Tube that connects the middle ear cavity to the throat; auditory tube

Eversion (e-VER-zhun) Turning outward, with reference to movement of the foot

Excretion (eks-KRE-shun) Removal and elimination of metabolic waste products from the blood

Exocrine (EK-so-krin) Referring to a gland that secretes through a duct

Extracellular (EK-strah-sel-u-lar) Outside the cell

Fascia (FASH-e-ah) Band or sheet of fibrous connective tissue

Fascicle (FAS-ih-kl) Small bundle, as of muscle cells or nerve cell fibers

Feces (FE-seze) Waste material discharged from the large intestine; excrement; stool

Feedback Return of information into a system, so that it can be used to regulate that system

Fertilization (fer-til-ih-ZA-shun) Union of an ovum and a spermatozoon

Fetus (FE-tus) Developing offspring from the third month of pregnancy until birth

Fibrin (FI-brin) Blood protein that forms a blood clot

Filtration (fil-TRA-shun) Movement of material through a semipermeable membrane under mechanical force

Fissure (FISH-ure) Deep groove

Flagellum (flah-JEL-lum) Long whiplike extension from a cell used for locomotion; pl., flagella

Flexion (FLEK-shun) Bending motion that decreases the angle between bones at a joint

Follicle (FOL-lih-kl) Sac or cavity, such as the ovarian follicle or hair follicle

Follicle-stimulating hormone (FSH) Hormone produced by the anterior pituitary that stimulates development of ova in the ovary and spermatozoa in the testes

Fontanelle (fon-tah-NEL) Area in the infant skull where bone formation has not yet occurred; "soft spot"

Foramen (fo-RA-men) Opening or passageway, as into or through a bone; pl., foramina (fo-RAM-in-ah)

Fornix (FOR-niks) A recess or archlike structure

Fossa (FOS-sah) Hollow or depression, as in a bone; pl., fossae (FOS-se)

Fovea (FO-ve-ah) Small pit or cup-shaped depression in a surface; the fovea centralis near the center of the retina is the point of sharpest vision

FSH See Follicle-stimulating hormone

Gamete (GAM-ete) Reproductive cell; ovum or spermatozoon

Gamma globulin (GLOB-u-lin) Protein fraction in the blood plasma that contains antibodies

Ganglion (GANG-le-on) Collection of nerve cell bodies located outside the central nervous system

Gastrointestinal (gas-tro-in-TES-tih-nal) **(GI)** Pertaining to the stomach and intestine or the digestive tract as a whole

Gene Hereditary unit; portion of the DNA on a chromosome

Genetic (jeh-NET-ik) Pertaining to the genes or heredity

Gestation (jes-TA-shun) Period of development from conception to birth

GH See Growth hormone

GI See Gastrointestinal

Gingiva (JIN-jih-vah) Tissue around the teeth; gum

Glial cells (GLI-al) The connective tissue cells of the nervous system; neuroglia

Glomerular (glo-MER-u-lar) **filtrate** Fluid and dissolved materials that leave the blood and enter the kidney nephron through Bowman's capsule

Glomerulus (glo-MER-u-lus) Cluster of capillaries in Bowman's capsule of the nephron

Glucose (GLU-kose) Simple sugar; main energy source for the cells; dextrose

Glycogen (GLI-ko-jen) Compound built from glucose molecules that is stored for energy in liver and muscles

Golgi (GOL-je) **apparatus** System of membranes in the cell that formulates special substances

Gonad (GO-nad) Sex gland; ovary or testis

Gonadotropin (gon-ah-do-TRO-pin) Hormone that acts on a reproductive gland (ovary or testis); *e.g.,* FSH, LH

Gram (g) Basic unit of weight in the metric system

Gray matter Nervous tissue composed of unmyelinated fibers and cell bodies

Growth hormone (GH) Hormone produced by anterior pituitary that promotes growth of tissues; somatotropin

Gustatory (GUS-tah-to-re) Pertaining to the sense of taste (gustation)

Gyrus (JI-rus) Raised area of the cerebral cortex; pl., gyri (JI-ri)

Helminth (HEL-minth) Worm

Hematocrit (he-MAT-o-krit) **(Hct)** Volume percentage of red blood cells in whole blood; packed cell volume

Hemoglobin (he-mo-GLO-bin) **(Hb)** Iron-containing protein in red blood cells that transports oxygen

Hemolysis (he-MOL-ih-sis) Rupture of red blood cells; v., hemolyze (HE-mo-lize)

Hemopoiesis (he-mo-poy-E-sis) Production of blood cells; hematopoiesis

Hemostasis (he-mo-STA-sis) Stoppage of bleeding

Heparin (HEP-ah-rin) Substance that prevents blood clotting; anticoagulant

Heredity (he-RED-ih-te) Transmission of characteristics from parent to offspring by means of the genes; the genetic makeup of the individual

Hilum (HI-lum) See hilus

Hilus (HI-lus) Area where vessels and nerves enter or leave an organ

Histamine (HIS-tah-mene) Substance released from tissues during an antigen–antibody reaction

Histology (his-TOL-o-je) Study of tissues

HIV See Human immunodeficiency virus

Homeostasis (ho-me-o-STA-sis) State of balance within the body; maintenance of body conditions within set limits

Hormone Secretion of an endocrine gland; chemical messenger that has specific regulatory effects on certain other cells

Human immunodeficiency virus (HIV) The virus that causes AIDS

Hydrolysis (hi-DROL-ih-sis) Splitting of large molecules by the addition of water, as in digestion

Hydroxycholecalciferol (hy-drok-se-ko-le-kal-SIF-eh-rol) The active form of vitamin D; promotes absorption of calcium in the small intestine to increase blood calcium levels

Hyperglycemia (hi-per-gli-SE-me-ah) Abnormal increase in the amount of glucose in the blood

Hypertonic (hi-per-TON-ik) Describing a solution that is more concentrated than the fluids within a cell

Hypophysis (hi-POF-ih-sis) Pituitary gland

Hypothalamus (hi-po-THAL-ah-mus) Region of the brain that controls the pituitary and maintains homeostasis

Hypotonic (hi-po-TON-ik) Describing a solution that is less concentrated than the fluids within a cell

ISH See Interstitial cell-stimulating hormone

Ileum (IL-e-um) The last portion of the small intestine

Immunity (ih-MU-nih-te) Power of an individual to resist or overcome the effects of a particular disease or other harmful agent

Immunization (ih-mu-nih-ZA-shun) Use of a vaccine to produce immunity

Implantation (im-plan-TA-shun) The embedding of the fertilized egg into the lining of the uterus

Inferior (in-FE-re-or) Below or lower

Inferior vena cava (VE-nah KA-vah) Large vein that drains the lower part of the body and empties into the right atrium of the heart

Insertion (in-SER-shun) End of a muscle attached to a movable part

Integument (in-TEG-u-ment) Skin; adj., integumentary

Intercellular (in-ter-SEL-u-lar) Between cells

Interleukin (in-ter-LU-kin) A substance released by a T cell or macrophage that stimulates other cells of the immune system

Interneuron (in-ter-NU-ron) A nerve cell that transmits impulses within the central nervous system

Interstitial (in-ter-STISH-al) Between; pertaining to spaces or structures in an organ between active tissues

Interstitial cell–stimulating hormone (ICSH) see Luteinizing hormone

Intracellular (in-trah-SEL-u-lar) Within a cell

Inversion (in-VER-zhun) Turning inward, with reference to movement of the foot

Ion (I-on) Charged particle formed when an electrolyte goes into solution

Iris (I-ris) Circular colored region of the eye around the pupil

Islets (I-lets) Groups of cells in the pancreas that produce hormones; islets of Langerhans (LAHNG-er-hanz)

Isometric (i-so-MET-rik) **contraction** Muscle contraction in which there is no change in muscle length but an increase in muscle tension, as in pushing against an immovable force

Isotonic (i-so-TON-ik) Describing a solution that has the same concentration as the fluid within a cell

Isotonic contraction Muscle contraction in which the tone within the muscle remains the same but the muscle shortens to produce movement

Isotope (I-so-tope) Form of an element that has the same atomic number as another but a different atomic weight

Jejunum (je-JU-num) Second portion of the small intestine

Joint Area of junction between two or more bones; articulation

Juxtaglomerular (juks-tah-glo-MER-u-lar) **(JG) apparatus** Structure in the kidney composed of cells of the afferent arteriole and distal convoluted tubule that secretes the enzyme renin when blood pressure decreases below a certain level

Keratin (KER-ah-tin) Protein that thickens and protects the skin; makes up hair and nails

Kidney (KID-ne) Organ of excretion

Kilocalorie (kil-o-KAL-o-re) A measure of the energy content of food. Technically, the amount of heat needed to raise l kg of water 1° centigrade

Lacrimal (LAK-rih-mal) Referring to tears or the tear glands

Lactation (lak-TA-shun) Secretion of milk

Lacteal (LAK-te-al) Capillary of the lymphatic system; drains digested fats from the villi of the small intestine

Lactic (LAK-tik) **acid** Organic acid that accumulates in muscle cells functioning without oxygen

Larynx (LAR-inks) Structure between the pharynx and trachea that contains the vocal cords; voice box

Lateral (LAT-er-al) Farther from the midline; toward the side

Lens Biconvex structure of the eye that changes in thickness to accommodate for near and far vision; crystalline lens

Leukocyte (LU-ko-site) White blood cell

LH See Luteinizing hormone

Ligament (LIG-ah-ment) Band of connective tissue that connects a bone to another bone; thickened portion or fold of the peritoneum that supports an organ or attaches it to another organ

Lipid (LIP-id) Type of organic compound, one example of which is a fat

Liter (LE-ter) **(L)** Basic unit of volume in the metric system.

Lumen (LU-men) Central opening of an organ or vessel

Lung Organ of respiration

Luteinizing (LU-te-in-i-zing) **hormone (LH)** Hormone produced by the anterior pituitary that induces ovulation and formation of the corpus luteum in females; in males, it stimulates cells in the testes to produce testosterone and is called *interstitial cell–stimulating hormone (ICSH)*

Lymph (limf) Fluid in the lymphatic system

Lymphatic duct Vessel of the lymphatic system

Lymph node Mass of lymphoid tissue along the path of a lymphatic vessel that filters lymph and harbors white blood cells active in immunity

Lymphocyte (LIM-fo-site) Agranular white blood cell that functions in immunity

Lysosome (LI-so-some) Cell organelle that contains digestive enzymes

Macrophage (MAK-ro-faj) Large phagocytic cell that develops from a monocyte

Macula (MAK-u-lah) Spot; flat, discolored spot on the skin, such as a freckle or measles lesion; small yellow spot in the retina of the eye that contains the fovea, the point of sharpest vision; also called macule

Magnetic resonance imaging (MRI) Method for studying tissue based on nuclear movement after exposure to radio waves in a powerful magnetic field

Major histocompatibility complex Group of genes that codes for specific proteins (antigens) on the surface of cells. These antigens are important in cross-matching for tissue transplantation. They are also important in immune reactions.

Malnutrition (mal-nu-TRISH-un) State resulting from lack of food, lack of an essential component of the diet, or faulty use of food in the diet

Mastication (mas-tih-KA-shun) Act of chewing

Matrix (MA-triks) The nonliving background material in a tissue; the intercellular material

Medial (ME-de-al) Nearer the midline of the body

Mediastinum (me-de-as-TI-num) Region between the lungs and the organs and vessels it contains

Medulla (meh-DUL-lah) Inner region of an organ; marrow

Medulla oblongata (ob-long-GAH-tah) Part of the brain stem that connects the brain to the spinal cord

Megakaryocyte (meg-ah-KAR-e-o-site) Very large cell that gives rise to blood platelets

Meiosis (mi-O-sis) Process of cell division that halves the chromosome number in the formation of the reproductive cells

Melanin (MEL-ah-nin) Dark pigment found in skin, hair, parts of the eye, and certain parts of the brain

Membrane Thin sheet of tissue

Mendelian (men-DE-le-en) **laws** Principles of heredity discovered by an Austrian monk named Gregor Mendel

Meninges (men-IN-jeze) Three layers of fibrous membranes that cover the brain and spinal cord

Menopause (MEN-o-pawz) Time at which menstruation ceases

Menses (MEN-seze) Monthly flow of blood from the female reproductive tract

Mesentery (MES-en-ter-e) Membranous peritoneal ligament that attaches the small intestine to the dorsal abdominal wall

Mesocolon (mes-o-KO-lon) Peritoneal ligament that attaches the colon to the dorsal abdominal wall

Metabolic rate Rate at which energy is released from nutrients in the cells

Metabolism (meh-TAB-o-lizm) Physical and chemical processes by which an organism is maintained

Meter (ME-ter) **(m)** Basic unit of length in the metric system

MHC See major histocompatibility complex

Micrometer (MI-kro-me-ter) **(μm)** 1/1000th of a millimeter; micron; also an instrument for measuring through a microscope (pronounced mi-KROM-eh-ter)

Microorganism (mi-kro-OR-gan-izm) Microscopic organism

Micturition (mik-tu-RISH-un) Act of urination; voiding of the urinary bladder

Midbrain Upper portion of the brainstem

Mineral (MIN-er-al) Inorganic substance; in the diet, an element needed in small amounts for health

Mitochondria (mi-to-KON-dre-ah) Cell organelles that manufacture ATP with the energy released from the oxidation of nutrients; sing., mitochondrion

Mitosis (mi-TO-sis) Type of cell division that produces two daughter cells exactly like the parent cell

Mitral (MI-tral) **valve** Valve between the left atrium and left ventricle of the heart; bicuspid valve

Mixture Blend of two or more substances

Molecule (MOL-eh-kule) Particle formed by chemical bonding of two or more atoms; smallest subunit of a compound

Monocyte (MON-o-site) Agranular white blood cell active in phagocytosis

Motor (MO-tor) Describing structures or activities involved in transmitting impulses away from the central nervous system; efferent

MRI See Magnetic resonance imaging

Mucosa (mu-KO-sah) Lining membrane that produces mucus; mucous membrane

Mucus (MU-kus) Thick protective fluid secreted by mucous membranes and glands; adj., mucous

Murmur Abnormal heart sound

Mutation (mu-TA-shun) Change in a gene or a chromosome

Myelin (MI-el-in) Fatty material that covers and insulates the axons of some neurons

Myocardium (mi-o-KAR-de-um) Middle layer of the heart wall; heart muscle

Myoglobin (MI-o-glo-bin) Compound that stores oxygen in muscle cells

Myometrium (mi-o-ME-tre-um) The muscular layer of the uterus

Myosin (MI-o-sin) One of the two contractile proteins in muscle cells, the other being actin

Negative feedback Self-regulating system in which the result of an action is the control over that action; a method for keeping body conditions within a normal range and maintaining homeostasis

Nephron (NEF-ron) Microscopic functional unit of the kidney

Nerve Bundle of neuron fibers outside the central nervous system

Nerve impulse Electrical charge that spreads along the membrane of a neuron; action potential

Neurilemma (nu-rih-LEM-mah) Thin sheath that covers certain peripheral axons; aids in regeneration of the axon

Neuroglia (nu-ROG-le-ah) Supporting and protective cells of the central nervous system; glial cells

Neuromuscular junction Point at which a nerve fiber contacts a muscle cell

Neuron (NU-ron) Conducting cell of the nervous system

Neurotransmitter (nu-ro-TRANS-mit-er) Chemical released from the ending of an axon that enables a nerve impulse to cross a synapse

Neutrophil (NU-tro-fil) Phagocytic granular white blood cell; polymorph; poly; PMN; seg

Node Small mass of tissue, such as a lymph node; space between cells in the myelin sheath

Norepinephrine (nor-epi-ih-NEF-rin) Neurotransmitter similar to epinephrine; noradrenaline

Nucleotide (NU-kle-o-tide) Building block of DNA and RNA

Nucleus (NU-kle-us) Largest organelle in the cell, containing the DNA, which directs all cell activities; group of neurons in the central nervous system; in chemistry, the central part of an atom

Olfactory (ol-FAK-to-re) Pertaining to the sense of smell (olfaction)

Ophthalmic (of-THAL-mik) Pertaining to the eye

Organ (OR-gan) Body part containing two or more tissues functioning together for specific purposes

Organelle (or-gan-EL) Specialized subdivision within a cell

Organic (or-GAN-ik) Referring to compounds found in living things and containing carbon, hydrogen, and oxygen

Organism (OR-gan-izm) Individual plant or animal; any organized living thing

Organ of Corti (KOR-te) Receptor for hearing located in the cochlea of the internal ear

Origin (OR-ih-jin) Source; beginning; end of a muscle attached to a nonmoving part

Osmosis (os-MO-sis) Movement of water through a semipermeable membrane

Osmotic (os-MOT-ik) **pressure** Tendency of a solution to draw water into it; is directly related to the concentration of the solution

Ossicle (OS-ih-kl) One of three small bones of the middle ear: malleus, incus, or stapes

Ossification (os-ih-fih-KA-shun) Process of bone formation

Osteoblast (OS-te-o-blast) Bone-forming cell

Osteoclast (OS-te-o-clast) Cell that breaks down bone

Osteocyte (OS-te-o-site) Mature bone cell; maintains bone but does not divide

Osteoporosis (os-te-o-po-RO-sis) Abnormal loss of bone tissue with tendency to fracture

Ovary (O-vah-re) Female reproductive gland

Ovulation (ov-u-LA-shun) Release of a mature ovum from a follicle in the ovary

Ovum (O-vum) Female reproductive cell or gamete; pl., ova

Oxidation (ok-sih-DA-shun) Chemical breakdown of nutrients for energy

Oxygen (OK-sih-jen) **(O_2)** The gas needed to break down nutrients completely for energy within the cell

Oxygen debt Amount of oxygen needed to reverse the effects produced in muscles functioning without oxygen

Pacemaker Sinoatrial (SA) node of the heart; group of cells or artificial device that sets the rate of heart contractions

Pancreas (PAN-kre-as) Large, elongated gland behind the stomach; produces digestive enzymes and hormones (*e.g.,* insulin)

Papilla (pah-PIL-ah) Small nipplelike projection or elevation

Parasite (PAR-ah-site) Organism that lives on or within another (the host) at the other's expense

Parasympathetic nervous system Craniosacral division of the autonomic nervous system

Parathyroid (par-ah-THI-royd) Any of four small glands embedded in the capsule enclosing the thy-roid gland; produces hormone that regulates calcium in the blood

Parietal (pah-RI-eh-tal) Pertaining to the wall of a space or cavity

Parturition (par-tu-RISH-un) Childbirth; labor

Pelvis (PEL-vis) Basinlike structure, such as the lower portion of the abdomen or the upper flared portion of the ureter (renal pelvis)

Penis (PE-nis) Male organ of urination and sexual intercourse

Pericardium (per-ih-KAR-de-um) Fibrous sac lined with serous membrane that encloses the heart

Perichondrium (per-ih-KON-dre-um) Layer of connective tissue that covers cartilage

Perineum (per-ih-NE-um) Pelvic floor; external region between the anus and genital organs

Periosteum (per-e-OS-te-um) Connective tissue membrane covering a bone

Peripheral (peh-RIF-er-al) Located away from a center or central structure

Peripheral nervous system (PNS) All the nerves and nervous tissue outside the central nervous system

Peristalsis (per-ih-STAL-sis) Wavelike movements in the wall of an organ or duct that propel its contents forward

Peritoneum (per-ih-to-NE-um) Serous membrane that lines the abdominal cavity and forms outer layer of abdominal organs; forms supporting ligaments for some organs

pH Symbol indicating hydrogen ion (H^+) concentration; scale that measures the relative acidity and alkalinity (basicity) of a solution

Phagocytosis (fag-o-si-TO-sis) Engulfing of large particles through the cell membrane

Pharynx (FAR-inks) Throat; passageway between the mouth and esophagus

Physiology (fiz-e-OL-o-je) Study of the function of living organisms

Pia mater (PI-ah MA-ter) Innermost layer of the meninges

Pineal (PIN-e-al) **gland** Gland in the brain that is regulated by light; involved in sleep–wake cycles

Pinocytosis (pi-no-si-TO-sis) Intake of small particles and droplets by the cell membrane

Pituitary (pih-TU-ih-tar-e) **gland** Endocrine gland located under and controlled by the hypothalamus; releases hormones that control other glands; hypophysis

Placenta (plah-SEN-tah) Structure that nourishes and maintains the developing individual during pregnancy

Plasma (PLAZ-mah) Liquid portion of the blood

Plasma cell Cell that produces antibodies; derived from a B cell

Plasma membrane Outer covering of a cell; regulates what enters and leaves cell; cell membrane

Platelet (PLATE-let) Cell fragment that forms a plug to stop bleeding and acts in blood clotting; thrombocyte

Pleura (PLU-rah) Serous membrane that lines the chest cavity and covers the lungs

Plexus (PLEK-sus) Network of vessels or nerves

PNS See Peripheral nervous system

Pons (ponz) Area of the brain between the midbrain and medulla; connects the cerebellum with the rest of the central nervous system

Portal system Venous system that carries blood to a second capillary bed before it returns to the heart

Posterior (pos-TE-re-or) Toward the back; dorsal

Prime mover Muscle that performs a given movement; agonist

Progeny (PROJ-eh-ne) Offspring

Progesterone (pro-JES-ter-one) Hormone produced by the corpus luteum and placenta; maintains the lining of the uterus for pregnancy

Proprioceptor (pro-pre-o-SEP-tor) Sensory receptor that aids in judging body position and changes in position; located in muscles, tendons, and joints

Prostaglandins (pros-tah-GLAN-dinz) Group of hormones produced by many cells; these hormones have a variety of effects

Protein (PRO-tene) Organic compound made of amino acids; contains nitrogen in addition to carbon, hydrogen, and oxygen (some contain sulfur or phosphorus)

Prothrombin (pro-THROM-bin) Clotting factor; converted to thrombin during blood clotting

Proton (PRO-ton) Positively charged particle in the nucleus of an atom

Proximal (PROK-sih-mal) Nearer to point of origin or to a reference point

Pulse Wave of increased pressure in the vessels produced by contraction of the heart

Pupil (PU-pil) Opening in the center of the eye through which light enters

Radiograph (RA-de-o-graf) Image produced by passage of x-rays through the body onto sensitized film

Receptor (re-SEP-tor) Specialized cell or ending of a sensory neuron that can be excited by a stimulus; also, a site in the cell membrane to which a special substance (*e.g.,* hormone, antibody) may attach

Recessive (re-SES-iv) Referring to a gene that is not expressed if a dominant gene for the same trait is present

Reflex (RE-flex) Simple, rapid, automatic response involving few neurons

Reflex arc (ark) A pathway through the nervous system from stimulus to response; commonly involves a receptor, sensory neuron, central neuron(s), motor neuron, and effector

Refraction (re-FRAK-shun) Bending of light rays as they pass from one medium to another of a different density

Renin (RE-nin) Enzyme released from the juxtaglomerular apparatus of the kidneys that indirectly increases blood pressure by activating angiotensin

Resorption (re-SORP-shun) Loss of substance, such as that of bone or a tooth

Respiration (res-pih-RA-shun) Exchange of oxygen and carbon dioxide between the outside air and body cells

Reticuloendothelial (reh-tik-u-lo-en-do-THE-le-al) **system** Protective system consisting of highly phagocytic cells in body fluids and tissues, such as the spleen, lymph nodes, bone marrow, and liver

Retina (RET-ih-nah) Innermost layer of the eye; contains light-sensitive cells (rods and cones)

Retroperitoneal (ret-ro-per-ih-to-NE-al) Behind the peritoneum, as are the kidneys, pancreas, and abdominal aorta

Ribonucleic (RI-bo-nu-kle-ik) **acid (RNA)** Substance needed for protein manufacture in the cell

Ribosome (RI-bo-some) Small body in the cytoplasm of a cell that is a site of protein manufacture

RNA See Ribonucleic acid

Rugae (RU-je) Folds in the lining of an organ, such as the stomach or urinary bladder; sing., ruga (RU-gah)

Saliva (sah-LI-vah) Secretion of the salivary glands; moistens food and contains an enzyme that digests starch

SA node See Sinoatrial node

Schwann cell (shvahn) Cell in the nervous system

that produces the myelin sheath around peripheral axons

Sclera (SKLE-rah) Outermost layer of the eye; made of tough connective tissue; "white" of the eye

Scrotum (SKRO-tum) Sac in which testes are suspended

Sebum (SE-bum) Oily secretion that lubricates the skin; adj., sebaceous (se-BA-shus)

Semen (SE-men) Mixture of sperm cells and secretions from several glands of the male reproductive tract

Semicircular canal Bony canal in the internal ear that contains receptors for the sense of dynamic equilibrium; there are three semicircular canals in each ear

Sensory (SEN-so-re) Describing cells or activities involved in transmitting impulses toward the central nervous system; afferent

Sensory adaptation Gradual loss of sensation when sensory receptors are exposed to continuous stimulation

Septum (SEP-tum) Dividing wall, as between the chambers of the heart or the nasal cavities

Serosa (se-RO-sah) Serous membrane; epithelial membrane that secretes a thin, watery fluid

Serum (SE-rum) Liquid portion of blood without clotting factors; thin, watery fluid; adj., serous (SE-rus)

Sex-linked Referring to a gene carried on a sex chromosome, usually the X chromosome

Sinoatrial (si-no-A-tre-al) **(SA) node** Tissue in the upper wall of the right atrium that sets the rate of heart contractions; pacemaker of the heart

Sinusoid (SI-nus-oyd) Enlarged capillary that serves as a blood channel

Solute (SOL-ute) Substance that is dissolved in another substance (the solvent)

Solution (so-LU-shun) Mixture, the components of which are evenly distributed

Solvent (SOL-vent) Substance in which another substance (the solute) is dissolved

Somatic nervous system The division of the nervous system that controls voluntary activities and stimulates skeletal muscle

Spermatozoon (sper-mah-to-ZO-on) Male reproductive cell or gamete; pl., spermatozoa

Sphincter (SFINK-ter) Muscular ring that regulates the size of an opening

Sphygmomanometer (sfig-mo-mah-NOM-eh-ter) Device used to measure blood pressure

Spleen Lymphoid organ in the upper left region of the abdomen

Stasis (STA-sis) Stoppage in the normal flow of fluids, such as blood, lymph, urine, or contents of the digestive tract

Stenosis (sten-O-sis) Narrowing of a duct or canal

Sterilization (ster-ih-li-ZA-shun) Process of killing every living microorganism on or in an object; procedure that makes an individual incapable of reproduction

Steroid (STE-royd) Category of lipids that includes the hormones of the sex glands and the adrenal cortex

Stethoscope (STETH-o-skope) Instrument for conveying sounds from the patient's body to the examiner's ears

Stimulus (STIM-u-lus) Change in the external or internal environment that produces a response

Subcutaneous (sub-ku-TA-ne-us) Under the skin

Sudoriferous (su-do-RIF-er-us) Producing sweat; referring to the sweat glands

Sulcus (SUL-kus) Shallow groove, as between convolutions of the cerebral cortex; pl., sulci (SUL-si)

Superior (su-PE-re-or) Above; in a higher position

Superior vena cava (VE-nah KA-vah) Large vein that drains the upper part of the body and empties into the right atrium of the heart

Surfactant (sur-FAK-tant) Substance in the alveoli that prevents their collapse by reducing surface tension of the fluids within

Suspension (sus-PEN-shun) Mixture that will separate unless shaken

Suture (SU-chur) Type of joint in which bone surfaces are closely united, as in the skull; stitch used in surgery to bring parts together or to stitch parts together in surgery

Sympathetic nervous system Thoracolumbar division of the autonomic nervous system

Synapse (SIN-aps) Junction between two neurons or between a neuron and an effector

Synarthrosis (sin-ar-THRO-sis) Immovable joint

Synovial (sin-O-ve-al) Pertaining to a thick lubricating fluid found in joints, bursae, and tendon sheaths; pertaining to a freely movable (diarthrotic) joint

System (SIS-tem) Group of organs functioning together for the same general purposes

Systemic (sis-TEM-ik) Referring to a generalized infection or condition

Systole (SIS-to-le) Contraction phase of the cardiac cycle; adj., systolic (sis-TOL-ik)

Tachycardia (tak-e-KAR-de-ah) Heart rate more than 100 beats per minute

Tachypnea (tak-IP-ne-ah) Excessive rate of respiration

Target tissue Tissue that is capable of responding to a specific hormone

T cell Lymphocyte active in immunity that matures in the thymus gland; destroys foreign cells directly; T lymphocyte

Tendon (TEN-don) Cord of fibrous connective tissue that attaches a muscle to a bone

Testis (TES-tis) Male reproductive gland; pl., testes (TES-teze)

Testosterone (tes-TOS-ter-one) Male sex hormone produced in the testes; promotes the development of sperm cells and maintains secondary sex characteristics

Tetanus (TET-an-us) Constant contraction of a muscle; infectious disease caused by a bacterium (*Clostridium tetani*); lockjaw

Tetany (TET-an-e) Muscle spasms due to abnormal calcium metabolism, as in parathyroid deficiency

Thalamus (THAL-ah-mus) Region of the brain located in the diencephalon; chief relay center for sensory impulses traveling to the cerebral cortex

Thorax (THO-raks) Chest; adj., thoracic (tho-RAS-ik)

Thrombocyte (THROM-bo-site) Blood platelet; cell fragment that participates in clotting

Thymus (THI-mus) Endocrine gland in the upper portion of the chest; stimulates development of T cells

Thyroid (THI-royd) Endocrine gland in the neck

Thyroid-stimulating hormone (TSH) Hormone produced by the anterior pituitary that stimulates the thyroid gland

Thyroxine (thi-ROK-sin) Hormone produced by the thyroid gland; increases metabolic rate and needed for normal growth; T_4

Tissue Group of similar cells that performs a specialized function

Tonsil (TON-sil) Mass of lymphoid tissue in the region of the pharynx

Tonus (TO-nus) Partially contracted state of muscle; also, tone

Toxin (TOK-sin) Poison

Toxoid (TOK-soyd) Altered toxin used to produce active immunity

Trachea (TRA-ke-ah) Tube that extends from the larynx to the bronchi; windpipe

Tract Bundle of neuron fibers within the central nervous system

Trait Characteristic

Tricuspid (tri-KUS-pid) **valve** Valve between the right atrium and right ventricle of the heart

Triiodothyronine (tri-i-o-do-THI-ro-nin) Thyroid hormone that functions with thyroxine to raise cellular metabolism; T_3

TSH See Thyroid-stimulating hormone

Tympanic (tim-PAN-ik) **membrane** Membrane between the external and middle ear that transmits sound waves to the bones of the middle ear; eardrum

Umbilical (um-BIL-ih-kal) **cord** Structure that connects the fetus with the placenta; contains vessels that carry blood between the fetus and placenta

Umbilicus (um-BIL-ih-kus) Small scar on the abdomen that marks the former attachment of the umbilical cord to the fetus; navel

Urea (u-RE-ah) Nitrogen waste product excreted in the urine; end product of protein metabolism

Ureter (U-re-ter) Tube that carries urine from the kidney to the urinary bladder

Urethra (u-RE-thrah) Tube that carries urine from the urinary bladder to the outside of the body

Urinary bladder Hollow organ that stores urine until it is eliminated

Urine (U-rin) Liquid waste excreted by the kidneys

Uterus (U-ter-us) Muscular, pear-shaped organ in the female pelvis within which the fetus develops during pregnancy

Uvea (U-ve-ah) Middle coat of the eye, including the choroid, iris, and ciliary body; vascular and pigmented structures of the eye

Uvula (U-vu-lah) Soft, fleshy, V-shaped mass that hangs from the soft palate

Vaccine (vak-SENE) Substance used to produce active immunity; usually, a suspension of attenuated or killed pathogens given by inoculation to prevent a specific disease

Vagina (vah-JI-nah) Lower part of the birth canal that opens to the outside of the body; female organ of sexual intercourse

Valve Structure that prevents fluid from flowing backward, as in the heart, veins, and lymphatic vessels

Vas deferens (DEF-er-enz) Tube that carries sperm cells from the testis to the urethra; ductus deferens

Vasectomy (vah-SEK-to-me) Surgical removal of part or all of the ductus (vas) deferens; usually done on both sides to produce sterility

Vasoconstriction (vas-o-kon-STRIK-shun) Decrease in the diameter of a blood vessel

Vasodilation (vas-o-di-LA-shun) Increase in the diameter of a blood vessel

Vector (VEK-tor) An insect or other animal that transmits a disease-causing organism from one host to another

Vein (vane) Vessel that carries blood toward the heart

Vena cava (VE-nah KA-vah) A large vein that carries blood into the right atrium of the heart; superior vena cava or inferior vena cava

Venous sinus (VE-nus SI-nus) Large channel that drains deoxygenated blood

Ventilation (ven-tih-LA-shun) Movement of air into and out of the lungs

Ventral (VEN-tral) Toward the front or belly surface; anterior

Ventricle (VEN-trih-kl) Cavity or chamber; one of the two lower chambers of the heart; one of the four chambers in the brain in which cerebrospinal fluid is produced; adj., ventricular (ven-TRIK-u-lar)

Venule (VEN-ule) Very small vein that collects blood from the capillaries

Vertebra (VER-teh-brah) A bone of the spinal column; pl., vertebrae (VER-teh-bre)

Vestibule (VES-tih-bule) Part of the internal ear that contains receptors for the sense of equilibrium; any space at the entrance to a canal or organ

Villi (VIL-li) Small fingerlike projections from the surface of a membrane; projections in the lining of the small intestine through which digested food is absorbed; sing., villus

Viscera (VIS-er-ah) Organs in the ventral body cavities, especially the abdominal organs

Vitamin (VI-tah-min) Organic compound needed in small amounts for health

Vitreous (VIT-re-us) **body** Soft, jellylike substance that fills the eyeball and holds the shape of the eye; vitreous humor

White matter Nervous tissue composed of myelinated fibers

X-ray Ray or radiation of extremely short wavelength that can penetrate opaque substances and affect photographic plates and fluorescent screens

Zygote (ZI-gote) Fertilized ovum; cell formed by the union of a sperm and an egg

Biologic Terminology

Biologic terminology is based on an understanding of a relatively few basic elements. These elements—roots, prefixes, and suffixes—form the foundation of almost all biologic terms. A useful way to familiarize yourself with each term is to learn to pronounce it correctly and say it aloud several times. Soon it will become an integral part of your vocabulary.

The foundation of a word is the word root. Examples of word roots are *abdomin-,* referring to the belly region; and *aden-,* pertaining to a gland. A word root is often followed by a vowel to facilitate pronunciation, as in *abdomino-* and *adeno-.* We then refer to it as a "combining form." The hyphen added to a combining form indicates that it is not a complete word; if the hyphen precedes the combining form, then it commonly appears as the ending, as in -cyte, meaning "cell."

A prefix is a part of a word that precedes the word root and changes its meaning. For example, the prefix *sub-* in *subcutaneous* means "below." A suffix, or word ending, is a part that follows the word root and adds to or changes its meaning. The suffix *-ase* means "enzyme", as in *lipase,* an enzyme that digests fat.

Many biologic words are compound words; that is, they are made up of more than one root or combining form. Examples of such compound words are *histology* (study of tissues), *erythrocyte* (red blood cell), and many more difficult words, such as *sternoclavicular* (indicating relations to both the sternum and the clavicle).

A general knowledge of language structure and spelling rules is also helpful in mastering biologic terminology. For example, adjectives include words that end in *-al,* as in *sternal* (the noun is *sternum*), and words that end in *-ous,* as in *mucous* (the noun is *mucus*).

The following list includes some of the most commonly used word roots, combining forms, prefixes, and suffixes, as well as examples of their use.

a-, an- absent, deficient, lack of: *amorphous, atrophy, anaerobic.*

ab- away from: *abduction, aboral*

abdomin-, abdomino- belly or abdomen: *abdominal, abdominopelvic*

acou- hearing, sound: *acoustic*

acr-, acro- extreme ends of a part, especially of the extremities: *acromion, acrosome*

ad- (sometimes converted to *ac,-, af-, ag-, ap-, as-, at-,*) toward, added to, near: *adrenal, accretion, agglomerated, afferent*

aden-, adeno-, gland: *adenoid, adenocyte*

-agogue inducing, leading, stimulating: *chologogue, galactagogue*

amb-, ambi-, both, on two sides: *ambidextrous, ambivalent*

angio- vessel: *angiogram, angiotensin*

ant-, anti- against; to prevent, suppress, or destroy: *antibiotic, anticoagulant, antihistamine*

ante- before, ahead of: *antecedent, antenatal, antepartum*

antero- position ahead of or in front of (*i.e.,* anterior to) another part: *anterolateral, anteroventral*

arthr-, arthro- joint or articulation: *arthritis, arthroscope, arthrosis*

-ase enzyme: *lipase, protease*

audio- sound, hearing: *audiogenic, audiometry, audiovisual*

aur- ear: *aural, auricle*

aut-, auto- self: *autodigestion, autoimmune, autonomic*

bi- two, twice: *bifurcate, bisexual*

bio- life, living organism: *antibiotic, biochemistry, biology*

blast-, blasto-, -blast early stage, immature cell or bud: *blastula, blastophore, erythroblast*

bleph-, blephar-, blepharo- eyelid, eyelash: *blepharoptosis, blepharospasm*

brachi- arm: *brachial, brachiocephalic*

brady- slow: *bradycardia*

bronch-, broncho-, bronchi- windpipe or other air tubes: *bronchiole, bronchoscope*

bucc- cheek: *buccal*

cardi-, cardia-, cardio- heart: *cardiac, cardiologist, cardiovascular*

centi- relating to 100 (used in naming units of measurements): *centigrade, centimeter*

cephal-, cephalo- head: *cephalic, cephalopelvic*

cervi- neck: *cervical, cervix*

cheil-, cheilo-, lips; brim or edge: *cheilitis, cheilosis*

cheir-, cheiro- (also written **chir-, chiro-**) hand: *cheiromegaly, chiropractic*

chol-, chole-, cholo- bile, gall: *chologogue, cholecyst, cholecystokinin*

chondr-, chondri-, chondro- cartilage: *chondrocyte, hypochondrium, perichondrium*

circum- around, surrounding: *circumorbital, circumrenal, circumduction*

-clast break: *osteoclast*

colp-, colpo- vagina: *colposcope, colpotomy*

contra- opposed, against: *contraindication, contralateral*

cost-, costa-, costo- ribs: *intercostal, costosternal*

counter- against, opposite to: *counteract, counterirritation, countertraction*

crani-, cranio- skull: *craniosacral, cranium*

crypt-, crypto- hidden, concealed: *cryptic, cryptogenic*

cut- skin: *cuticle, subcutaneous*

cysti-, cysto- sac, bladder: *cystic, cystitis, cystoscope*

cyt-, cyto-, cyte cell: *cytoplasm, cytology, osteocyte*

dactyl-, dactylo- digits (usually fingers, but sometimes toes): *dactylitis, polydactyly*

de- remove: *decompose, deoxygenate, detoxify*

dendr- tree: *dendrite*

dent-, denti- dento-, tooth: *dentition, dentin, dentifrice*

derm-, derma-, dermo-, dermat-, dermato- skin: *dermatitis, dermatology, dermis*

di-, diplo- twice, double: *dimorphism, diarthrosis*

dia- through, between, across, apart: *diaphragm, diaphysis*

dis- apart, away from: *dissect, dissolve, distal*

dors-, dorsi-, dorso- back (in the human, this combining form refers to the same regions as postero-): *dorsiflexion, dorsonuchal*

-ectasis expansion, dilation, stretching: *angiectasis, bronchiectasis*

ecto- outside, external: *ectoderm, ectogenous, ectoplasm*

-emia blood: *anemia, glycemia, hyperemia*

encephal-, encephalo- brain: *diencephalon, encephalogram*

end-, endo- within, innermost: *endarterial, endocardium, endothelium*

enter-, entero- intestine: *enteric, mesentery*

epi- on, upon: *epidermis, erythropoiesis*

eryth-, erythro- red: *erythrocyte, erythropoiesis*

-esthesia sensation: *anesthesia, paresthesia*

eu- well, normal, good: *euphoria, eupnea*

ex-, exo- outside, out of, away from: *excretion, exocrine, exophthalmic*

extra- beyond, outside of, in addition to: *extracellular, extrasystole, extravascular*

fascicle- fibrous connective tissue layers: *fascia, fascicle*

-fer to bear, to carry: *afferent, efferent, transfer*

fibr-, fibro- threadlike structures, fibers: *fibrillation, fibroblast, myofibril*

galact-, galacta-, galacto- milk: *galactagogue, galactose*

gastr-, gastro- stomach: *gastric, gastrointestinal*

gen-, geno- a relationship to reproduction or sex: *genetic, genotype, regenerate*

-gen an agent that produces or originates: *allergen, fibrinogen, pepsinogen*

-genic produced from, producing: *psychogenic, neurogenic*

genito- organs of reproduction: *genitoplasty, genitourinary*

-geny manner of origin, development or production: *ontogeny, progeny*

glio-, -glia gluey material; specifically, the connective tissue of the central nervous system: *gliogenous, neuroglia*

gloss-, glosso- tongue: *glossal, glossopharyngeal*

gly-, glyco- sweet, relating to sugar: *glycogen, glycolytic, glycosuria*

-gnath, gnatho- related to the jaw: *agnathous, prognathic*

gon- seed, knee: *gonad, gonarthritis*

-gram   record, that which is recorded: *electrocardiogram, hologram, tomogram*

-graph   instrument for recording: *electroencephalograph, sonograph*

gyn-, gyne-, gyneco-, gyno-   female, woman: *gynecology, gynandromorph*

hem-, hema-, hemato-, hemo-   blood: *hematology, hemoglobin, hemostasis*

hemi-   one half: *hemisphere, hemilateral, hemiplegia*

hepat-, hepato-   liver: *hepatic, hepatogenous*

heter-, hetero-   other, different: *heterogeneous, heterosexual, heterozygous*

hist-, histo-, histio-   tissue: *histology, histiocyte*

homeo-, homo-   unchanging, the same: *hemeostasis, homosexual*

hydr-, hydro-   water: *dehydration, hydrolysis*

hyper-   above, over, excessive: *hyperglycemia, hypersecretion, hypertonic*

hypo-   deficient, below, beneath: *hypochondrium, hypodermic, hypogastrium*

hyster-, hystero-   uterus: *hysterectomy*

-ia   state of: *myopia, hypochondria, phobia*

idio-   self, one's own, separate, distinct: *idiopathic, idiosyncrasy*

im-, in-   in, into, lacking: *implantation, inanimate, infiltration*

infra-   below: *infraspinous, infracortical*

inter-   between: *intercostal, interstitial*

intra-   within a part or structure: *intracranial, intracellular, intraocular*

iso-   equal: *isotonic, isometric*

juxta-   next to: *juxtaglomerular*

karyo-   nucleus: *karyotype, karyoplasm*

kerat-, kerato-   cornea of the eye, certain horny tissues: *keratin, keratoplasty*

lacri-   tear: *lacrimal*

lact-, lacto-   milk: *lactation, lactogenic*

later-   side: *lateral*

leuk-, leuko-   (also written as *leuc-, leuco-*) white: *leukemia, leukocyte, leukoplakia*

lig-   bind: *ligament, ligature*

-logy   study of: *cytology, endocrinology, physiology*

lyso-, -lysis   flowing, loosening, dissolution (dissolving of): *hemolysis, paralysis, lysome*

macro-   large, abnormal length: *macrophage, macroblast.* See also **-mega, megalo-**

mast-, masto-   breast: *mastectomy, mastitis*

meg-, mega-, megal-, megalo-   unusually or excessively large: *megacolon, megaloblast, megakaryocyte*

men-, meno-   physiologic uterine bleeding: *menses, menopause*

mening-, meningo-   membranes covering the brain and spinal cord: *meninges, meningitis*

mes-, mesa-, meso-   middle, midline: *mesencephalon, mesoderm, mesothelium*

meta-   change, beyond, after, over, near: *metabolism, metacarpal, metaplasia*

-meter   measure: *hemocytometer, sphygmomanometer*

micro-   very small: *microscope, microbiology, micrometer*

mono-   single: *monocular, monocyte, mononucleosis*

my-, myo-   muscle: *myenteron, myocardium, myometrium*

myel-, myelo-   marrow (often used in reference to the spinal cord): *myelin, myeloid, myeloblast, myoglobin*

neo-   new, strange: *neocortex, neonatal, neoplasm*

neph-, nephro-   kidney: *nephrology, nephron*

neur-, neuro-   nerve: *neurilemma, neuroglia, neuron*

noct-, nocti-   night: *noctambulation, noctiphobia, nocturnal*

ocul-, oculo-   eye: *ocular, oculist, oculomotor*

odont-, odonto-   tooth, teeth: *odontogenesis, orthodontics*

-oid   likeness, resemblance: *lymphoid, myeloid*

olig-, oligo-   few, a deficiency: *oligodendrocyte, oligospermia, oliguria*

onych-, onycho-   nails: *eponychium, hyponychium*

oo-, ovi-, ovo-   ovum, egg: *oocyte, oviduct, ovoplasm* (do not confuse with **oophor-**)

oophor-, oophoro-   ovary: *oophorectomy, oophoritis, oophoron.* See also **ovar-**

ophthalm-, ophthalmo-   eye: *ophthalmia, ophthalmologist, ophthalmoscope*

orth-, ortho-   straight, normal: *orthopedics, orthopnea, orthosis*

oscillo-   to swing to and fro: *oscilloscope*

oss-, osseo-, ossi-, oste-, osteo-   bone, bone tissue: *osseous, ossicle, osteocyte*

ot-, oto-   ear: *otolith, otology*

ovar-, ovario-   ovary: *ovarian, ovariotomy.* See also **oophor-**

ox-, oxia   pertaining to oxygen: *anoxia, hypoxemia*

para-   near, beyond, apart from, beside: *paramedical, parametrium, parathyroid, parasagittal*

ped-, pedia-   child, foot: *pedal, pedicel, pediatrician*

per-   through, extremely: *percutaneous, perfusion*

peri-   around: *pericardium, perichondrium*

phag-, phago-   to eat, to ingest: *phage, phagocyte*

-phagia, -phagy   eating, swallowing: *aphagia, dysphagia*

-phasia   speech, ability to talk: *aphasia, dysphasia*

-phil, -philic   to be fond of, to like (have an affinity for): *eosinophil, chromophilic, hydrophilic*

phot-, photo-   light: *photoreceptor, photophobia*

pile-, pili-, pilo-   hair, resembling hair: *pileous, piliation, pilonidal*

pleur-, pleuro-   pleura; serous membrane covering the lung and lining the chest cavity: *pleural, pleurisy*

-pnea   air, breathing: *dyspnea, eupnea*

pneum-, pneuma-, pneumo-, pneumon-, pneumato-   lung, air: *pneumatic, pneumograph, pneumonia*

pod-, podo-   foot: *podiatry, podocyte*

-poiesis   making, forming: *erythropoiesis, hematopoiesis*

poly-   many: *polychromic, polymer, polymorphic*

post-   behind, after, following: *postnatal, postocular, postpartum*

pre-   before, ahead of: *premature, premolar, prenatal*

pro-   in front of, before: *prosencephalon, prolactin, prothrombin*

proct-, procto-   rectum: *proctoscope, proctologist*

pseud-, pseudo-   false: *pseudopod, pseudostratified*

psych-, psycho-   mind: *psychosomatic, psychotherapy*

pulmo-, pulmono-   lung: *pulmonic, pulmonology*

pyel-, pyelo-   kidney pelvis: *pyelitis, pyelogram*

rachi-, rachio-   spine: *rachidial, rachicentesis*

radio-   emission of rays or radiation: *radioactive, radiography, radiology*

re-   again, back: *reabsorption, reaction, regenerate*

ren-, reno-   kidney: *renal, renin*

retro-   backward, located behind: *retrocecal, retroperitoneal*

rheo-   flow of matter, or of a current of electricity: *rheostat, rheoscope*

rhin-, rhino-   nose: *rhinencephalon, rhinitis, rhinoplasty*

salping-, salpingo-   tube: *salpingitis, salpingoscopy*

scler-, sclero-   hardness: *sclera, sclerosis*

-scope   instrument used to look into or examine a part: *bronchoscope, endoscope, arthroscope*

semi-   mild, partial, half: *semiflexion, semilunar, semipermeable*

-sis   condition or process, usually abnormal: *dermatosis, osteoporosis*

somat-, somato-   body: *somatic, somatotype*

sono-   sound: *sonogram, sonography*

splanchn-, splanchno-   internal organs: *splanchnic, splanchnoptosis*

sta-, stat-   stop, stand still, remain at rest: *stasis, static*

sthen-, stheno-, sthenia, -sthenic   strength: *asthenic, calisthenics*

stomato-   mouth: *stomatitis*

sub-   under, below, near, almost: *subclavian, subcutaneous, subluxation*

super-   over, above, excessive: *superego, supernatant, superficial*

supra-   location above or over: *supranasal, suprarenal*

sym-, syn-   with, together: *symbiotic, symphysis, synapse*

tacho-, tachy-   rapid, fast, swift: *tachycardia, tachypnea*

tars-, tarso-   eyelid, foot: *metatarsal, tarsitis, tarsoplasty*

tax-, -taxia, -taxis   order, arrangement: *chemotaxis, taxonomy*

tens-   stretch, pull: *extension, tensor*

therm-, thermo-, -thermy   heat: *thermometer, thermotaxis*

tox-, toxic-, toxico-   poison: *toxemia, toxicology, toxin*

trache-, tracheo-   trachea, windpipe: *tracheal, tracheotomy*

trans-   across, through, beyond: *transorbital, transpiration, transplant, transport*

tri-   three: *triad, triceps*

trich-, tricho-   hair: *trichology, trichosis*

-trophic, -trophy   nutrition (nurture): *atrophic, hypertrophy*

-tropic   turning around, influencing, changing: *corticotropic, gonadotropic, thyrotropic*

ultra-   beyond or excessive: *ultrasound, ultraviolet, ultrastructure*

uni-   one: *unilateral, uniovular, unicellular*

-uria   urine: *glycosuria, hematuria, pyuria*

vas-, vaso-   vessel, duct: *vascular, vasectomy, vasodilation*

viscer-, viscero-   internal organs, viscera: *visceral, visceroptosis*

Appendices

Appendix 1. Metric Measurements

UNIT	ABBREVIATION	METRIC EQUIVALENT	U.S. EQUIVALENT
Units of length			
Kilometer	km	1000 meters	0.62 miles; 1.6 km/mile
Meter*	m	100 cm; 1000 mm	39.4 inches, 1.1 yards
Centimeter	cm	1/100 m; 0.01 m	0.39 inches; 2.5 cm/inch
Millimeter	mm	1/1000 m; 0.001 m	0.039 inches; 25 mm/inch
Micrometer	μm	1/1000 mm; 0.001 mm	
Units of weight			
Kilogram	kg	1000 g	2.2 lb
Gram*	g	1000 mg	0.035 oz.; 28.5 g/oz
Milligram	mg	1/1000 g; 0.001 g	
Microgram	μg	1/1000 mg; 0.001 mg	
Units of volume			
Liter*	L	1000 mL	1.06 qt
Deciliter	dL	1/10 L; 0.1 L	
Milliliter	mL	1/1000 L; 0.001 L	0.034 oz., 29.4 mL/oz
Microliter	μL	1/1000 mL; 0.001 mL	

*Basic unit.

365

Appendix 2. Celsius–Fahrenheit Temperature Conversion Scale

CELSIUS TO FAHRENHEIT

Use the following formula to convert Celsius readings to Fahrenheit readings:

$$°F = 9/5°C + 32$$

For example, if the Celsius reading is 37°

$$°F = (9/5 × 37) + 32$$
$$= 66.6 + 32$$
$$= 98.6°F \text{ (normal body temperature)}$$

FAHRENHEIT TO CELSIUS

Use the following formula to convert Fahrenheit readings to Celsius readings:

$$°C = 5/9 (°F − 32)$$

For example, if the Fahrenheit reading is 68°:

$$°C = 5/9 (68 − 32)$$
$$= 5/9 × 36$$
$$= 20°C \text{ (a nice spring day)}$$

temperature
conversion
scale

Index

Note: Page numbers followed by *f* indicate figures; those followed by *t* indicate tables; those followed by *b* indicate boxed material.

A

Ab (antibody), 182, 188, 239–240
abdomen
    muscles of, 105
    regions of, 9, 9*f*
abdominal aorta, 212, 214–215
abdominal cavity, 8, 8*f*
abdominopelvic cavity, 8, 8*f*, 262–263,
    264*f*
abducens nerve, 142*f*, 143, 154
abduction, 85*f*, 86
ABO blood group system, 188*t*, 188–189,
    189*f*
abortions, 337–338
    induced, 338
    spontaneous, 337–338
    therapeutic, 338
absorption, 261, 273
accessory nerve, 142*f*, 143
accessory organs
    of digestive system, 261, 269–271,
        270*f*
    of reproductive system, 313
accommodation, 153
acetabulum, 78
acetylcholine (ACh), 93, 117, 126*b*
Achilles tendon, 106
acid(s), 20
acid-base balance, 307
    kidneys in, 298
acidity, 20, 21*f*
acoustic nerve, 142*f*, 143, 156
acromion, 76
acrosome, 317, 317*f*
ACTH (adrenocorticotropic hormone),
    167*t*, 169
actin, 94, 94*f*
action potential, 93, 116*f*, 116–117
active transport, 35
Adam's apple, 249
adaptation
    dark, 150
    sensory, 161
adduction, 85*f*, 86
adductor muscles, 106
adenoids, 234
adenosine triphosphate (ATP), 5
ADH (antidiuretic hormone), 167*t*, 169,
    300, 307
adipose capsule, 294
adipose tissue, 44–45
adrenal cortex, 167*t*, 171
adrenal glands, 167*t*, 170–171
adrenaline, 117, 171
adrenal medulla, 167*t*, 171
adrenergic system, 125
adrenocorticotropic hormone (ACTH),
    167*t*, 169
aerobic exercise, 96*b*

aerobic phase, of cellular respiration,
    279–280, 280*t*
afferent arteriole, 296*f*, 297, 298*f*
afferent nerves, 116
afferent neurons, 116, 119
afterbirth, 336
Ag. *See* antigen(s) (Ag)
agglutination, 188, 189*f*
agglutinins, 188
agglutinogens, 188
aging
    body temperature with, 287–288
    digestive system with, 275
    endocrine system with, 175
    eyes with, 153
    heart with, 203*f*, 204
    integumentary system with, 60–61
    male reproductive system with, 318
    muscles with, 106–107
    nervous system with, 143
    nutrition with, 285
    respiratory system with, 257
    skeletal changes with, 67–68, 80–81
    urinary system with, 303–304
agranulocytes, 185
air passageways, lining of, 250–251, 251*f*
air pollution, 254*b*
albumin, 182
alcohol, 284
aldosterone, 167*t*, 171
alimentary tract. *See* digestive tract
alkaline phosphatase, 191
alkalinity, 20–21, 21*f*
allergies, food, 284
alveolus(i), 251–252, 252*f*
amino acid(s), 22
    in blood plasma, 182
    for energy, 281
    nonessential and essential, 281
amino acid compounds, 165
amniotic fluid, 334, 335*f*
amniotic sac, 334, 335*f*
amphiarthrosis, 81
amylase, 272
anabolism, 5, 279, 281
anaerobic metabolism, 95–96
anaerobic phase, of cellular respiration,
    279, 280*t*
anal canal, 269
anaphase, 33, 33*f*
anastomosis(es), 215–217, 216*f*
anatomic position, 6
anatomy, 3
androgens, 173
angiotensin, 298
anions, 18, 306–307
ANP (atrial natriuretic peptide), 173
ANS. *See* autonomic nervous system
    (ANS)

antagonist, 98
anterior, defined, 6, 6*f*
anterior fontanel, 72, 72*f*
anterior lobe, of pituitary, 167, 167*t*, 169
anterior superior iliac spine, 78
anti-A serum, 188, 189*f*
antibody(ies) (Ab), 182, 188, 239–240
anti-B serum, 188, 189*f*
anticoagulants, 187
antidiuretic hormone (ADH), 167*t*, 169,
    300, 307
antigen(s) (Ag), 188, 237
    human leukocyte, 238
    major histocompatibility complex, 238
antigen-antibody reaction, 240
antigen-presenting cells (APCs), 238
antiserum, 188, 189*f*, 241
anus, 269
aorta, 210, 212–215, 213*f*
    abdominal, 212, 213–214
    ascending, 212
    thoracic, 212, 213
aortic arch, 212
aortic bodies, 257
aortic valve, 198*f*, 199
APCs (antigen-presenting cells), 238
apex, 198
aponeurosis, 97
appendages, 55, 58
appendicitis, 269
appendicular skeleton, 69, 70*t*, 76*f*–81*f*,
    76–79
appendix, 269
appetite, 274–275
aqueous humor, 150
arachnoid, 132, 133*f*
arachnoid villus(i), 132, 133*f*
areola, 338*f*
areolar tissue, 44
arm
    arteries to, 215
    bones of, 76–77, 77*f*
    muscles of, 102–103
arrector pili, 58
arterial arches, 216
arterioles, 209, 210–211
arteriovenous anastomoses, 216*f*, 217
arteriovenous shunt, 216*f*, 216–217
artery(ies)
    defined, 209
    systemic, 212–217, 215*f*
    walls of, 210–211, 211*f*, 212*f*
articular cartilage, 84
articulation. *See* joint(s)
ascending aorta, 212
ascending colon, 269
ascending tracts, 121
ascorbic acid, 283*t*
association neurons, 115–116

Give them roots.
Watch them grow.